THE ROUTLEDGE INTERNATIONAL HANDBOOK OF MAD STUDIES

By drawing broadly on international thinking and experience, this book offers a critical exploration of Mad Studies and advances its theory and practice.

Comprised of 34 chapters written by international leading experts, activists and academics, this handbook introduces and advances Mad Studies, as well as exploring resistance and criticism, and clarifying its history, ideas, what it is, and what it can offer. It presents examples of mad studies in action, covering initiatives that have been taken, their achievements and what can be learned from them. In addition to sharing research findings and evidence, the book offers examples and insights for advancing understandings of experiences of madness and distress from the perspectives of those who have (had) those experiences, and also explores ways of supporting people oppressed by conventional understandings and systems.

This book will be of interest to all scholars and students of Mad Studies, disability studies, sociology, socio-legal studies, mental health and medicine more generally.

Peter Beresford OBE is Visiting Professor at the University of East Anglia, UK and Co-Chair of Shaping Our Lives, the national disabled people's and service users' organization and network.

Jasna Russo is a long-term activist in the international psychiatric survivor movement. She is Visiting Professor at Alice Salomon University of Applied Sciences in Berlin, Germany where she lectures in Research Methods as well as in Critical Diversity and Community Studies. Together with Angela Sweeney, Jasna Russo is a co-editor of *Searching for a Rose Garden. Challenging Psychiatry, Fostering Mad Studies* (2016).

THE ROUTLEDGE INTERNATIONAL HANDBOOK OF MAD STUDIES

Edited by Peter Beresford and Jasna Russo

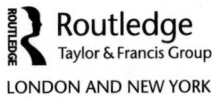

LONDON AND NEW YORK

First published 2022
by Routledge
2 Park Square, Milton Park, Abingdon, Oxon OX14 4RN

and by Routledge
605 Third Avenue, New York, NY 10158

Routledge is an imprint of the Taylor & Francis Group, an informa business

British Library Cataloguing-in-Publication Data
A catalogue record for this book is available from the British Library

Library of Congress Cataloging-in-Publication Data
Names: Beresford, Peter, editor. | Russo, Jasna, editor.
Title: The Routledge international handbook of mad studies /
edited by Peter Beresford and Jasna Russo.
Description: Milton Park, Abingdon, Oxon; New York, NY: Routledge, 2022. |
Series: Routledge international handbooks |
Includes bibliographical references and index.
Identifiers: LCCN 2021014615 (print) | LCCN 2021014616 (ebook) |
ISBN 9781138611108 (hardback) | ISBN 9781032024226 (paperback) |
ISBN 9780429465444 (ebook)
Subjects: LCSH: Psychiatry–Handbooks, manuals, etc. |
Mental illness–Handbooks, manuals, etc.
Classification: LCC RC456 .R66 2022 (print) |
LCC RC456 (ebook) | DDC 616.89–dc23
LC record available at https://lccn.loc.gov/2021014615
LC ebook record available at https://lccn.loc.gov/2021014616

ISBN: 978-1-138-61110-8 (hbk)
ISBN: 978-1-032-02422-6 (pbk)
ISBN: 978-0-429-46544-4 (ebk)

DOI: 10.4324/9780429465444

Typeset in Bembo
by Newgen Publishing UK

I want to dedicate this book to the disabled people's and service user led organization, Shaping Our Lives (www.shapingourlives.org.uk), which I am proud of being involved in from its beginnings now more than twenty years ago. We all identify as disabled people or service users. We have had many struggles over the years as individuals and as an organization. We have come close to closing because of the problems facing such user controlled organisations in being granted resources and legitimacy. But we are still going and still I hope supporting people to have more control over their lives and over the policies and politics that impact on them – the same aim I have for this book.

Peter Beresford

I dedicate this work to all people who have come in contact with psychiatry and learned that they should expect less from life, not trust what they feel and doubt what they know. I hope for this book to show that that is not the way things are.

Jasna Russo

CONTENTS

TABLE

CONTRIBUTORS

Victoria Armstrong, Ph.D., is Chief Executive of Disability North – a user-led organisation based in Newcastle upon Tyne in the North of England.

Joanne Azevedo is Lecturer in Social Work at Algoma University, Timmins, Ontario, Canada.

Rebecca Ballen is a clinical social worker in private practice and an activist with the Coalition Against Psychiatric Assault, Toronto, Ontario, Canada.

Fleur Beaupert is an independent researcher based in Sydney, Australia. Fleur has researched and written on mental health law and disability justice for over a decade, focusing on developments since the advent of the Convention on the Rights of Persons with Disabilities.

Liz Brosnan has a Medical Sociology Ph.D. researching the dynamics of service-user involvement. After 10 years in academia, including postdocs at NUI Galway and Kings College London, she returned to real-world implementation in Irish mental health services and remains an Independent Survivor Researcher.

Peter Campbell was born and raised in the Scottish Highlands and has lived in London since 1973. He was a founder member of Survivors Speak Out, Survivors Poetry and Survivors History Group and has worked for many years as a freelance trainer. He has Honorary Doctorates in Education at Anglia Ruskin University and The Open University.

María Isabel Cantón is a Mad activist, constantly seeking deconstruction for transformation, struggling with her own ignorance and anthropocentrism.

Sarah Carr is Senior Fellow in Mental Health Policy at the University of Birmingham, UK. As an academic specialising in service user and survivor knowledge and research, Sarah has experience of mental distress and service use and uses this to inform her work.

Chris Chapman is Associate Professor and Co-Chair SexGen at the York School of Social Work, York University, Toronto, Ontario, Canada.

Andrea Daley is Associate Professor at the School of Social Work, Renison University College (affiliated with University of Waterloo), Waterloo, Canada. Her research interests include the ways in which psychiatric discourses are implicated in cultural representations of gender(s).

Bhargavi V. Davar, Ph.D., is a person with psychosocial disability. She founded the Bapu Trust for Research on Mind & Discourse in 1999, to give an organisational framework to her human rights work (www.baputrust.com). She is an International trainer in the UN CRPD; a trained Arts Based Therapist, an Arts Based Therapy teacher.

Femi Eromosele is a postdoctoral fellow at the Centre for the Advancement of Scholarship, University of Pretoria. His research is largely situated at the intersection of literature and discourses of illness and health. He is also interested in African popular culture, especially the music video.

Jana-Maria Fey is a doctoral candidate in the Department of Politics, University of Sheffield. Her current research concerns the global politics of mental health and the relationships between mental health, governance, and the global political economy.

Abir Gebara, MSW, was Research Assistant at the School of Social Work, Ryerson University, Toronto, Ontario, Canada.

Nargis Hussaini is a clinical case manager at Kinark Child and Family Services, Toronto, Ontario, Canada.

Richard Ingram is Instructor in Continuing Studies at Simon Fraser University, Canada.

Ameil Joseph MSW, RSW, Ph.D., is Associate Professor at the School of Social Work, McMaster University in Hamilton, Ontario, Canada.

Pan Karanikolas (BA/LLB, UNSW) is a Ph.D. candidate in the Department of Social Inquiry, School of Humanities and Social Sciences at La Trobe University, Australia.

Colin King Ph.D., was diagnosed with schizophrenia at 17, established as a mental health practitioner, commissioner, teacher and black survivor research activist, setting up the Whiteness and Race Equality network for the illegal imprisonment of black men.

Naoyuki Kirihara, Ph.D., is running committee member of the Japan National Group of Mentally Disabled People, starting researcher of the Graduate School of Core Ethics and Frontier Sciences of Ritsumeikan University. He participated in the deliberation on revision of the Mental Health Act at the 193rd ordinary session of the Japanese Diet as the sole witness with psychosocial disabilities. Subsequently, the Bill of Mental Health Act was abolished.

Brenda A. LeFrançois, PhD, is a University Research Professor at Memorial University of Newfoundland in Canada. Their activist scholarship focuses on psychiatrisation, sanism and anti-sanist praxis, from mad studies and critical childhood studies perspectives.

Billie Lever Taylor is a Research Clinical Psychologist based at Kings College London. Informed also by her personal experiences, her work has focused on perinatal mental health, parent–infant work, and systemic family approaches.

Reima Ana Maglajlić is Senior Lecturer in Social Work at the University of Sussex in the United Kingdom.

Sonia Meerai is a Ph.D Student, working on Gender, Feminist and Women Studies at the Faculty of Graduate Studies, York University, Toronto, Ontario, Canada.

China Mills is Senior Lecturer in Public Health and Programme Director of the Masters of Public Health (MPH) at City, University of London. China's research traces different facets of the global mental health assemblage.

Hannah Morgan is Senior Lecturer in Disability Studies in the Department of Sociology at Lancaster University, UK. Hannah is Director of the Centre for Disability Research (CeDR) and hosts the biennial Lancaster Disability Studies Conference. Her work focuses on disabled people's experience of health, social care and welfare services and professional practice and education.

Daniel Mwesigwa Iga, Mental Health Uganda, World Network of Users and Survivors of Psychiatry, Pan African Network of Persons with Psychosocial Disabilities, My Story Initiative, Like Minds Uganda, International Disability Caucus, International Disability Alliance.

Essya M. Nabbali is an English/French bilingual researcher, educator, and advocate; a self-described de/organiser, data storyteller, and occasional poet. She is a faculty member of Capilano University and adjunct instructor to the Justice Institute of British Columbia in Canada.

Mary O'Hagan was a key initiator of the psychiatric survivor movement in New Zealand in the late 1980s and was the first chairperson of the World Network of Users and Survivors of Psychiatry between 1991 and 1995. She has been an advisor to the United Nations and the World Health Organization.

Darby Penney, M.L.S., Senior Research Associate, Advocates for Human Potential, Inc., Sudbury, Massachusetts, USA. She serves on the Boards of the National Association for Rights Protection and Advocacy and the Campaign for Trauma-Informed Policy and Practice.

Jennifer Poole is Associate Professor at the School of Social Work, Ryerson University, Toronto, Ontario, Canada.

Geoffrey Reaume is Associate Professor in the Critical Disability Studies program at York University, Toronto, Canada. He established the first university credit course on Mad People's History beginning in 2000.

David Reville was Adjunct Professor at Ryerson University, Toronto, Canada; he taught A History of Madness and Mad People's History, 2004–2014. He has been a mad activist for over 50 years.

Prateeksha Sharma, Ph.D., is a researcher, 'peer therapist' based out of Haryana in North India. Her website is at prateekshasharma.com. She is a classical musician and self-trained researcher, working in three areas: music, counselling and mental 'health'.

Irit Shimrat is a writer and editor and co-founded and co-ordinated the Ontario Psychiatric Survivors' Alliance and edited the national magazine *Phoenix Rising: The Voice of the Psychiatrized*.

Angela Sweeney is a trauma survivor researcher and Senior Lecturer in User-Led Research at King's College London where she undertook her Ph.D in the 2000s. Angie's interests include trauma, gender-based violence and parenting.

Danny Taggart is Academic Director of the Doctorate in Clinical Psychology at the University of Essex. He is currently seconded to the Independent Inquiry into Child Sexual Abuse where he is the Principal Psychologist/Clinical Lead for the Truth Project.

Lynn Tang is Assistant Professor in the Department of Sociology and Social Policy at Lingnan University, Hong Kong. Her core research areas include mental health, social inequalities, suicide prevention and related policies.

Lauren J. Tenney, Ph.D, MPhil, MPA, BPS, Psychiatric Survivor.

Brenda Del Rocio Valdivia Quiroz has training and experience in psychology, art therapy, neurodiversity, activism, project management and research. She works at SODIS, Society and Disability (Sociedad y Discapacidad) in Peru, and is also involved in Coalition for Mental Health and Human Rights, Collective Feminist Madness and Latin American Sphere Network of Psychosocial Diversity.

Trish Van Katwyk is Associate Professor at the School of Social Work, Renison University College (affiliated with University of Waterloo), Waterloo, Canada. Her research focuses on community-based, participatory, and arts-based ways of knowing, being, and doing.

David Webb, Ph.D. (Victoria University, Melbourne, 2005), is an Australian suicide survivor and retired academic/activist.

Wilda L. White is the founder of MadFreedom, a U.S.-based, human and civil rights membership organisation whose mission is to secure political power to end discrimination and oppression based on perceived mental state.

Caroline Yeo is a researcher, activist and reflector who works at the University of Nottingham in England. She is a poet and artist who studied Architecture. She was inspired by her lived experience of trauma as a child and psychiatric abuse to become a survivor researcher and self-identify as mad.

ACKNOWLEDGEMENTS

Editing this book has been a complex and demanding task and it means that we have a big debt of gratitude to many people. Trying to stay true to our aim of reaching out globally to people who identify as survivors and as people with psychosocial disabilities has meant that we have had to rely on the help, support, knowledge and effort of many people and organisations in many places in order to identify and make contact with the contributors. We thank them for their trust, kindness and commitment to this project.

We also owe a massive debt to all contributors for the generosity and effort with which they have followed through our invitation and supported the development of the book over a period of years. We thank them for the time and the ideas they invested as well as for their patience throughout the process. We also want to thank Kasumi Ito for her generous support and translation from Japanese. And finally, we thank the anonymous reviewers and our publisher for their belief in this book project from its proposal stage. We owe a particular debt to Routledge and the team who have brought the book to fruition, particularly Catherine Jones and Claire Jarvis, who have gone the extra mile to support our project.

We are aware that our reach is likely to have exceeded our grasp and that there are inevitably gaps and shortcomings in what we were able to achieve. We take responsibility for this but hope nonetheless that we have helped make it possible for more people to become familiar with the debates we explore. We also hope that the book will help people in their struggles to gain more visibility and respect and for these to be strengthened and reinforced for the future.

Our book highlights the complexity of action by survivors/people with psychosocial disabilities and the many barriers we face. For this reason, we want to thank all those who have inspired us over the years as well as those directly helping us in this work. Thank you.

Peter Beresford would like to thank my partner Suzy Croft for all her support through the production of this book, all my friends and colleagues at Shaping Our Lives, the UK disabled people's and user-led organisation (www.shapingourlives.org.uk) and our third editor, who sadly wasn't able to remain in the role, but I am pleased to say she remains my friend.

Jasna Russo wishes to thank the people who gave her advice and support and helped her get through difficult times throughout the course of putting together and editing this book. These are Vanessa Jackson, Rea Maglajlić, Isidora Randjelović, Zofia Rubinsztajn and Nebojša Tabački. I also warmly thank Stephanie Wooley for her feedback and the copy editing of my chapters, as well as Katharina Dieckmann and Elisa Strauch for their assistance with the formatting of the whole manuscript.

INTRODUCTION

Peter Beresford

A new opportunity

This book has grown out of our belief that Mad Studies represents a unique opportunity to rethink human mental wellbeing and to renew understandings and responses to it. The reality is that we live in a world that generates madness and distress, fails frequently to address them adequately or appropriately and often can even make them worse. There also seems to be a growing informal alliance between psychiatry, the lead discipline that is meant to help us in our distress and neoliberalism, with its rejection of state intervention and preoccupation with market economics. Both are increasingly powerful, both individualise explanations and both pathologise the subjects of social problems.

We believe that Mad Studies offers, for the first time, a real prospect of effective opposition to the marginalisation and oppression of people experiencing madness and distress, which is strongly philosophically and intellectually grounded. This gives it the chance to challenge the present dominance of reactionary and over-medicalised thinking. In one sense, Mad Studies is not unprecedented. There have been mad people/survivor movements and paradigms clearly challenging prevailing understandings of distress, madness and mental illness for many years. But until Mad Studies there has not been a significant initiative which has combined these two characteristics – of being survivor-led and theoretically grounded.

Although psychiatry has always had enormous power over people's lives, from its foundation it has created controversy and its scientific basis called into question. This is perhaps hardly surprising given that its 'treatment' repertoire has included large-scale institutionalisation, forced 'treatment' and restraint, and dangerous interventions like insulin shock therapy, brain surgery and electroconvulsive therapy (ECT) (Porter, 2003; Whitaker, 2004). More modern expressions of such concerns have been the anti-psychiatry and critical-psych and radical social work movements from the 1960s on the one hand, and on the other, the mental health service user/survivor movement emerging particularly from the 1980s.

Distrust of and opposition to psychiatry emerged as an international phenomenon. The diagnosis of political dissidents in the Soviet Union as 'mentally ill' cast an additional worrying spotlight on psychiatry's failings (Fulford et al, 1993). There was also support from other movements. The emerging gay rights movement challenged the classification of homosexuality

DOI: 10.4324/9780429465444-1

as a mental illness in the DSM (Diagnostic and Statistical Manual of Mental Disorders), eventually largely achieving its goal (Porter op cit).

The professional challenge

The developments loosely lumped together as 'anti-psychiatry' in the 1960s had many things in common as well as some significant differences. They offered critiques of psychiatry and mainstream 'psych' and their world views, and different understandings of madness and distress. Most closely associated with anti-psychiatry were UK psychiatrists R.D. Laing and David Cooper, from Italy, Franco Basaglia and in the US, Theodore Lidz. They were concerned with making sense of madness, highlighting its personal and social relations and the deficiencies of psychiatry. Other thinking associated with the movement ranged from Goffman's critiquing of 'total institutions' and their damaging effects, Foucault's understanding of psychiatry as primarily repressive and controlling, to the sociologist, Thomas Scheff's interpretation of 'mental illness' as a label of deviance imposed by society (Goffman, 1961; Scheff, 1966; Donnelly, 1992; Crossley, 1998; Foucault, 1988 and 2006).

While some psychiatric system survivors welcomed these professional critiques and in some cases allied with and have subsequently drawn on them, their initiators were not necessarily natural allies of survivors and our movement. Thus another key figure associated with the anti-psychiatry movement was the American psychiatrist Thomas Szasz. Some survivors have valued him as a critic of the moral and scientific foundations of psychiatry, who argued that mental illnesses are not illnesses in the same way that physical illnesses are (Szasz, 1961). But few would likely be sympathetic to his support for and work with scientology (a group which also rejected psychiatry) or sign up to what has been seen as his provision of 'a rationale for regressive social policies' (Goldstein, 1980).

The anti-psychiatrists were involved in reform and challenging abuse, as well as counter-theory building, so their appeal to a nascent survivor movement is hardly surprising. Basaglia played a central part in the closure of Italy's big psychiatric institutions. Laing and Cooper set up more than 20 therapeutic communities, including the famous London East End Kingsley Hall, where staff and residents were intended to have equal status and medication was only used on a voluntary basis (Nasser, 1995).

The anti-psychiatry movement was also being driven by individuals with adverse experiences of psychiatric services. This included those who felt they had been harmed by psychiatry or who thought that they could have been helped more by other approaches, including those compulsorily (including via physical force) admitted to psychiatric institutions and subjected to compulsory medication or procedures. During the 1970s, the anti-psychiatry movement was involved in promoting restraint from many practices seen as psychiatric abuses.

Some survivors linked up with the anti-psychiatry movement and others have subsequently been inspired by it. While many of the professionals involved in anti-psychiatry, radical social work and critical psychology may have challenged conventional devaluing of mental health service users, generally they do not seem to have turned to mental health service users/survivors as equal collaborators or see their work as one of co-production giving equal value to the experiential knowledge of the people on the receiving end of the systems they were exploring. An exception has been the radical social work movement of the twenty-first century. Crucially anti-psychiatry, like the critical psychiatry and psychology that came after it was essentially led by mental health professionals and academics and grew out of their agendas and preoccupations.

Leaders and key figures in the anti-psychiatry movement largely operating as clinicians and professionals, legitimated by their qualifications and status. One thing they largely had in common was being positioned as acknowledged 'experts'. As we have seen, they mainly worked under the auspices of the psychiatric system that they attacked and rejected, empowered by the privilege and status it gave them. While they might share with survivors what they were against (although certainly not always), this does not necessarily mean they necessarily sought the same things or in the same way. As far as their discourse was concerned, whatever their proposals, power largely stayed where it was (Crossley, op cit; Nasser, op cit).

The asymmetrical situation of service users/survivors

The anti-psychiatry movement and indeed the radical and critical psych organisations that followed in its footsteps, may look like the equivalent of Boy David against the Goliath of the psychiatric system it was challenging. But it was able to draw on academic and professional resources and privilege to provide a strong intellectual and philosophical grounding for its position. It was able to generate a library of texts as justification and rationale for its critique of psychiatry and mainstream interpretations of madness and distress. It's hardly surprising that the mental health service user/survivor movements that began tentatively to emerge from the 1960s turned to high profile anti-psychiatry for moral support and inspiration. It was one of the few potential allies it had, even their interests weren't necessarily shared.

The situation for service users/survivors, on the other hand, was very different. Here was a group characterised by poverty, isolation and disempowerment, whose identities were seen as spoiled and whose rationality was also likely to be called into question. Who was likely to listen to them? Already in the 1960s in the UK, for example, the scale of neglect in big institutions for older and disabled people and mental health service users was becoming clear through the work of campaigners and academics like Barbara Robb and Peter Townsend (Robb, 1967; Townsend, 1962). In the 1970s, the then legal officer of UK Mind, Larry Gostin (2010) won landmark rulings in the European Court of Human Rights over widespread abuse in psychiatric services (Beresford, 2016a, pp. 113–114). All these reports from independent sources were initially dismissed as exaggerated and unreliable, so it is not difficult to imagine what response service users would get when they tried to bring them to official attention.

The mental health service user/survivor movement that flowered from the 1980s onwards (Campbell, 2009), does not seem to have shared a clear underpinning philosophy of its own. This is not to say that it did not articulate, was not guided by and highlighted a number of principles that were shared internationally. Such principles were made explicit in the founding charter of the radical UK survivors organization, Survivors Speak Out in the mid-1980s. They included that:

- The lives of mental health service users are of equal value to those of others
- Mental health service users have a right to speak for themselves
- There is a need to provide non-medicalised services and support
- Service users' first-hand experience should be valued
- Discrimination against people with experience of using mental health services must end (Survivors Speak Out, 1987).

The international survivor movement can be seen as one of the 'new social movements' emerging globally in the second half of the twentieth century, largely based on shared identity and common experiences of oppression. Thus, there is the existence of black civil rights, women's, LGBTQ and grey power movements. Certainly welfare state user movements like those of survivors and disabled people highlighted their links and overlaps with these movements (Lent,

2002). The disabled people's movement, however, was significantly different to the survivors movement. In some ways, it was a separatist movement, arguing for different kinds of support to what was generally provided and developing its own underpinning model or theory – the social model of disability and its related philosophy for change – independent living (Campbell and Oliver, 1996). The same does not seem to have been true of the survivors movement (Barnes et al, 1999). The many groups and user organisations that emerged often operated within the psychiatric system and its services and related voluntary organisations and were sometimes linked with and funded by them. That the movement did not have the same kind of distinct philosophical basis or perhaps independence as the disabled people's movement, made it particularly vulnerable and dependent.

Reform not revolution

While the disabled people's movement prioritised supporting people to live in mainstream society outside the service system, it was difficult for survivors to do the same, both because that was where they could often expect to return to and because they were reluctant to abandon other service users languishing in its backwards, custodial and forensic provision. If the disabled people's movement was constantly seeking ways of helping disabled people escape traditional services, the survivor movement was often having to focus on engaging with them to safeguard the rights of their peers within them. This meant that they needed to get into the system, needed its collaboration to do so and were often dependent on it and associated voluntary organisations for their funding. This could impose further constraints on the movement's independence. Such charitable/voluntary organisations have largely been consensual and their rationale has generally been to speak *for* service users rather than to enabling them to speak for *themselves*. They tend to be deeply enmeshed in the psychiatric system, its values and philosophy, frequently relying on its funding for their continuing existence.

As well as its justifiable fears around adopting a separatist strategy, the survivor movement faced other obstacles in the way of developing its own independence and independent philosophy Three convincing arguments have been offered to explain mental health service users' frequent reluctance to distance themselves from conventional psychiatry and why they might shy away from adopting a radical philosophy for their movement – even though their movement offered an implicit philosophical challenge to the prevailing biomedical model (Beresford et al, 2016). First, seems to have been the fear of many involved that if they challenged the underpinning medical model, then service users would be dismissed as in denial about their own pathology and lack of rationality (Campbell, 1996). Second, as mental health service users, their rationality would always be regarded as open to question and therefore their ideas seen as suspect. Third, there seems to have been a more generalised reluctance to sign up to any monolithic theories about themselves for fear that these again might dominate and damage them in the same way that they feel psychiatric thinking long has done (Plumb, 1994).

It is perhaps not surprising therefore, that there was essentially a hole in the survivors movement where a philosophy might have been. However, there does seem to have been at least two major exceptions to this, although qualifications apply in both cases.

Exceptions to the rule?

One of these was the development of the international hearing voices movement. Again this challenged assumptions that hearing voices was necessarily a manifestation of a 'mental illness' or 'psychosis', instead regarding it as an expression of the diversity of human perception and experience to be explored and understood. In this it can be seen an extension of the search for meaning of anti-psychiatrists like Cooper and Laing, supporting people to understand and manage such voices or problems underpinning them. Significantly though, the movement was established by the Dutch psychiatrists Marcus Romme and Sandra Escher, although it has generated networks of voice hearers internationally operating on the basis of offering peer support (Romme and Escher, 1992, 1993). Thus, this was a development initiated by psychiatrists but clearly centrally involving the people with direct experience and their understandings.

The other was the emergence in the 1990s of *Mad Pride*. Originating in Canada it spread internationally and was based on 'reclaiming' the language, meaning and ownership of madness. It rejected the biomedical model and was deliberately confrontational. It sought to 'visibilise' the history and realities of psychiatry and the experience of survivors through protests, demonstrations, cultural events walking tours and mass media campaigns. Its emphasis on 'pride', meant that it came to be associated with the idea of being 'mad positive' (Curtis, 2003; Glaser, 2008). In the UK it was a minority part of the survivors movement. By no means all survivors feel positive about their madness and distress or necessarily see it as something positive to celebrate. So in our view, however important Mad Pride is, and while acknowledging its contribution in challenging the never-ending devaluing of survivors and our identities by recasting words like 'mad', 'nutter', 'loony' and 'psycho', it does not really speak to many survivors, for whom their experience as well as the reactions to such experience and perceptions, continue to be as a vale of tears.

A survivor-led ideological challenge

There was also an important exception to the general lack of clear philosophical base to the survivor movement and its tendency to be reformist rather than revolutionary; embedded rather than separatist. This was the work of survivor writer and activist Peter Sedgwick. He published his defining book *Psychopolitics* in 1982 and significantly it was republished more than 30 years later amid emerging interest in Mad Studies. His book is not only a rare example of an explicit ideological challenge to prevailing biomedical understandings, from a survivor perspective. It was both forged independent of anti-psychiatry professionals and directly from lived experience. Sedgwick could identify as a service user, academic and professional (educational psychologist), but what most seemed to motivate him were his left wing politics. These were something he shared with founders of the international disabled people's movement like Mike Oliver and Vic Finkelstein. His writings have much more in common with the political than the anti-psychiatry or social policy writings of his time. He was suspicious of professional critiques and of some of the big anti-psychiatry names that are now often seen as key to the development of the survivor movement. He saw them as regressive and individualizing, instead calling for a renewal of policy and understanding (Beresford, 2016b).

Sedgwick was not optimistic about the development of a survivors' movement – and perhaps in some senses he was right. Not only has it been unduly dependent on the service system it has wanted to change, but it has often been co-opted by it and the ideas which it has espoused like 'recovery', peer support', 'personalisation' and 'mindfulness' have been subverted to reinforce neoliberal social policy goals and used to force service users into low grade employment, under the continuing dominance of the medical model in mental health policy and practice. As Sedgwick understood, both intellectually and from his own experience, there was no golden age of psychiatry in the NHS before Mrs Thatcher's 1980s reforms.

Sedgwick rejected the prevailing individualistic medicalised model of 'mental illness' and saw societies as driving people into madness and distress. Perhaps the first lesson to learn from him is the importance of having a political understanding and addressing ideological issues if a helpful and successful challenge is to be made to the dominant model of psychiatry now operating within neoliberal politics. Even if times have changed, the present heavily politicised context of mental health issues gives added relevance to Sedgwick's approach and understanding.

Perhaps a second lesson that Sedgwick offers comes from the fact that he was as critical of many of the opponents of conventional mental health policy and thinking as he was of those then prevailing. He did not make the easy assumption that the enemies of damaging policy were necessarily the friends of mental health service users/survivors. *Psychopolitics* is largely made up of an analysis of what he saw as the shortcomings of contemporary radicals and associated interpretations of madness and distress.

One of Sedgwick's preoccupations was with how we can approach issues of madness and distress in ways that are less likely to impose and perpetuate divisions between mind and body? This was a fundamental failing of psychiatry when Sedgwick was writing and now it continues to be a major problem. His concerns were holistic in other senses too. He was preoccupied with the 'victory of humanity' and saw the way to achieve this as a 'socialised and organised' humanity. He saw the attainment of this as 'the central problem of psychiatric care' and 'central problem of social liberation' (op cit, p. 256). Thus he combined a concern with the political, the psychological and self-liberation.

The emergence of Mad Studies

In this Sedgwick prefigures Mad Studies, which has similar concerns. What connects them is the underpinning concern of Mad Studies and its advocates to develop a philosophically and ideologically grounded movement with the capacity to take effective action based on survivor-led understandings of madness and human wellbeing. While Mad studies, has emerged in the twenty-first century as a pioneering new development, it is directly linked to values and principles first emphasised by Sedgwick. This is not to say that there may not be tensions between the two. However, these core values are of central importance. They certainly seem to be shared by Sedgwick and Mad Studies as currently delineated. These are commitments to prioritising:

- being ideologically positioned
- collectivity
- building on alliances.

The recent emergence of Mad Studies can be seen to herald a new direction of travel for survivor self-organisation and involvement. However, it can also be seen as less a change in direction for survivor activists and researchers as a return to first principles and their original ways of working. The Mad Studies movement is committed to a praxis for radical survivor-led change that seeks to unify learning and action (Le Francois et al, 2013; Costa, 2014). It is committed to remain accountable to the mad community and to stay connected with their struggles (LeFrançois, 2015; LeFrancois et al, 2013, p17). While its origins can be traced to Canada, in recent years it has begun to emerge as an international movement, albeit being one that is still largely situated in the Global North. This introductory chapter reflects the history of Mad Studies. It strongly refers to the UK context as well as introducing European developments. We have however sought in the body of the text to go beyond this, putting Mad Studies in its much more truly global context. Mad Studies offers a lens to make sense of the increasingly maddening effects of the world in which all of us live. Its focus is being brought to bear on a widening range of issues confronting us all, from art to violence (Netchitailova, 2019; Daley et al, 2019). Thus as has been said, it:

> can ask wider questions about society and culture. For example, it can explore mad people's histories, cultures, politics, and communities, including *before* the invention of psychiatry; and use mad-centred knowledge to critique existing cultures and practices.
>
> *(Spandler and Poursanidou, 2019, p. 9)*

Mad Studies is not only reflected in the sweep of its focus, but also its commitment to being philosophically grounded and broad based. This is reflected in three of its defining characteristics. These are:

1. Mad Studies is based on an explicit divorce from a simplistic biomedical model and all the theoretical and treatment premises associated with it. Instead it values and draws on other understandings and disciplines to come into it, rejecting a solely medical dominance. This includes sociology, anthropology, social work, cultural studies, feminist, Queer studies, disability studies and history. It prioritises social understandings and interpretations of Madness and distress, as has the disabled people's movement before it.
2. Mad Studies values and places an emphasis on first person or experiential knowledge, treating it with equality and returning to the founding values of the survivor movement; that survivors' experience, lives, viewpoints and knowledge must be treated with equality. At the same time it gives value to the first-person knowledge of everyone, not just those psychiatrised, acknowledging the complexity of our identities and all that each of us experience and can bring to bear.
3. Moving on from this, Mad Studies is survivor-led but it is not limited to survivors. Because Mad Studies has a place for *all* our first hand experiential knowledge, it makes it possible for a wide range of roles and standpoints to contribute equally to Mad Studies – if they accept its core principles. It isn't only us as survivors/mental health service users, but allies, professionals, researchers, loved ones, and so on that people can be part of Mad Studies. This is a venture we can all work for together in alliance (Beresford and Russo, 2016). As the editors of the first collection of writings on Mad Studies, *Mad Matters*, published in 2013, wrote:

> We are not locating 'Mad Studies' as originating solely within the community of people deemed Mad, but also as including allies, social critics, revolutionary theorists, and radical professionals who have sought to distance themselves from the essentialising biological determinism of psychiatry whilst respecting, valuing and privileging the Mad thoughts of those whom conventional psychiatry would condemn to a jumble of diagnostic prognostications.
>
> *(Le Francois et al, 2013, p. 2)*

Helen Spandler and Dina Poursanidou see Mad Studies:

> as a 'project' in an existential sense: that is, it is not fixed but in the process of becoming; and is an on-going concern for both of us. In this sense, it is a personal and political, as well as an intellectual project.
>
> *(Spandler and Poursanidou, 2019, p. 2)*

As survivor researcher Angela Sweeney has said, Mad Studies can offer a:

> unifying theoretical framework that has as its central goal the critique of biomedical psychiatry and the development of critical and radical counter-discourses.
>
> *(Sweeney, 2016, p. 47)*

So Mad Studies is everyone's business. In our view it offers a real possibility of displacing prevailing discourses on madness and wellbeing. But the challenge it faces is a massive one. More than 30 years of international neoliberal politics, underpinned by a notion of human nature as selfish rather than altruistic, have been linked with an accelerating commitment to the market rather than the state, increasing social inequality and a trend to make cuts in public services and spending, internationally. One consequence of the emergence of Western neoliberal governments is that they have formed a powerful alliance with traditional, dominant and expanding psychiatry. Mental health services may be under attack but 'psych-thinking' is on the upsurge.

Mad Studies is not narrowly concerned with psychiatry or other conventional and Western responses to people's madness and distress. But these can't be ignored because of their global reach and ambitions. This expansion of psychiatry is reflected in: the massively growing range of psychiatric diagnostic categories (APA, 2014); their application to more groups and the routine use of associated psychotropic drugs for a widening range of people, issues and situations, for example, children and young people experiencing difficulties in school and the family; older people in institutional settings and people with learning difficulties identified as having 'challenging behaviour'; as well as increasing interest in organic, genetic and bioethical approaches to madness and distress (Johnstone, 2014). Both neoliberalism and mainstream psychiatry individualise responsibility and frame understanding in terms of individual rather than social causes and analysis. In the UK, mental health policy and services have been chronically underfunded, community and support services have suffered increasing cuts, and there has been a shift to more control and forensic services and away from support services.

Such policies seem committed to the *generation* of mental ill health and distress, rather than to reducing it. There is now strong evidence that the increasing inequality associated with such neoliberal politics and ideology has damaging effects on the physical and mental health of most, if not all, of us (Wilkinson and Pickett, 2009). While the consequences of such inequality are widely felt across social groups, it is particularly damaging to those on lower incomes and included in the lower socio-economic groups, being associated with higher morbidity and mortality rates (Dorling, 2013).

So, we can hardly look to this as a global politics that is likely to take seriously mental health policy and practice when it is one that is essentially distressing and maddening. It is a politics that seeks to make you deny who you are and hate everyone else by othering them. We believe that this makes it a politics of madness.

Question marks over Mad Studies

Having said this, we must also be clear about issues already identified, which indeed we will be seeking to explore and address in this book, of exclusions and biases which threaten Mad Studies and put it at risk of failing in its large, ambitious task.

What is interesting is that such criticisms of Mad Studies have not only come from non-survivors and the psych-system but also from some survivors themselves and indeed some prominent survivor activists. They also significantly came at a surprisingly early stage in the development of the movement, once it became more internationalised. Thus at an early UK conference on Mad Studies, Brenda LeFrancois (2015), one of the Canadian co-editors of *Mad Matters*, 'called attention to the "potential undoing" of this emerging field unless those who were engaged in teaching and "disciplining" it actively sought to decenter whiteness and to be accountable to mad communities outside of academia' (cited in Kalathil and Jones, 2016, p. 187). Similarly Spandler and Poursandiou have highlighted the need for Mad Studies to be 'more attuned to potential exclusions' (op cit, 2019, p. 1).

Indeed it is in relation to its perceived 'exclusions' that Mad Studies has mainly come under attack. Thus the main criticisms of Mad Studies so far have been that it is elitist, academicised, racialised, tied to the Global North at the expense of the Global South, inadequately addresses diversity and is based on exclusionary language. Diana Rose, herself a survivor academic at the UK Institute of Psychiatry, describing Mad Studies as the 'new orthodoxy in mental health research' has argued that it runs the risk of being 'elitist', and 'leaving others behind', noting that 'most of the prominent writers have PhDs or are candidates' (Rose, 2018). Both she and Kalathil and Spandler, who cite others, also relate this to the fact that such 'spaces for knowledge production' have perpetuated barriers in the way of 'user/survivor students and researchers from marginalized and minoritized backgrounds, including people from racialized communities and individuals with particular clusters of "mad" experiences putatively deemed unacceptable' (Kalathil and Jones, 2016, p. 185). Survivor consultant Alison Faulkner has highlighted the need for Mad Studies to develop a 'mature capacity to deal with difference and diversity within its constituency' (Faulkner, 2017).

Another key criticism made of Mad Studies is that following in the footsteps of the old anti-psychiatry movement, it has been narrowly focused on opposing psychiatry (Spandler and Poursanidou, 2019). This is not only a problem in itself, but also seen as particularly unhelpful in relation to the Global South where psychiatry is much more marginal and people 'with mental health conditions' are reported as being treated with great harshness and cruelty, including being chained up and maltreated (Read et al, 2009; Human Rights Watch, 2019). The use of Mad terminology has also been seen as particularly damaging and offensive to Black and minority ethnic groups and people in the Global South – another expression of the imposition of western ideas upon them (Beresford, 2019).

There is one more concern raised about Mad Studies and it is indeed one we have raised ourselves. This is the way in which it, like other progressive developments from marginalised groups, including disabled people and survivors are susceptible to being subverted by the very forces they seek to oppose (Beresford and Russo, 2016). Thus we have seen mainstream survivor activity developing innovative ideas like 'peer support', 'self-management' and 'recovery' restructured and used to support neoliberal and psych-system goals. We shall try and explore here what can be done to safeguard Mad Studies from this external threat and how its particular contribution can be fostered despite this.

Writing this book

These all seem important concerns to us and we hope here to begin the process of seriously addressing them. We also hope that this book will give this task further impetus. We believe that it is all our responsibility to seek to address these possible shortcomings as well as to highlight them and that this is a key part of the Mad Studies project. From our experience these are problems that tend to beset all New Social Movements, and which limit their potential if left unchallenged. Then they run the risk of being reduced to abstracted academic areas, narrowly tied to the preoccupations of their Western initiators. For us, supporting and strengthening the

Mad Studies movement globally, which we see as the most positive and potentially effective expression of collective survivor struggle so far, is critical.

At the same time, while we have worked hard to challenge these exclusions, in putting this book together we have to acknowledge that our reach has often outstripped our grasp. We have tried hard to avoid seeing this as any kind of excuse. However, it is hardly surprising given that the issues we are concerned with here are structural as well as personal ones that are tied to some of the most entrenched barriers, inequalities and discriminations that operate in our world. Thus our task has always been to challenge these, recognising that we too are subject to their effects, without being weakened in our resolve to try to transcend them.

While we have put together a number of publications between us, this book has perhaps been the most difficult, demanding and complex. It has taken much longer to produce than might have been expected. We made a commitment early on that we would work to access the widest range of survivor voices to create as full and inclusive a picture of Mad Studies as possible. This included reaching out to try and address difference with equality, supporting people to contribute who might not feel confident to do so on their own, helping them to put together what they wanted to say and seeking to be flexible in the kind of contributions we included. We wanted to extend our engagement equally to the Global South, without making any assumptions that what happens and matters in the North, including Mad Studies itself, is the same for the South and without imposing another model or theory from the Global North.

We started with a familiarity and networks with both the international survivor and the Mad Studies movement. However, the demands of commercial publishers and the lives of many survivors do not sit comfortably together. Deadlines, madness and distress are not necessarily ready partners. We haven't had money to pay people for their efforts and while this might not be a problem for those working as academics who could count it as part of their work, it certainly could be for many others, trying to keep their heads above water on low incomes and with few safeguards. Quite simply, if you need money to live, you can't take on tasks that divert you from making a living.

People have contributed despite having really difficult times, in one way or another, despite frequent problems of low income, poor health and in some cases the difficulties their madness faced them with. Not all the people we would have liked to contribute to the book were able to; they were already over-committed, weren't well enough physically or mentally, or just didn't respond to our enquiries. Others for one reason or another may not have wanted to. Certainly we believe that putting together the knowledge of survivors on this and other subjects is not something that can adequately be done through commercial processes. Grant givers must in future pay more attention to levelling up the playing field to ensure more equal access for the accounts and experiential knowledge of survivors and indeed other marginalised groups.

The book's structure and contents

The book is organised into five parts which explore the past, present and future of Mad Studies; and analyse its personal, political, cultural, social, academic and geographic relations.

Part 1: Mad Studies and political organising of people with psychiatric experience

In Part 1 we explore the nature of Mad Studies globally, tracing its origins and relations with the survivor and related movements that began to emerge internationally in the last quarter of the twentieth century. In an opening chapter Jasna Russo provides an overview for these global developments that examines the challenge posed by the new survivor knowledges generated by collective action and self-organisation. This is followed by a series of chapters by survivor activists involved in such developments in both the Global South and North, examining both their personal and local experience and what role, if any, Mad Studies has played and is playing in relation to survivor activism and resistance.

In Chapter 2 long-term activist Mary O'Hagan begins the process with an historical analysis of the situation in New Zealand, highlighting the hesitant progress of the survivor movement compared for example with that of the LGBTQ movement. Next, Bhargavi Davar writing about the Indian experience highlights both her personal experience and the progress made by survivors against the background of a subcontinent that was the subject of psychiatrisation under British imperial and colonising power. In the fourth chapter, Brenda Valdivia Quiroz highlights the connections between the personal and the political as she charts her experience as a survivor and engagement in the survivor movement as a woman from an indigenous community in what she identifies as a discriminatory society. Writing from Canada, Irit Shimrat next focuses on the role of experiential survivor knowledge in challenging what she calls the 'mental health pseudo-sciences', its role in finding better ways of coping with difference and distress and the part that Mad Studies informed by such knowledge can play in rethinking ourselves and the politics we live under.

This is followed by Chapter 6, an account by one of the founders of the UK survivor movement, Peter Campbell, setting out some of its key concerns and the establishment of the founding organisation Survivors Speak Out. In Chapter 7, Daniel Mwesigwa Iga reports on the development of survivor-led activism in Uganda guided by the provisions of the United Nations Convention on the Rights of People with Disabilities (UNCRPD) and how this has offered both activists and policymakers an alternative paradigm mobilising communities to support people with psycho-social disabilities and challenge traditional stigmatising understandings of them in the Global South. Next, Derby Penney, a long-term activist focuses on using survivor knowledge to influence public policy in the USA. She highlights first-hand the problems of trying to work in and against the system, the way in which survivor demedicalised roles have been remedicalised and the need for a Mad Studies movement in US academia. In Chapter 9, Naoyuki Kirihara offers an account of the past and present history of the survivor movement in Japan and drawing on his own involvement in it, highlighting its engagement with the UNCRPD and exploring strategies for effectively extending its influence in the academy. Finally, in this section of the book, Wilda White who identifies as a Mad activist and independent researcher, against a backdrop of a psychiatric medical malpractice trial, draws on the concept of epistemic injustice to argue the importance of focusing Mad scholarship and advocacy beyond psychiatry and the mental health system to challenge the broader denial of survivors' basic human and civil rights.

Part 2: Situating Mad Studies

In Part 2 of the book we are concerned with situating Mad Studies in its broader contexts. These include its historical, disciplinary, philosophical and legal contexts. In the opening Chapter 11, Richard Ingram traces the evolution of the concept 'Mad Studies' in the academic world and in particular its relationship with the Canadian 'Mad movement'. After that, Geoffrey Reaume discusses the differences between anti-psychiatry, critical psychiatry and Mad Studies, and the extent to which knowledge has been reclaimed that was more often about rather than by mad people. He also argues that Mad Studies has the potential to be more relevant than the other two because its origins lie *within* the mad community. In Chapter 13, Hannah Morgan from the UK, with long-term experience of convening the Lancaster biennial international Disability Studies conference, explores the close, complex and sometimes fractious relationship between Disability Studies and Mad Studies. She considers their similarities and differences and the complex and uncertain role of the social model of disability in relation to Mad Studies as well as the importance of the two disciplines maintaining dialogue with each other. Finally in this section of the book, in Chapter 14, Fleur Beaupert and Liz Brosnan draw us back to the role of the UN CRPD and focus on the damaging and violent consequences of conventional mental health law. They draw on the idea of 'absent knowledges', in this case the experiential knowledge of survivors and point to the potential of international human right law to draw in such absent knowledges.

Part 3: Mad Studies and knowledge equality

The contribution of survivors' lived experience and experiential knowledge and their centrality in Mad Studies figures large in this part of the book. First in his chapter on 'The Subjects of Oblivion', Amiel Joseph focuses on 'racial erasure' within Mad Studies, its continuities and implications, as well as ways to work against that. He engages with 'obliviousness' to highlight at both individual and structural levels how this idea is used to ignore and collude with ableism, sanism, eugenics, white supremacy and other forms of oppression and discrimination. He argues that instead Mad Studies, can be applied in practice, in teaching, for transformative ends. In Chapter 16, survivor researcher Sarah Carr calls into question the possibility of meaningful co-production in the context of mental health under the structural constraints currently operating. Despite what she describes as power asymmetries, her conclusions are not pessimistic, but emphasise that transformative co-production will not work without thorough attention being paid to underlying epistemic injustices that continue in psychiatric systems.

In Chapter 17 trauma survivor and psychologist Danny Taggart considers how the increased sharing of 'experiential knowledge' in the structures of mental health 'impacts on us' and what happens when our experience becomes a form of commodity that can be traded, debated and discarded. He concludes by discussing what the implications might be of different interpretations for 'experiential knowledge' producers in mental health. Angela Sweeney and Billie Lever Taylor make the focus of their chapter, 'De-pathologising Motherhood'. They critique the pathologising and discriminatory consequences of clinical interpretations of maternal distress. They make the case for foregrounding mothers' experiential knowledge to avoid neglecting the interpersonal and sociocultural contexts of maternal distress and to respond helpfully to them. In their Chapter 19, Jennifer Poole and her colleagues offer an analysis of the professional regulation of madness for social workers, social service workers and nurses in Canada, informed by Mad Studies, institutional ethnography and critical disability studies. They highlight the damaging consequences of existing processes, discussing epistemic injustice and problematising 'public safety'. The last chapter in this section of the book subjects the global rise of 'mental health anti-stigma' campaigns to scrutiny. Authors Jana-Maria Fey and China Mills draw on scholarship from Mad Studies, survivor research and user-controlled research, to offer an anti-sanist analysis of the deployment of (anti-)stigma as a dominant narrative in global effort to tackle ever-rising numbers of diagnosable mental disorders. More broadly, the chapter highlights the importance of continued reflection on the legitimation of knowledge through academic discourse and the kind of voices being heard in the process.

Part 4: Doing Mad Studies

In Part 4 of the book we focus on *doing* Mad Studies; what adopting this paradigm means in practical day-to-day terms. We look at what it means for how to understand and address

Madness and distress in a wide range of contexts; from the medicalisation of distress and the maddening effects of war and conflict, through to rethinking suicide and the relationship of Madness and violence (Webb, 2010 and Maglajlic. 2016).

In the opening chapter survivor activist María Isabel Cantón raises the question of why we must talk about demedicalisation in the context of her own direct experience and her country, Nicaragua. In social settings where the medicalisation of 'mental illness' is the norm, she explores the personal and social problems of adopting this understanding which challenges the systemic oppression of some of the most marginalised groups. In Chapter 22, Amber Karanikolas, writing from Australia, discusses the historic institutionalisation of mental health service users and recent deinstitutionalisation policy which resulted in many more coming the way of police, prisons and criminal legal system. It calls for closer conversation between abolitionist and anti-carceral activists, psychiatric survivors and scholars within Mad Studies, seeking an end to carceral approaches to managing Madness and mental distress. In her chapter, Reima Ana Maglajlic explores the relationship between madness and political conflict through the lens of Mad Studies, using auto-ethnography and broader thinking to shape an analysis of her experiences of madness and political conflict, primarily in Bosnia and Herzegovina. She concludes that more knowledge at the intersection of Mad Studies and political conflict is needed but has yet to be developed. In Chapter 24, 'The Architecture Of My Madness', activist Caroline Yeo explores the meanings of physical spaces in which her own lived experience as well as experiences more generally take place. Through the use of narrative and poetry she describes different types of building and space from the home and hospital to the University and the part they played in the abuse, which now informs her work. She offers the concept of guesthouse as a place of retreat, reflection and of asylum.

In the next chapter, suicide survivor David Webb explores suicide and suicidality from the perspective of those who have undertaken, considered and attempted it. He highlights the exclusion, rejection and neglect of these perspectives in suicidology, challenging this and attempting to address it. Bringing together the evidence from his survivor-led analysis of suicide, he offers an alternative to psychiatric ways of thinking about it, based on valuing subjective and inter-subjective lived experience and the knowledge that comes from it. Chapter 26 explores the high profile and contentious relationship between violence and Madness. Authors Andrea Daley and Trish Van Katwyk examine the de-coupling of old assumptions about this relationship and the re-coupling of new first-hand understandings, which relocate violence away from Mad people and on to political and social structures and processes that govern social institutions, including those that are charged with managing madness. They stress the importance of Mad Studies retaining its grassroots associations, even as it becomes an academic field of study.

In Chapter 27, academic Lynn Tang reviews the debate about the contentious idea of 'recovery'. She draws on a research project on Chinese communities in the UK to argue that recovery's progressive potential can still be achieved through a shift from seeing it as a project of individuals to a project of communities, envisioning possible alliances of recovery, inequality and Mad Studies movements. Essya Nabbali's chapter pivots on the 2019 date when the final report of the Canadian National Inquiry into Missing and Murdered Indigenous Women and Girls and 2SLGBTQQIA people (see her chapter for an explanation) was released. Through highlighting a nexus of reactionary developments it draws out the relationship between critical race, Indigenous, and Mad studies, contending that the pursuit of 'difference', historically for structural adjustment, can be flipped to lend itself to problem definition and agenda-setting for contemporary policy purposes. Finally in this section, we hear from Lauren Tenney on the subject of Spirituality, Psychiatry and Mad Studies. Evidencing the oppressive potential of psychiatry and its inheritance of religion's social control role, she introduces feminist, anti-psychiatry and survivor-led frameworks and research, making the case for developing research about spirituality through the lens of Mad Studies.

Part 5: Inquiring into the future for Mad Studies

In this final part of the book contributors both offer their own ideas, insights and cautions about the future of Mad Studies internationally and we consider the lessons learned from pulling together the enormous diversity of experience and knowledge emerging from the process of putting this book together.

In the opening chapter, Chapter 30, Canadian pioneer survivor activist and educator David Reville, having helped Mad Studies develop in the academy, now calls for Mad Studies to be taken back 'into the community'. Given that Mad Studies is 'founded in the stories of Mad people', he argues that it is wrong to 'sequester' their stories, denying them their own history of resistance and suggests ways to reverse this. In their chapter, Victoria Armstrong and Brenda LeFrançois pick up this theme, calling for the bridging of the community/academy divide. Drawing on their experiences of bringing Mad Studies into the university, the authors elaborate their vision(s) for the democratic potentials of Mad Studies as well as their concerns over neoliberal co-option. They offer their own insights into the construction of a Mad Studies that bridges the academy/community divide.

In Chapter 32, in his examination of 'Madness, Decolonisation and Mental Health Activism in Africa', Femi Eromosele highlights the way that Africa-based advocacy groups have drawn on the provisions of the UN CRPD, within an historical context circumscribed by wide-ranging calls for decolonisation. He considers different discourses for decolonisation in Mad Studies, including the African communitarian notion 'Ubuntu', as an alternative conception of personhood and justice to that enshrined in human rights. Prateeksha Sharma, reporting on the situation in India calls for a move beyond identity politics embedded in linguistic categories, to recognise resource differences inherent in the world, who gets to speak for whom and acknowledge class privilege among those who are audible. The author urges building an emancipatory resistance by conceding to differences between the Global North and South, building culturally responsive tools, instead of simply transposing ideas developed elsewhere on societies lacking opportunities to counteract authority, rhetoric and discrimination. In Chapter 34 survivor Colin King focuses on the central importance of Mad Studies fundamentally challenging white privilege if it is to represent a truly progressive alternative to the psychiatrisation and devaluing of madness and distress. He offers a lived experience Afro-centric model and approach as the basis of political and power equality for co-production working across the colour line for race equality in mental health.

In the Afterword, Jasna Russo highlights some key issues and concerns emerging from the book. These relate to the way we approach and work with differences, as well as where to find room for Mad Studies in and outside the academic world. In a Postscript Peter Beresford puts the book and Mad Studies into the broader context of a maddening world and global futures.

Conclusion

We hope this book has helped readers gain a more in-depth understanding of the development of and prospects for Mad Studies internationally. We hope we have been able to convey the richness of this development as well as its different relationships and the different strands at work in different parts of the world. We hope particularly that we have done justice to the diversity of experience, experiential knowledge and especially the innovative developments taking place in the Global South and low income countries. Mad Studies is a discipline and field of action that is crucially about making change – progressive change in line with empowerment, social justice and anti-discrimination. We hope very much that this book can play a part in that, helping mobilise people and build alliances in relation to these goals.

References

APA (2014), *DSM-5 - Diagnostic and Statistical Manual of Mental Disorders*, Arlington, US, American Psychiatric Association.

Barnes, M., Harrison, S., Mort, M., and Shardlow, P. (1999), *Unequal Partners: User Groups and Community Care*, Bristol, Policy Press.

Beresford, P. (2016), *All Our Welfare: Towards Participatory Social Policy*, Bristol, Policy Press.

Beresford, P. (2016b), From Psycho-Politics To Mad Studies: Learning the legacy of Peter Sedgwick, *Critical And Radical Social Work*, Volume 4, Number 3, November, pp. 343-355).

Beresford, P. (2019), 'Mad', Mad Studies And Advancing Inclusive Resistance, *Disability & Society*, DOI: 10.1080/09687599.2019.1692168

Beresford, P., Perring, R., Nettle, M., and Wallcraft, J. (2016), *From Mental Illness to a Social Model of Madness and Distress?: Exploring What Service Users Say*, London, Shaping and Lives and National Survivor User Network (NSUN).

Beresford, P., and Russo, J. (2016), Supporting the Sustainability of Mad Studies and Preventing Its Co-option, *Disability & Society*, Volume 31, Issue 2, February, pp. 270–274.

Campbell, P. (1996), The History of the User Movement in the United Kingdom, in T. Heller, J. Reynolds, R. Gomm, R. Muston, and S. Patterson (editors), *Mental Health Matters: A Reader*, Basingstoke, Macmillan in association with the Open University.

Campbell, P. (2009), The Service User/Survivor movement, in J. Reynolds, R. Muston, T. Heller, J., Leach, M. McCormick, J. Wallcraft, and M. Walsh (editors), *Mental Health Still Matters*, Basingstoke, Palgrave, pp. 46–52.

Campbell, J., and Oliver, M. (1996), *Disability Politics: Understanding Our Past, Changing Our Future*, London, Routledge.

Costa, L. (2014), *Mad Studies - What it is and Why You Should Care* [Online]. Available: https://madstudies2014.wordpress.com/2014/10/15/mad-studies-what-it-is-and-why-you-should-care-2/ accessed 24 May 2020.

Crossley, N. (1998), R.D. Laing and the British Anti-Psychiatry Movement: A Socio-historical Analysis, *Social Science And Medicine*, Vol 47, No 7, pp. 877–889.

Curtis, T.R. (2003), *Mad Pride: A Celebration of Mad Culture*, London, Spare Change Books.

Daley, A. Costa, L., and Beresford, P. (2019), *Madness, Violence And Power: A Critical Collection*, Toronto, University of Toronto Press.

Donnelly, M. (1992), *The Politics Of Mental Health In Italy*, London, Routledge, pp. 39–82.

Dorling, D. (2013), *Unequal Health: The Scandal of Our Times*, Bristol, Policy Press.

Faulkner, A. (2017), Survivor Research And Mad Studies: The Role and Value of Experiential Knowledge in Mental Health Research, *Disability and Society*, Vol 32, No 4, pp. 500–520.

Foucault, M. (1988), *Madness and Civilization: A History of Insanity in the Age of Reason*, New York, Vintage Books.

Foucault, M. (2006), *History of Madness* (first published 1961), New York, Routledge.

Fulford, K., Smirnov, A., and Snow, E. (1993), Concepts of Disease and the Abuse of Psychiatry in the USSR, *The British Journal of Psychiatry*, Vol 162, No 6, pp 801–810.

Glaser, G. (2008), Mad Pride Fights A Stigma, 11 May, *New York Times*, https://www.nytimes.com/2008/05/11/fashion/11madpride.html, accessed 10 May 2020.

Goffman, E. (1961), *Asylums: Essays on the Social Situation of Mental Patients and Other Inmates*, New York, Doubleday.

Goldstein, M.S. (1980), The Politics of Thomas Szasz: A Sociological View, *Social Problems*, Vol 27, No 5, June, pp. 570–583.

Gostin, L.O. (2010), *From A Civil Libertarian To A Sanitarian: 'A Life of Learning'*, Presidential Address for the Faculty Convocation, Georgetown University Law Center, Washington, October, Washington DC, Georgetown University Law Center.

Human Rights Watch, (2019), Nigeria: People With Mental Health Conditions Chained, Abused, *Human Rights Watch*, https://www.hrw.org/news/2019/11/11/nigeria-people-mental-health-conditions-chained-abused, accessed 25 May 2020.

Johnstone, L. (2014), *A Straight-Talking Introduction To Psychiatric Diagnosis*, Wyastone Leys, PCCS Books.

Kalathil, J., and Jones, N. (2016), Unsettling Disciplines: Madness, Identity, *Research, Philosophy, Psychiatry and Psychology*, Vol 23, No 3/4, September/December, pp. 183–188.

LeFrancois, B.A., Menzies, R., and Reaume, G. (editors) (2013), *Mad Matters: A Critical Reader in Canadian Mad Studies*, Toronto, Canadian Scholars Press.

LeFrançois, B.A. (2015), Acknowledging the Past and Challenging the Present, in Contemplation of the Future: Some (Un) Doings of Mad Studies, Paper presented at the *Making Sense of Mad Studies Conference*, 30 September–1 October, Durham University.

Lent, A. (2002), *British Social Movements Since 1945: Sex, Colour, Peace and Power*, Basingstoke, Macmillan/Palgrave.

Maglajlic, R.A. (2016), Co-creating The Ways We Carry Each Other: Reflections on Being an Ally and a Double Agent, in J. Russo, and A. Sweeney (editors) *Searching for a Rose Garden. Challenging Psychiatry, Fostering Mad Studies*, Monmouth, PCCS Books, pp. 210–217.

Nasser, M. (1995), The Rise And Fall Of Anti-psychiatry, *Psychiatric Bulletin*, Vol 19, No 12, pp. 743–746.

Netchitailova, E. (2019), The Mystery Of Madness Through Art And Mad Studies. *Disability & Society*, Vol 34, Issue 9–10, pp. 1509–1515.

Plumb, A. (1994), *Distress Or Disability?: A Discussion Document*, Manchester, Greater Manchester Coalition of Disabled People.

Porter, R. (2003), *Madness: A Brief History*, Oxford, Oxford University Press.

Read, U.M., Adibokah, E., and Nyame, S. (2009), Local Suffering and the Global Discourse of Mental Health And Human Rights: An Ethnographical Study of Responses to Mental Illness in Rural Ghana, *Globalization and Health*, Vol 5, No 13, https://link.springer.com/article/10.1186%2F1744-8603-5-13/metrics accessed 23 May 2020.

Robb, B. (1967), *Sans Everything: A Case to Answer*, Edinburgh, Nelson.

Romme, M.A.J. and Escher, S.D. (1992), *Accepting Voices*, London, Mind Publications.

Romme, E.. and Escher, S. (editors), (1993), *Accepting Voices: A New Analysis of the Experience of Hearing Voices*, London, MIND.

Rose, D. (2018), Renewing Epistemologies: Service User knowledge, in P. Beresford, and S. Carr (editors), *Social Policy First Hand: An International Introduction to Participatory Social Welfare*, Bristol, Policy Press, pp. 132–141.

Scheff, T.J. (1966), *Being Mentally Ill: A Sociological Theory*, Chicago, Aldine Press.

Sedgwick, P. (1982), *Psychopolitics*, London, Pluto Press.

Spandler, H., and Poursanidou, K. (2019), Who is Included in the Mad Studies Project, 15 July, Open Volume 10, pp. 1–20, https://jemh.ca/issues/v9/documents/JEMH%20Inclusion%20iii.pdf accessed 22 May 2020.

Survivors Speak Out (1987), Charter of Needs and Demands (Edale Conference Charter), agreed and presented at the Survivors Speak Out conference, London, 18–20 September 1987, London, Survivors Speak Out.

Sweeney, A. (2016), Why Mad Studies Needs Survivor Research and Survivor Research Needs Mad Studies, *Intersectionalities: A Global Journal of Social Work Analysis, Research, Polity, and Practice*, Vol 5, No 3, pp. 36–61.

Szasz, T.S. (1961), *The Myth Of Mental Illness: Foundations of a Theory of Personal Conduct*, New York, Harper Row.

Townsend, P. (1962), *The Last Refuge: A Survey of Residential Institutions and Homes for the Aged in England and Wales*, London, Routledge and Kegan Paul.

Webb, D. (2010) *Thinking About Suicide: Contemplating and Comprehending the Urge to Die*, Ross-on-Wye, PCCS Books.

Whitaker, R. (2004), *Mad in America: Bad Science, Bad Medicine, and the Enduring Mistreatment of the Mentally Ill*, New York, Basic Books.

Wilkinson, R., and Pickett, K. (2009), *The Spirit Level: Why More Equal Societies Almost Always Do Better*, London, Penguin Books.

PART 1

Mad Studies and political organising of people with psychiatric experience

1

THE INTERNATIONAL FOUNDATIONS OF MAD STUDIES

Knowledge generated in collective action

Jasna Russo

Introduction

Besides contributing my own experiences and reflections on international activism in the mental health service user/psychiatric survivor movement[1] through this chapter, I have also attempted to bridge the other contributions in this first section of the book. As editors, we want to demonstrate the centrality of political organizing of people with psychiatric experience in the emergence and further development of Mad Studies. The chapters that follow document different starting points and various directions of advocacy and political struggles of people who come together and organize themselves most often under the name of survivors of psychiatry or people with psychosocial disabilities. These accounts chart a non-unified, diverse movement and provide a range of standpoints. Operating under different socio-political circumstances, emerging at different points in time and with different priorities and terminologies – what all organizations and networks clearly have in common is their struggle for human rights. But there is also another, less explored aspect that I wish to focus on: the process of joint knowledge making that takes place alongside mutual support and political action. This way of generating knowledge is neither purposefully initiated nor represents an end in itself. Similar processes transpire in emancipatory and liberation movements that preceded the formation of Women, Black, Queer or Disability Studies. The constantly expanding and diversifying knowledge base realized by people who come together around a specific social justice issue is also key to understanding Mad Studies as activist scholarship that started long before the term Mad Studies was coined. The vast and collective body of knowledge assembled by people deemed mad themselves endures, deepens and grows regardless of its official recognition. Or as Brenda LeFrançois puts it:

> Mad Studies […] takes place within or without academia, but never without community.
>
> *(2016: v)*

I would add that Mad Studies also takes place with or without being named Mad Studies.

DOI: 10.4324/9780429465444-3

In this chapter, I explore some features of knowledge formation that I think are foundational for Mad Studies. In the first step, I describe the entry points and the geographies of the organizations I personally joined and my own processes of becoming that were taking place within and outside of those organizations. The remainder of this chapter describes the way I see the link between Mad Studies and our diverse political organizing and why I think that Mad Studies can (and should) do what our movements have not been able to.

Movements as a place to be

It is commonly being said that movements are made up of people. Less is being said about the ways in which movements also make us as people. That includes both those great as well as those not so great experiences and encounters which shape our background and become part of who we are. Like many other activist-authors I cannot write about our movement without writing about myself and my own commitment. The intimate link between our own lives and our political work and the impossibility to separate the two seems to be at the heart of all social movements as powerfully described by Alicia Garza, a co-founder of Black Lives Matter:

> We inherit movements. We recommit to them over and over again, even when they break our hearts because they are essential to our survival.
>
> *(2020: xiii)*

The first political group I joined was a feminist group at the Student Cultural Center in Belgrade, my home town in former Yugoslavia. I was 22 and my first forced psychiatric hospitalization and treatment were already behind me. As this was the only women's group in the city at that time, the obvious focus of our work was violence against women. And even though we were welcome to share our own experiences under the slogan 'personal is political' I could only partially share mine. The mysteries and chaos of 'personal' somehow could not fit the clarity and straightforwardness of the 'political'. The prevailing activist narrative did not really leave room for the option of becoming broken or losing one's mind. This was acceptable for those 'other' women that we were supposed to support in sisterhood or theorize about. But the unspoken expectations of the 'feminist self' quickly made me understand that my own account of violence needed to be limited to a certain point and that I should keep its real ending for myself. There was some understanding of psychiatry as part of 'patriarchal' regime, but the actual personal experience of being diagnosed and forcibly treated was something better left undisclosed. Years later in the course of my employment as a counsellor in a shelter for women and children survivors of domestic violence in Germany, I faced similar impossibilities and saw how 'political' can edit or simply filter out parts of 'personal' that overwhelm and upset the 'cause' for which we have come together. I do not mean to undermine the sense of belonging and purpose that I found in women's groups and organizations, but often I felt limits and longings wonderfully described by Dorothy Allison when she writes about sexual abuse:

> Behind the story I tell is the one I don't. Behind the story you hear is the one I wish I could make you hear.
>
> *(1995: 39)*

Discovering and joining the psychiatric survivor movement came as a huge relief to me. Nothing seemed so mysterious and chaotic anymore that it couldn't be shared, understood but also tolerated and sometimes even carried together. That instant easiness and normality that I felt – if I may at all use such word in this context – opened up worlds for me. The first organization I joined was the European Network of (ex)Users and Survivors of Psychiatry that I am still an individual member of. What followed are almost 30 years of meeting different people, having all kinds of encounters and exchanges, including very intense and close ones. Even though constrained to one continent – the European Network was a meeting point of considerable differences in the early 1990s, probably more than today. One difference that I vividly remember was between Western and Eastern Europe, which then gradually dissolved with the political and economic changes that followed. The fact that my entry point into the movement was not local meant that from the very beginning I could see my personal experiences in a much broader framework. I didn't have a cultural context to share and not even a common language. After all these years, the situation remained pretty much the same for me, meaning that I am always in a position to focus on other connections, sometimes very far away from historical and other circumstances in which I grew up. I can't say that it was difficult to find such connections internationally. Intra-nationally though, things felt rather different. My immigration to Berlin accompanied by the struggle for residence and work permit turned me into a second-class citizen. In local survivor organizations I found myself part of an almost non-existent minority group within dominant German culture and among native speakers. I could share my experiences of madness and psychiatry but not the kind of acute existential struggles that I was going through. Those struggles lasted for several years and got their happy ending at some point, but my 'comrades' could not really relate to how that situation was affecting my mental and emotional state. In this matter I received far more understanding and support from my colleagues in the previously mentioned shelter where I worked. They didn't know about my psychiatric history, but they knew the troubles I was going through as the majority were migrants themselves. Obviously, no matter how politicized each of these spaces was, there were always unspoken norms that encircled the realm of familiar and imaginable and ruled communication. I will later come back to this phenomenon and its implications for Mad Studies.

My involvement in the German survivor movement continues in different ways and with some breaks, but international settings still remain the most natural and comfortable for me. It is almost as if places without a particular geographical location offer me more grounding and feel more like actual places to me. Perhaps this comes from the coincidence that my discovery of the survivor movement and joining the European Network happened soon after the war broke out in my country. In the course of my first years as a member of the Network, Yugoslavia was falling apart while I was gradually building my psychiatry-free life elsewhere. Looking backwards, I can clearly see how international survivor activism actually offered me a home and helped me build that life. More than simply giving me somewhere to belong to when I was kind of displaced in every sense, the survivor movement also became the most important learning place for me. That ongoing learning is unlike any education I have received so far, including my latest degree in the field of Mad Studies. Yet certainly, things were not only cosy and rosy and this chapter will not turn into a love letter to the survivor movement. There were too many arguments, hurts, divides and bitter lessons learned as well.

My experiences of 'international' are confined to the organizations in the Global North. Here I do not mean personal contacts only but also published sources and older movement documents from those parts of the world. I have had encounters with activists from Asia, Africa and Latin America, but to a much lesser extent and much more through learning about their work than through actually working and thinking together. It seems to me that despite an always growing number of means to communicate and overcome geographical distance we are not really coming closer. Sometimes it feels that we are even falling further apart. When I read how Alicia Garza says that "[m]ovements are the story of how we've come together when we've come apart" (2020: xiv) – I wish our movement were such story. On local and sometimes country levels – it might be the case; globally it isn't, with the exception of a few episodes of successful international action. This is of course just the way I see it. Coming together across geographical and other borders takes time, above all to listen and get to know each other and understand each other's realities, if possible without applying one's own cultural, political and other lenses. That is easier said than done in the speedy and profoundly divided world we inhabit.

But even though being aware of many limits and weaknesses of our political organizing at all levels, I cannot objectively judge the movement that has given me a home for many years or distance myself from it by any kind of rational decision. Distance grows with time and by getting closer to people whom the movement didn't really offer a home and by understanding why that was. Distance also grows as I keep finding other connections and more ways to be and intervene in the world. Still, I cannot write about survivor activism from an unengaged place or as if it weren't part of myself. I can also not criticize it as if it were a foreign body or without seeing my own doings as part of its many failures. To me, Mad Studies means a continuation of activism and political work that deepens and shifts that work to another level and entails a valuable chance to address the limits and failures inherent in many social movements. Mad Studies has the potential to stop us from falling further apart and help us connect on a different ground.

Overcoming single-issue politics

The most common failure of many social movements is their single-issue struggle, as famously expressed by Audre Lorde (1982). Here, the survivor movement is no exception. One reason for sure is 'strategic essentialism' (Voronka, 2016) exercised in many organizations by virtue of pushing forward one type of discrimination and oppression at the cost of all others. As we know, identities built around one form of injustice and the enactment of a collective self-definition are powerful emancipatory acts that can become a force to drive social change. But as we also know, such collective identities inevitably create a deadlock: they are never big or suitable enough to capture the many layers of social experience and therefore prove incapable of addressing them. The limitations inherent to identity politics commonly result in agendas that appeal to and are owned by the dominant groups within movements. Social justice movements can become places of injustice that create their own 'others'. The second-waves of the feminist and the disability movements made that clear. Mad Studies holds the potential of being such a second wave, hopefully strong enough to revise and enhance the agenda of political organizing that began in response to psychiatric oppression. As contributions in this section show, that oppression operates differently across the globe: in places where psychiatry is just one among a number of institutions of colonial heritage, the movements unite around other, more pressing issues and kick off with broader agendas for change (see TCI Asia Pacific[2] as well as contributions from Bhargavi Davar, Brenda Valdivia and Daniel Mwesigwa Iga in this section). Mad Studies opens up avenues to contextualize and de-center psychiatric oppression and avoid dead-end roads of identity politics.

Having said this – and even with the 'mad' adjective – Mad Studies does not imply embracing mad identity. For many contributors in this book and beyond, including myself – identifying as mad is not an option. It is important to remember this distinction for want of a better word and in the meantime not to confuse Mad Studies with the Mad Pride movement (see

Chapters 33 and 34 by Prateeksha Sharma and Colin King for deeper consideration of this critical issue). The human rights activist and author, Tina Minkowitz, points to the traps of ontologizing our experiences of discrimination or in other words – turning those experiences into who we are:

> Paradoxically in naming the discrimination and calling attention to the needs there is a risk of a discriminatory, violent, and objectifying response, an essentializing of our identity that diminishes our full humanity. This is the challenge faced by every equality seeking movement and it is not the end of the story but, rather, is an ongoing call for humanity to grapple with injustice.
>
> *(Minkowitz, 2014: 131)*

In another text that offers a comprehensive outline and discussion of different identities that emerge in relation to psychiatric experience, Minkowitz (2020) concludes that "we don't need a complete theory of identities, we need theory that is useful for the purposes at hand". Without this demand to serve a particular purpose and as a knowledge-making project, Mad Studies does not require the kind of strategizing typical of political action. This gives us an important opportunity to take a break from focusing on what is useful and invites us to further explore and get to the core of those uncomfortable and impractical questions that (we think) pose a threat to our collective action. This kind of joint effort could expand our understanding of political beyond claims for legal equality and help us develop a sense of togetherness that does not cement our relationship with psychiatry. I don't mean this as a call to 'overcome' and 'get by' with experiences that determined us in so many ways. I mean this as a call to foster our ability to see, feel and act beyond those experiences rather than wed ourselves and our politics to the version of injustice that we were personally subjected to. On an individual level this means that if we are to re-write the stories of our lives, we need to break free not only from demographic categories that position and arrange us in the world but also from categories of our experiences that are making us into less of who we are and can be. After all, psychiatric experience is just one such category. However intense our encounters with psychiatric regimes are, however decisive for our life trajectories and no matter how central to our political organizing, the exclusive focus on psychiatrization remains insufficient and inadequate to understand the world we live in, let alone change it. This doesn't mean that our movement does not matter or that our struggles for fundamental freedoms and human rights are outdated. Unfortunately, far and wide that is not the case. But it means that we can do more and do better and that Mad Studies might help us to move that way.

The words of Eli Clare, a queer disability activist and author vividly illustrate how none of us "leads a single-issue life" (Lorde, 1982):

> Gender reaches into disability; disability wraps around class; class strains against abuse; abuse snarls into sexuality; sexuality folds on top of race … everything finally piling into a single human body. To write about any aspect of identity, any aspect of the body, means writing about this entire maze. This I know, and yet the question remains: where to start?
>
> *(Clare, 2015: 143)*

Rather than having to prioritize any of these aspects, doing Mad Studies means freedom – and also responsibility – to start from nothing less than precisely that entire maze.

Situating first-person knowledge

Our movements are places where first-person knowledge or knowledge coming from our many experiences gets articulated, exchanged and gathered. This is more than sharing personal experiences. It is a joint process of making sense of the experiences that are commonly being psychiatrized and pushed into social exile; it is a process of legitimizing those experiences, giving them a status, finding a language to communicate them. The movement did not come up with any unifying theory of madness but it brought about many viable and sustainable answers on how to respect human crises and respond to them:

> We may gain understanding from each other but no one should assume that we are all the same; that we react the same, experience the same and that the same things work for us. Being a mental health service user, in both positive and difficult senses, really is about the difference and the fact that we are all of us as human beings different.
>
> *(Beresford, 2010:10–11)*

In the course of many years of coming together, supporting each other and organizing we not only resolved many individual situations, we also found some important answers to broader questions faced by the societies we live in. We developed ideas, concepts and practices that profoundly challenge the 'scientific' evidence base, as well as conventional evidence and policy-making about us and our lives. Our movements gave birth to approaches and methodologies that are just and better suited to understand and respond to what is being diagnosed and treated as mental illness or perceived as madness. Though integral to political activism, these underpinning processes of joint knowledge production are often not recognized as legitimate epistemic practices.

In his outline of the history of the Japanese movement, Naoyuki Kirihara (Chapter 9) describes (successful) action against an amendment of the Japanese Mental Health Act that intended to further restrict the human rights of people with psychosocial disabilities:

> We concentrated our biggest efforts on developing theories to oppose the Bill.
>
> *(000)*

This is one of rare accounts that actually mentions theory building as part of political action. The intellectual labor that takes place as a matter of course in many groups and organizations is commonly not associated with theoretical work. This certainly has to do with our internalized institutional views about what such work looks like and who is designated to perform it. However, there are also powerful mechanisms in place that actively exclude our collective knowledge from the realm of social science. In her essay "Theory as Liberatory Practice", bell hooks (1991: 4) describes devaluation and marginalization of certain types of knowledge as practice that serves to establish the academic notion of 'theory':

> It is evident that one of the many uses of theory in academic locations is in the production of an intellectual class hierarchy where the only work deemed truly theoretical is work that is highly abstract, jargonistic, difficult to read, and containing obscure references that may not be at all clear or explained.

Rather than theorizing from 'academic locations', the processes of knowledge generation within political movements are situated in lived realities of their members. First-person knowledge does not emerge in an attempt to mirror different realities or come closer to social worlds in order to understand them better. Coming from *within* the reality that it seeks to understand, first-person knowledge has a different grounding and enables different epistemology than knowledge coming from any third-person, *outside* perspective. Kate Millet actually uses the term 'reality model' when exposing the wrongfulness of medical theories about us and our lives:

> In other words, life is very difficult: death is hard to endure, bereavement, the death of love, love's labour lost, hard economic times, lost employment, lost opportunities, the embittering frequency of every form of disappointment in life. This is a reality model, built upon reality. The medical model, on the other hand, is not based upon any reality, nor is it medical, though it uses the prestige of physical medicine and the reality of physical disease to mystify us and to command a general social consent, lay or legal.
>
> *(Millet, 2007: 32)*

The value of insider perspectives in knowledge-making is attracting more attention in some fractions of social and even medical science that seek to involve multiple voices and come closer to lived realities that they study. But typically qualified as subjective, first-person perspectives are not seen as valid, self-sufficient knowledge-making locations. Such status is also commonly denied to perspectives from the first-person plural that are at the heart of political organizing: while they cannot be dismissed as subjective, our perspectives are being qualified as biased and over-involved. Collective first-person knowledge by its nature is in sharp contrast to academic dis-engagement, individualism and the competitiveness of social science. This incompatibility of jointly and horizontally (non-hierarchically) assembled knowledge with the academic notions of authorship and scientific 'discovery' is familiar to other scholarship that began outside of the 'ivory tower'. In her above-mentioned essay, bell hooks (1991: 3) writes that "the production of feminist theory is complex, that it is less the individual practice than we often think and usually emerges from engagement with collective sources"

Movements are collective endeavors and so are their respective knowledge-making processes. The collective bodies of knowledge they produce involve the powerful fusion of ideas, histories and wisdom passed on among many different people, places and generations:

> Movements do not have official moments when they start and end, and there is never just one person who initiates them. Movements are much more like waves than they are like light switches. Waves ebb and flow but they are perpetual, their starting point unknown, their ending point undetermined, their direction dependent upon the conditions that surround them and the barriers that obstruct them.
>
> *(Garza, 2020: xiii)*

Knowledge gathered in organizations of psychiatric survivors and people with psychosocial disabilities comes as a result of many conversations and thinking together in order to act upon the issues that concern us. As distinct from places of education where people come to receive knowledge – our movements are places where people contribute their knowledge. Based on the initial premise that everybody has valid knowledge, we focus instead on what we can do with that knowledge, with what we know together. Knowledge making within movements is inseparable from acting upon what we know and this proximity between the two is very different from reserved and hesitant evidence-making patterns of social science. Mad Studies has therefore inherited considerable disillusionment in conventional and particularly in medical science and a lot of justified distrust in the notion of a knowing 'expert'. If it is to stay true to its own self-conception of 'activist scholarship' (LeFrançois, 2016) Mad Studies must be careful about not turning into another third-person enterprise, that takes on the role of knowledge making about 'others'. Mad Studies has good prospects to insist on the fact that everybody has 'lived experience' and that in that sense there can be no such thing as 'us' who know (better) as opposed to those ('others') whom we study. Building on the knowledge making traditions of our movements, Mad Studies opens up a space for each and every one to join knowledge production precisely from where and who they are.

Taking responsibility for our collective knowledge

In her essay "Mad Studies – What it is and why you should care", Canadian activist and author Lucy Costa (2014) powerfully invites everybody to become part of, but at the same time not take ownership of, Mad Studies project:

> Mad Studies has grown out of the long history of consumer/survivor movements organised both locally and internationally. […] Together, we can cultivate our own theories/ models/ concepts/ principles/ hypotheses/ and values about how we understand ourselves, or our experiences in relationship to mental health system(s), research and politics. No one person, or school, or group owns Mad Studies or defines its borders.

At the time of writing, seven years have passed since Lucy Costa wrote this. In the meantime, the term Mad Studies has become more well-known and is branding itself inside and outside university courses. This also includes approaches to Mad Studies as an academic field that is by default separate from activism and at the most just seen in historical connection with our movements. I will come back to these developments in the afterword to this collection. Here I wish to focus briefly on the question of (non)ownership.

The fact that the vast body of knowledge of people deemed mad is out there, at everybody's disposal certainly makes that knowledge an important and accessible emancipatory source for many.[3] But it also readies that knowledge for distortion and co-optation of different kinds. We can't pretend that we haven't already witnessed and analyzed such developments (Costa et al., 2012; Penney and Prescott, 2016; McWade, 2016; Fabris, 2016). The truth is that our collective achievements are not being collectively owned. This means that the ideas and practices that we develop, continue to be detached from the contexts in which they emerge and disentangled from their original meaning and intention. The destiny of our collective first-person knowledge largely depends on those who make use of it. Putting a Mad Studies or any other kind of label on that body of knowledge will certainly not stop such projects. Also, collective ownership is still an uncommon concept and not easy to establish in the type of world we live in. But if we are to disrupt the long tradition of erasure of knowledge of people deemed mad, then we might begin thinking about taking more responsibility for what we know and what generations before us have assembled. By this, I don't mean 'defining borders' or any bureaucratic act of 'sealing' ownership. One of the best features of our collective knowledge is its resistance to definition and control and the ability to always find itself anew outside such ambitions. What I mean is taking on the task of building on that knowledge base *independently and regardless* of the momentary agendas and currencies of psychiatry and mental health that surround it. Taking our knowledge responsibly means engaging in complex tasks of researching, connecting, extending and deepening the international pool of knowledge created by people considered mad or disordered so that it gradually becomes more and more difficult to turn that knowledge into something else. I am aware that this implies a continuous battle on an extremely uneven playing field. What we are dealing with are not differences between perspectives and schools of thought. We are dealing with the systematic epistemic erasure that has lasted for centuries. The forms of epistemic injustice (Fricker, 2010) differ according to the historical epochs in the ways societies and their ruling regimes (mis)understand and approach 'madness'. These traditions range from active silencing, ignorance, belittlement, re-interpreting, overwriting, appropriating up to the level of issuing glossy invitations to 'co-production' or subtle remaking of 'survivor-control' into 'consumer-leadership'. It is without a doubt that these developments will continue with always more sophisticated methods but it makes a difference whether we stand in their way or seek to make some profit from what is on offer. In practice this is hardly ever a question of either / or and many times we find ourselves trying to do both. I am certainly not positioned to suggest any universal 'right' or 'wrong' but have a sincere hope that Mad Studies provides space in which we can leave the exhausting and risky subversion labor behind us and turn to further exploring, diversifying and deepening our first-person epistemologies to see where that will lead us. Indian activist and scholar Bhargavi Davar uses the powerful metaphor of unveiling when calling for our own responsibility towards alternative knowledge that is already there:

> I think that it is important to open the veil created by medical professionals in mental health, and look what else is already there. Otherwise, we tend to become the perpetrators who we are opposing. We ignore who they ignore. We repeat their rhetoric. We become victims of ourselves. That oppression is more difficult to combat.
>
> *(WNUSP, 2014: 12–13)*

Concluding remarks

Reflecting on my own experiences and personal learnings, I have attempted to explore in this chapter the processes of knowledge making that take place alongside activism and political action. Overshadowed by those more-pressing-things that movements are all about and by not corresponding to conventional understandings of 'intellectual labor' as well, knowledge-making traditions within movements of psychiatric survivors and people with psychosocial disabilities often go unnoticed. Generally, the ideas and concepts that we develop attract more attention than the joint knowledge-making processes that underpin them. However, the latter are the key to understanding Mad Studies and the potential contribution of this field. I have tried to highlight both the emancipatory aspects of these processes as well as their limitations and weaknesses, arguing that Mad Studies has a good chance of addressing these and moving collective knowledge making to another level. Most importantly, I hope I have demonstrated how the organizing of psychiatric survivors and people with psychosocial disabilities is central to Mad Studies and that this connection is not just a thing of the past. In my view, Mad Studies carries on the movements' work without the constraints and beyond current political agendas, including our own. It is about valuing and deepening our own knowledge and continuing to learn from each other as well as from other liberation movements and scholarship. It is not so much about where we get to exactly in our different contexts but more about how we get there and who we become on the way. Our knowledge should of course keep traveling in all possible directions while Mad Studies and collective action remain organically intertwined. Different in their scope, both of these projects belong together and can only improve and strengthen each other. It is the responsibility of all of us to keep this link alive and mutual.

Notes

1 This is a term used in the organizations that I was personally involved with. I often use the shortened form 'survivor movement' to express my own preference and affinity. None of the terms I use are meant as any kind of universal umbrella expression to subsume political organizing and stances described by other contributors to this book.
2 TCI Asia Pacific stands for Transforming Communities for Inclusion of persons with psychosocial disabilities – Asia Pacific. See more at https://www.tci-asia.org/
3 Besides oral histories that are kept alive within our respective movements there are also a number of written sources ranging from personal accounts, anthologies, newsletters and archives to research reports and conceptual work. What is considered to be the first written document of political organizing of people deemed mad dates back to 1620 (*The Petition of the Poor Distracted People in the House of Bedlam*). See the Opal Project (2007) for many more documents.

References

Allison, D (1995) *Two or Three Things I Know for Sure.* New York: Dutton.

Beresford, P (2010) *A Straight-Talking Introduction to Being a Mental Health Service User.* Ross-on-Wye: PCCS Books.

Clare, E (2015) *Exile and Pride: Disability, Queerness, and Liberation*, 16th anniversary edition. Durham and London: Durham University Press.

Costa, L (2014) Mad Studies – What It Is and Why You Should Care. https://madstudies2014. wordpress.com/2014/10/15/mad-studies-what-it-is-and-why-you-should-care-2/ Accessed: 24 February 2021.

Costa, L, Voronka, J, Landry, D, Reid, J, McFarlane, B, Reville, D and Church, K (2012) Recovering Our Stories: A Small Act of Resistance. *Studies in Social Justice* 6 (1): 85–101.

Fabris, E (2016) Community Treatment Orders: Once a Rosy Deinstitutional Notion? In Russo, J and Sweeney, A (eds.) *Searching for a Rose Garden. Challenging Psychiatry, Fostering Mad Studies.* Monmouth: PCCS Books. 97–105.

Fricker, M (2010) *Epistemic Injustice. Power and the Ethics of Knowing.* New York: Oxford University Press.

Garza, A (2020) *The Purpose of Power. How to Build Movements for the 21st Century.* London: Penguin Random House UK.

hooks, b (1991) Theory as Liberatory Practice. *Yale Journal of Law and Feminism*, 4 (1), Article 2.

LeFrançois, B (2016) Foreword. In Russo, J and Sweeney, A (eds.) *Searching for a Rose Garden. Challenging Psychiatry, Fostering Mad Studies.* Monmouth: PCCS Books. v–vii.

Lorde, A (1982) "Learning from the 60s" a Speech Delivered at the Celebration of the Malcolm X Weekend at Harvard University. https://www.blackpast.org/african-american-history/1982-audre-lorde-learning-60s/ Accessed: 24 February 2021.

McWade, B (2016) Recovery-as-Policy as a Form of Neoliberal State Making. *Intersectionalities. A Global Journal of Social Work Analysis, Research, Polity, and Practice* 5 (3): 62–81.

Millet, K (2007) The Illusion of Mental Illness. In Stastny, P and Lehmann, P (eds.) *Alternatives Beyond Psychiatry.* Berlin: Peter Lehmann Publishing. 29–37

Minkowitz, T (2014) Convention on the Rights of Persons with Disabilities and Liberation from Psychiatric Oppression. In Burstow, B, LeFrançois, B A and Diamond, S (eds.) *Psychiatry Disrupted: Theorizing Resistance and Crafting the (R)evolution.* Montreal and Kingston: McGill-Queen's University Press. 129–144.

Minkowitz, T (2020) Identities and Who Gets to Have Them https://tastethespring.wordpress.com/ 2020/12/17/identities-and-who-gets-to-have-them/?fbclid=IwAR0GvqlMZbqzcqjJfmzG7RmNSJ T4DQT_jWANGc79n3rrNONBsDJC_8YZifw Accessed: 24 February 2021.

Penney, D and Prescott, L (2016) The Co-optation of Survivor Knowledge: The Danger of Substituted Values and Voice. In Russo, J and Sweeney, A (eds.) *Searching for a Rose Garden. Challenging Psychiatry, Fostering Mad Studies.* Monmouth: PCCS Books. 35–45.

The Opal Project (2007) Our Story of Commitment: A Living History http://www.theopalproject.org/ ourstory.html. Accessed 15 February 2021.

Voronka, J (2016) The Politics of 'People with Lived Experience'. Experiential Authority and the Risks of Strategic Essentialism. *Philosophy, Psychiatry, & Psychology*, 23 (3/4): 189–201.

World Network of Users and Survivors of Psychiatry (WNUSP) (2014) WNUSP Board and Members Conversations: The Global Mental Health Movement and Us, the Global North Divide and Foucault https://wgwnusp2013.files.wordpress.com/2014/02/wnusp-conversation-from-the-margins-feb-2014.pdf Accessed 15 February 2021.

2

REFLECTIONS ON POWER, KNOWLEDGE AND CHANGE

Mary O'Hagan; based on a conversation with Peter Beresford

Introducing myself

From the age of 18 to about the age of 27 I was very involved in using mental health services, with countless admissions to hospital. It was the major feature of my life over those years. Like many people I found the services pretty bad. I thought they didn't understand my experience or respect what I was going through. They saw me as a bundle of deficits and held out little or no hope for my future.

When I came out of that experience, I felt very strongly that the people who run these services needed the help of people like us to make them better and more responsive. And in various guises I have been working on that project ever since to radically transform how people think about distress and deliver responses for people who are experiencing it.

I started as an advocate and began a peer-led organisation in Auckland called Psychiatric Survivors in the late 1980s – that's when the movement got going in New Zealand. In 1990 I started up a national network. And in 1991 I was elected the first Chairperson of the World Network of Users and Survivors of Psychiatry. I worked in London for a year as a user consultant, helping services change from an institutional to a more community base. Between 2000 and 2007 was a commissioner at New Zealand's Mental Health Commission, which was set up to monitor and help improve service delivery. When I left the Commission, I started up a social enterprise called PeerZone where we developed resources and peer support for people in one-to-one and group settings.[1] Over the last two years I have been working in the wellbeing promotion end of the spectrum at the Health Promotion Agency of New Zealand. All this time, alongside allies and others with lived experience, my big project has been to radically transform how services and society respond to people.

How much have we been able to achieve?

I sometimes think if I'd joined the gay rights movement as a young woman I might have felt a happier than I do today because so much has changed for lesbian and gay people in countries like ours. I'm not very happy about the progress we have made in the 'mad' movement and I've experienced a lot of sadness and anger about it. If I talked to a young person today who wants

DOI: 10.4324/9780429465444-4

to change the mental health system, I'd probably warn them that they might end up at my stage of life wondering what difference they made.

Why haven't we made that much difference? There's a number of things. One is the continuing dominance of psychiatry in health systems and the way psychiatry really still dominates the discourse, the knowledge base, the evidence and the resources. They run the show. It has become increasingly clear to me over the years that while we have a health-led system, that is dominated by clinical people, and uses most of the resources for pills and pillows services, we are doomed in terms of creating a system that really works for people.

The problem of psychiatry

Psychiatry doesn't have many tools – they are drugs, the Mental Health Act and hospitals. The trouble is they use these tools for everything. It's like only having a hammer when sometimes you need a screwdriver or a wrench. But it's not just that they don't have many tools – the tools themselves can be intrinsically harmful to people. I think compulsory treatment does more harm than good. I would love to see a world where people don't have compulsory legislation. I also think hospital-based services do far more harm than good. I have been advocating for years for community and home-based crisis support and the drastic downsizing of hospital beds. And of course, the medication is a double-edged sword. Some people feel helped by it and some feel harmed and a lot of people feel a bit ambivalent about it.

Psychiatry does routine harm, not just through the ethical lapses or the incompetence of a few, but because of standard practice and the whole paradigm that operates within.

Psychiatry needs to move away from the hub of the system and be just one of the spokes. Until that happens we won't see any big change.

Our survivor knowledge

We have done a lot as survivors over the last 50 years of the movement. But have we made much difference to the lives of people who are currently aged 14, 18, 20 or 25 who walk into a mental health service or who experience extreme distress? It may be that they have a better chance of getting a better deal today but there still are a lot of people getting a terrible deal. It's not just because services are under-resources – it's also where those resources sit and how they are used.

What are the indicators we have made a difference? The way services respond would be an indicator. But it's not just about the deal people get in services. We need to see a positive difference to people's life chances – their employment and housing prospects, and their prospects for having partners, children and friends.

Against a backdrop of psychiatric dominance, lived experience knowledge is very side-lined. It should be central to the whole thing. Our knowledge is optional clip-on whereby sometimes people think, 'Oh yes, we should have a lived experience perspective on this'.

We have a very interesting but tragic situation with the indigenous people in New Zealand. It's tragic that Maori were colonised by the Europeans who stole their land and suppressed their culture and language. There are many parallels because psychiatry has the same features of a colonising force on people with lived experience.

The Maori people have a very different worldview to the European derived culture in New Zealand. The Maori world view gets dropped and side-lined by the dominant white culture. People are so marinated in the dominant culture, that they can't even see that their goldfish bowl is one of many.

I think the same happens in psychiatry and the mental health system. People in the system are so indoctrinated into a particular world view that they have to make a huge effort to understand and absorb other world views, in this case the world view built up by people who experience distress.

The prospects for change?

Over my life, the power has stayed with psychiatry and increasingly with biological psychiatry. I read somewhere recently that 45 times as many research dollars are spent on biological research as on psycho-social research into what they call 'schizophrenia'. That tells you everything.

Despite my sadness I hold out hope for change. In New Zealand, we talk about the three baskets of knowledge – clinical, cultural and lived experience. We need to give each of these baskets an equal weighting. I don't necessarily subscribe to that, because I don't know if the clinical world view is that helpful, but some people say they have benefited from it.

In our country, we've got used to the challenge from Maori people saying, 'We've got a different way of knowing things'. So there's a parallel challenge to the one that we give as people with lived experience. I think it's quite helpful for people with lived experience, even though white people with lived experience can side-line the Maori world view as much as any other white people can. But in some ways Maori and lived experience world views have some things in common. The clinical European-derived scientific world view is about separating all the parts and examining them all in isolation from each other, splitting things off so your knowledge isn't contaminated with confounding variables. Whereas from a Maori world view that seems absurd because they have a very holistic, multi-dimensional view of life. Lived experience world views also favour the holistic and the subjective.

There is an increasing involvement of Maori in lived experience activities. There was some in the early days but it dropped off. Now they are a growing force with their own national network. This is important because Maori more often face intergenerational trauma and are much higher users of services. They are also subjected more to compulsory interventions.

Mad Studies

I'm all in favour of Mad Studies. I haven't gone down an academic route in my life although I guess I could have. I have quite high hopes for Mad Studies, but there's a network working in New Zealand and Australia, that calls themselves Service User Academia. Every time I go to one of their conferences I tell them, why don't you change your name because you're not in the role of service user when you are being academics. I can't understand why they don't change their name. They might think 'Mad Studies' is a bit provocative but other names have been suggested such as 'First Person Studies'.

What worries me is that quite often these lived experience academics are tagging on to other people's research, they are not setting the research agenda. We've got women's studies departments and disability studies departments. I don't know if there's a Mad Studies department anywhere in the world, though I think Ryerson University in Toronto is heading in that direction. I would like to see Mad Studies as a full discipline and not have lived experience academics hanging off the coat-tails of clinically trained academics. That worries me.

Psychiatry as a discipline has the service arena, but it also has academic arena and similar dynamics apply. Having said that, there are some very good psychiatrist and nurse academics who have really supported the development of academics with lived experience. They have cleared the way for lived experience academics to work in a self-determining way on their own projects.

I see hope with Mad Studies but I would like it to have been more developed by now. I'm getting to the point where a lot of the changes I would like to see may not happen in my lifetime.

Challenges to our movement

It's really interesting to see what's happened to our movement over the years. I think it's lost a lot of its edge. Movements start off with a hiss and a roar and they get under the establishment's skin. But what happened in New Zealand was the system said, 'Why don't you come and work for us?'. Initially we had a lot of independent survivor-led organisations which were weakened by the fact that a lot of the people in them ended up with jobs in the system. And now most of our contribution is not so much based on human rights or restoring our place in the world, it's about providing services within the service system.

It's good we have a place in the system, even if it is not a powerful place. But I do think there is a place for that more edgy, independent advocacy that in many countries it has receded. There is still an awful lot of advocacy needed for people who have ended up in the mental health system.

I don't have an answer to how you revive an independent movement. If we revived it today, it would be different. A social movement is a bit like spontaneous combustion. You can't plan or control a social movement.

Note

1 See more at https://www.peerzone.info/

3

SHIFTING IDENTITIES AS REFLECTIVE PERSONAL RESPONSES TO POLITICAL CHANGES

Bhargavi V. Davar

The political is personal: Beginnings of the Bapu Trust

I am 59 years old this year (2021) and so I go a long way back. I say that I started my work when I was five years old with my own childhood exposures to mental asylums of India. Around the time when I was exposed to those, India had just gotten independence so the colonial animal was just leaving our shores, so to speak. But the tail was still visible in many of our systems and in some systems, it continues to be fossilized. The colonial asylums and the laws deeply affected me, although of course at five, you don't know these things.

My mother was in that system. I saw this a lot. I have memories of her forced incarceration, of her being tied up, being strait-jacketed, tightly tied down in ropes or cloth, all those things, including direct shock (ECT without anaesthesia). It is a very visceral memory for me even today, after all these years. She was put away and circled between many such places, liberty deprived and treated inhumanely. It was my mother, but at five, she was an extension of me, so the effects rubbed off on me quite a lot.

It was the single most significant, enduring and impactful trauma of my life. No child should be exposed to involuntary commitment. It leaves an enduring trauma impact. My mother didn't live to tell that tale in full. It must have surely impacted her. When she ever remembered the doctors who did this to her, she would mouth profanities. I have built my complete life and work around just making sense, of well, what happened when I was five and six, what happened to her. My mom was in and out, and I kept seeing her coming in and going out of my life. These really bizarre things were happening in the name of care. It was quite paradoxical – I mean why would somebody be tied down and dragged into a mental asylum and why would that be called 'care'? So that question was very alive for me for dozens of years. I painted, wrote poetry, read books, but that question did not go away: And, hasn't till now!!

At 27, I pursued my PhD on a dialogue which I felt was at the core within the psychiatric 'sciences', so called. The science seriously compromised human freedom and human values, so my thesis was somewhat grandiosely called 'Psychoanalysis as a Human Science: Beyond Foundationalism' (Davar and Bhat, 1995). It was an obscure work in the philosophy of science, but really exploring what was going on with the mental and behavioural sciences – 'are they

DOI: 10.4324/9780429465444-5

even sciences?'; 'why they are constructed as they are?'; 'what constitutes proof of concept?'; 'did they not have a value base?', etc.

This was not so much from a colonial perspective, but from the perspective of philosophy of science. A 'disease' needed to have a bug, and this one didn't; so what kind of medical science was that? That psychiatry was deeply colonial in its practices was an understanding that came much later, when I realized that my mother lived in the cusp between a colonial regime and the new independent India. She occupied a cusp, like the families that were profoundly affected by the Partition (*when India and Pakistan separated*), but at the individual level. She was a victim of those changing times as India became post-colonial India, after a long period of hate and violence. Political incarceration, incarceration on the basis of economic, infectious, genetic and mental defects, to discard people identified as 'lunatic', 'idiots', 'lepers', 'paupers', 'vagrants', 'fakirs' and 'tribes' was normal for those times. Not that things are very different now: We have the new Mental Health Care Act, but the colonial asylums are still very much there in India with the same coercive design, even very much the same infrastructure, as they were all those years ago. The 'Leprosy Act' of yonder years is illegal, however 'leper colonies' remain.

The first time I ever made a presentation about my life and colonialism was just a few months ago, in December of 2019. My mother was wandering and homeless for a number of years because my family deserted her or put her away in these institutions. Over the years, I have seen my mother in different forms – a homeless person, a woman who was hearing voices, a spiritual woman, a disabled woman, a woman subject to extreme gender injustice, a saint possibly.... She left behind a lot of poems and her writings. She was a creative person. I saw her as a woman who was really anguished at not being allowed to be a mother – and here I was, being furious with her for deserting me and abandoning me and all of that. But she was not allowed to meet us. She was literally kicked out of the house. She was asked not to ever to come back. She also had a physical disability. It creates in me a great despair to think of her as a wandering mendicant: How did she move around? What did she eat? Where did she sleep? Were people kind to her? Did they abuse her? But the system is the same. We've had different formulations of the Mental Health Act over two centuries. We had the Lunatic Asylums Act of 1858, the Lunacy Act of 1912, all these other newer acts. The format has not changed. It is about arrest without a warrant and detention. I jokingly say that the British Raj gave us this fantastic railway system, but it also gave us these asylums.

I went through my own deep depression in my mid-thirties and by then I had finished my PhD, obsessed with my mother and her experiences. I think I lightened up a little bit in my late forties and that's a whole lifetime trying to make sense. I never lasted in any intimate relationship, so after a point, I just gave up on relationships. The trauma of the exposures was so high, my body was just reacting and getting triggered all the time.

I was largely working on my PhD and I was involved in other things: There was a sexual harassment campaign on campus. I led that campaign, things like that, but nothing big, no vision as such what I was doing. It was a kind of blundering along, reading, writing, painting, etc. I was focusing mostly on my studies, rationalizing. It helped me make sense of my life, what this 'psychiatry' was about. I was quite an introvert, you would not have noticed me in any room, a gathering or on any campus. I was quite silent and invisible.

Of course, the origin of my survivor identity is this experience, but it could pop up at the most unexpected times and cause conflict and harm. So I just focused on my life, on my work, of watching the things erupting out of my skin every now and then, trying to stay together enough to understand and make sense of exactly what happened to me when I was between 5 and 10 years old. That was that!

I had this deep sense of abandonment. My mother was not around for many years; and she was in and out of all these horrible places. Eventually, she settled in a temple in the south of India, so we hardly saw her for many years. So a part of the origin of my psychological distress is that I felt deeply abandoned and I carried that with me for many, many years. People can never give me enough love and care, enough hugs, because it was never enough.

We've done a lot of work on the lived experiences of women like me, going through psycho-social distress and disturbance. One strong learning from all of that is that we have neglected engagement with the body and the impact of trauma on our lived realities. And of course, we don't get enough hugs!! For me this is a big thing, I did not get much assistance from literature, what my body was telling me daily – 'unresolved trauma caused by the violence of incarceration'. And understanding the body as a way of healing the mind, for me, really came from sources very different from psychiatry – Peter Levine and Ann Frederick (1997), somatic healing, yoga, cycling, Buddhism, gardening, certain forms of arts-based therapies … all of that. I think in our contest for reclaiming our minds somewhere we have omitted what's happening in our bodies and I'd want to redirect our attention to that. Because trauma is here, it is in the skin, the scalp, it is everywhere in the body. That's the foundation for the Bapu Trust[1] and our work with body-based healing. The beginnings of the Trust was very much based on mad identity, and that was my own mad identity, and the vast sensory experiences that it opened up, allowing us to pursue another path of healing as well as advocacy.

Finding people like me with a mad identity

After I finished my PhD I started to look around and search for people who were critical of the 'psy' disciplines and it appeared as if I was the only one at that time in India. I didn't know much about the survivor movement and slowly I started to read. For my PhD I read a lot of works; David Cooper, women like Kate Millett, Germaine Greer, I read about Judi Chamberlin. One section of my PhD work was on anti-psychiatry and it was quite a revelation for me that I am not alone and there were so many people who have struggled with this. I got interested in the history of the user/survivor movement in the war period. Slowly I started identifying as a person who is a survivor of psychiatry, never a user, but a survivor of psychiatry. Since then I have named myself as a 'childhood survivor of psychiatric abuse with enduring trauma'! So this has been my identity, for the longest ever time. And of course, I met wonderful people between 1995 and 2000 and with whatever little money I had, I travelled. I met David Oaks, Judi Chamberlin, Sylvia Caras, Mary O'Hagan, Chris Hansen … . I met many, many wonderful people at this time. I read the movement archives – the *Madness Network News* archives, *Dendron*, Leonard Ray Frank and his fight against ECT, learned from the ex-patients' Liberation Movement, resistance poetry, art and installations. I read about the works of people like Iris Hölling, visited some projects on 'alternatives' and I learned about the Mad Pride movement. So I really spent a lot of my time reading and connecting with people. Of course, at that time we didn't have the internet and the computer entered our university a bit later during my study period. Connecting with people was in real time and space; sometimes a bit difficult, but then somehow, I managed! I gathered a lot of books and resources by writing letters to various folks around the world. It was always so exciting to have a paper or two trickle in, in the daily post.

After my PhD, with the first anti-psychiatry book in the country in my name, I met Jayasree Kalathil in Hyderabad during my different journeys, between 1995 and 2000. We shared a lot of critical ideas of our personal experiences of psychiatry. Jayasree had a strong feminist and human rights background, from which I drew inspiration and strength. We formed a very strong sisterhood at that time. I also met many other men and women who were running support groups or were coming together with a critical or anti-psychiatry perspective – very few, no more than a handful in India. Some of them have passed on. But there was a voice at that time. It was a very, very inaudible voice, but we were coming together. With Jayasree Kalathil we started a newsletter – called Aaina (meaning 'mirror'). The archives are still up on our website.[2] Jayasree Kalathil started it for the Bapu Trust and we kept it going for a good eight years. It gathered the voices of resistance to psychiatry in post-colonial India, the trauma and humiliation of forced incarceration, stories of abuse in the name of care and the ironic fact that all of this was legal!!

The systems haven't changed. In fact you see across Asia Pacific a very strong – what we call neocolonialism – particularly in the commonwealth countries. The World Health Organization (WHO) fuelled the case of creating more mental health laws, as if that was a sign of modernity. This trend to 'modernize' mental health care using colonial design of law is found across the Asia Pacific region. Neocolonial systems in mental health are typically two segments of law: (1) the mental health law with provision for violent incarceration; (2) incapacity law denying persons of their legal subjecthood. These laws are implemented through the asylums and through incapacity courts and case law.

We were recently in Timor Leste, for a country mission visit. They obtained independence very recently. They have extremely strong sentiments and anger towards the British, because their independence, just like the Indian independence, was driven by conflict – indigenous conflict, boundary conflicts, conflict with the empire – all of that. So their experiences of getting independence from the Raj was not so easy. There is one institution there, it is in the exact same form as it was in many years ago. And it is the same with India. We still have the large estates, bell tower structures, central surveillance, high wall security and triple detention (a large, prison-like gate around the periphery, lock up general wards and further inside, solitary confinement rooms).[3]

I was among the rare voices for Mad Studies for many years in India. Now people are calling themselves 'users' because globalizing psychiatry has brought in psycho-pharmaceuticals and medication and also private institutions in a very big way. People consider it modern to be 'mad' and on psych drugs, but the actual practices are brutally old and they continue to exist. A privately run institution for the insane – why would they have involuntary confinement, but they do. Why would a private agency take the power of the state and confine people against their will? But they do. So I jokingly say that the so-called mentally ill people are the only ones who pay to get arrested in this country and put away against their will! This is true for the Commonwealth. *Spoiler Alert* – the North Americas and Australia are a part of the Commonwealth too, so the same colonial game applies there as well, though the state may be paying for the violent incarceration of its own subjects.

But in some parts of Asia Pacific, it's different. My extensive travels helped me figure this out. Countries which were never colonized or were never colonized by the British have very different – and I would say, on a scale of zero to ten – much more liberal systems; or at least, they don't have classic mental health systems with a law and institutional infrastructure for restraint and solitary confinement. The WHO hasn't reached there yet, despite a lot of pressure over three decades from Geneva on making mental health legislations. It is a good thing because in those countries, communities can build support systems without having to pull something down. When colonialism has gone so deep as in India, into the mental health policy designs, pulling those institutions down is impossible. You cannot change the Indian railways and you cannot change these asylums and their format and design. I call it the 'intergenerational trauma' trap for policymakers, because they cannot imagine another kind of humane design (Davar and Ravindran, 2015).

The CRPD and how it changed our identity position

One of the good things that happened this millennium is the UN Convention on the Rights of Persons with disabilities. The CRPD is making a difference in India. Our advocacy has been framed under the CRPD, as a way to decolonize mental health. It is giving us a liberal perspective. Slowly people are turning to the CRPD. There is interest in a different narrative, a different approach. The user/survivor movement is not so popular as the women's movement. It is not known widely. The reason for that is, even if you take a country like India, you will not find so many angry users and survivors. I think that is partly because of the colonial mentality of saluting the authority, i.e. the doctors. The other reason is, we were just about forty institutions for the whole country some years ago. So the number of people who went in there and came out, or perished there, they were just too few and too scared, that they never mobilized. Many of the people who go into these institutions are also the most vulnerable; the urban poor, the women who have been kicked out of a difficult marriage, people like that. So they aren't going to gather together and rally at a Mad Pride march. We never had that.

In a typical Indian city today, if you are seen as behaving 'strangely', gender deviant, your family would push you to meet a mental health professional – a psychiatrist. And the psychiatrist, it depends, there are so many stories of gender bias and abuse. So if I was a woman in my twenties with tattoos and strange haircuts and hair colour, wearing torn jeans, (this is the modern young person of India), then I am likely to be asked if I am lesbian or if I am transgender. As if those are medical or mental problems, a lot of gender biases come in, even if I'm not saying anything about my sexuality. This is a big problem relating very much to the gender and mental health discourse in India, even now.

There is a big movement in recognition of psychosocial issues in relation to ethnicity and caste too. But what is happening there is that social injustice is getting converted algorithmically into psychiatric disorder. That's what happened with gender issues. That's what happened when I wrote about it way back in 1999 (Davar 1999). Psychiatrists hitched onto this bandwagon and now women are a big market for psychopharma. So the options for advocacy are – do you want to reform the mental health system, do you want to ask for better services? Do we want to say 'Oh well, we can build better mental institutions'. This is what a lot of well-intentioned people are thinking: we can actually do these things. They get into that and then they find that it's not possible, that it's a dead end. No one will be able to do that because that's the nature of the system. It is very old and it is not suited for modern society. You can't take a 400-year-old car and make it ok. You just have to put it in the museum and say 'Thank you for inventing this solution, but this is not for us today'. That's what we've got to do with the colonial asylum design, mental health laws and coercive treatment. It's not only in India, it's everywhere in the commonwealth.

I have been hounded down when I make public speeches based on my experiential knowledge. I have been laughed at, hooted, humiliated and openly insulted when I have made statements on public platforms, so it hasn't been easy. No way has it been easy. Even today, I am not very much included in much of the policy discussions going on in India. I am a very well recognized person internationally. I do lots of CRPD trainings. I am invited to United Nations forums. I do lots of training in the Asia Pacific region. People respect me and my writing, but not back home. These days it is getting better because people realize you cannot bypass the Convention and there are very few Convention experts in my country. 'Let's look up and see this person. Let's listen to what she has to say'.

Things here are changing. Even the governmental health movement is changing. The different offices of the United Nations are changing. We are getting amazing reports from different parts of the United Nations. Earlier it was just the CRPD committee. Now even the Convention against Torture officers are talking about forced treatment as torture. I think there are shifts. In my country and in the region, we don't have academia which recognizes Mad Studies. The best we might have is critical psychology done by psychologists. But you won't have people like me with very strong survivor or mad identity. I do think I harboured a mad identity for some time up to 2000–2001 but it changed after the Convention came in.

I think people move and shift in their identity positions. What was then was then and what is now is now. What has helped me and my peers in the movement is that the disabled person's identity is actually empowering because it opens the door to solutions for living a life on our own terms. The cross-disability movement and the CRPD gave us a wide range of solutions, particularly social and economic solutions for the problem of our basic issue in society – being in the margins. Inclusion in society will involve offers for various social, economic and other measures: work, housing, food, completing education, having access to sports and culture, etc. I think that's what is exciting with this Convention, the CRPD.

I'm comfortable identifying as having a psycho-social disability, because of what I have seen in these years after the CRPD came in. A lot of people argue that the Mad identity is an identity of resistance, but I also believe that it has been an identity of vulnerability. I have had deep experiences of this myself, of crashing and just bottoming-out and that's it. You just surrender to whatever this is, because traumas like that, they grab you, shake you and you can't make a response. A mad identity may not be very empowering because it pitches me only against psychiatry and that's the thing. I want to talk to people who have jobs to offer, who are in the school system, housing solutions for us. I want to talk to people who are in sports, food, arts… .

What I have seen for the Asia Pacific region, high income countries have too many lock up facilities – South Korea, Japan, China, to some extent Taiwan. Interestingly Thailand was never colonized by any country, they never had a mental health act or mental asylums. But because of the modernization process, and moving to a middle-income country from a poor country and becoming a booming economy, recently they brought in a mental health act. And of course, the number of institutions there rose phenomenally. China is very different of course, they have institutions for everybody, and for people with disabilities as well. I know that Hong Kong has a very, very strong, thriving survivor movement. Japan has one. These are people who have been in resistance for thirty or forty years. These are high income countries – very different from most of the countries of the Asia Pacific area, where these institutions do not exist and there is no mental health law. I would say the mental health law and asylum nexus is a commonwealth phenomenon. People in other countries are not very angry with psychiatrists because mental health institutions do not exist, so not many people are coming raging out of these institutions because they are not there.

Of course, things are changing. The Geneva based promoters of the mental health law betrayed us the most. They advocated for mental health law for far too long, seeing it as a human rights instrument. Eight years after the CRPD came in, recently they have withdrawn their resources and are creating new ideas about having a mental health law. Even the WHO is changing its tune on the mental health law.

We are now right behind the CRPD, working in the shadow of the CRPD. We place ourselves within the core of the disability movement. National, regional organizations of persons with disabilities (OPDs) are our closest partners for effecting a transformation. Our advocacy is not for a better psychiatry, inclusion in insurance etc. It is for inclusion in all policies relating to living a life independently with an adequate standard of living- inclusion in public housing policies, social protection, food security, poverty eradication, etc. This strategy is giving us a lot of gains, politically speaking. I suppose we don't see Mad Studies as central like that in the global north countries. There is a Latino group talking about psycho-social diversity, but there are many people there just as you have quite a few people here in the Asia region who harbour a Mad identity – a handful, but they are there. But this is not the bulk of us in the Global South.

One of the first regional conversations we had in the Asia Pacific network of persons with psychosocial disabilities was in 2013. That was after Gabor Gombos from Hungary visited us in 2008 or 2009. He taught us a lot about the CRPD. After that, I was trained in the CRPD by the International Disability Alliance and really soaked in it. I am so much part of the cross-disability movement here in India and more than me there are very strong leaders who are cross disability leaders, Yeni Rosa Damayanti, Alberto Vasquez, Liza Martinez and others. So we might have somewhere a 'Mad' identity and we may be part of some conversations around this. But we are strongly situated within the cross-disability movement. I think a part of the reason is not having these kinds of institutions and not having forced treatment to the extent that you have in the West or the Global North. The other reason is, that as I said, the very restricted nature of the dialogue between people who are being harmed by psychiatry and the psychiatrists. Within Mad Studies or within the anti-psychiatry movement or critical psychiatry movement, the dialogue never expands beyond whether psychiatry harmed, or not. Nothing more than that (at least, that is how we hear it in the Global South). In fact, generally we are more involved with the zero poverty movement, the caste resistance and the indigenous people's movement, the women's movement, the movement for strengthening primary education, etc. These are issues in our region and the disability discourse gives us several entry points into demanding change. We want inclusion into each and every one of the development agendas. We want to talk to all those actors who are creating empowering policies for social inclusion, and not just to health care professionals. I think that's the very big difference.

Notes

1 www.baputrust.com
2 https://baputrust.com/newsletter/
3 Such structures have remained intact in several places I have visited, though not all. Manila has one such institution with a triple lock up, and during my visit it was sad to see persons who were deaf and with intellectual disabilities in the inner confinement rooms.

References

Davar, B V and Bhat, P R (1995) *Psychoanalysis as a Human Science: Beyond Foundationalism*. New Delhi: Sage University Press.

Davar, B V (1999) *Mental Health of Indian Women: A Feminist Agenda*. New Delhi: Sage Publications.

Davar, B V and Ravindran, S (2015) 'Withdrawing justice, delivering care'. In Davar, B V and Ravindran, S (eds.) *Gendering Mental Health: Knowledges, Identities and Institutions*. New Delhi: Oxford University Press.

Levine, P and Frederick, A (1997) *Waking the Tiger: Healing Trauma. The Innate Capacity to Transform Overwhelming Experiences*. Berkeley: North Atlantic Books.

4

A CRAZY, WARRIOR AND "RESPONDONA" PERUVIAN

All personal transformation is social and political

Brenda Del Rocio Valdivia Quiroz

The connection and resistance of a sunflower

For as long as I can remember, I have been classified as someone who deviates from "the established norm" in various ways. Sometimes, being different and being able to raise my voice have led me to stand out, and receive social recognition for it. On other occasions, I was pressured to repress that and adjust to "being normal". It turns out that deviating from the norm is fine only as long as it does not go against the system.

One of my main characteristics since I was born, has been my (hyper) sensitivity with my perception thresholds quite sharp, both physically and emotionally. It could have started to develop with my first breaths. During my birth, I had my first problem in life: the umbilical cord tangled a couple of turns around my neck without letting me breathe and it was probably the first time in my life that I felt anguish. I think that from that experience on, I have kept a precedent in my body memory that made me feel endless anguish every time I felt that I was short of breath.

At three years old I was diagnosed with chronic asthma and since then, during my childhood, puberty and adolescence, I was (over)-medicalized with pills and inhalers, several times in emergencies with injections and oxygen, and hospitalized for weeks. I spent a long time on a bed in a completely white room; with bruises on my arms from the needles; without studying, playing, running or doing sports like other children; without seeing anyone for a long time (not even my family); and without knowing when I would go out. I felt alone and trapped. That is how since I was a child, not being able to breathe and feeling anguish, meant being isolated and losing freedom.

In my adolescence, being a woman in a country where gender violence is normalized from an early age was added to my respiratory issue. I went through some traumatic events that generated a lot of pain and anger for years, with a feeling of injustice that did not seem to be corrected by anything and I felt trapped once more. Then, I gradually realized that in my life I had been the victim of multiple abuses like one in every three women in my country, including symbolic, psychological and sexual violence many times. This, added to the long list of medical diagnoses, made me unconsciously disconnect from my body for a long time, since it seemed to be the cause of much of my pain. This caused my surrounding to see me as someone

DOI: 10.4324/9780429465444-6

weak, fragile and sick. In consequence, I was constantly excluded from almost everything. I ended up assuming that my sensitivity was a defect that I had to get rid of to stop experiencing so much pain and exclusion.

Another of my outstanding characteristics is my rationalization mechanism and its process of over-thinking. Since I was a child I always heard "you are very mature for your age", and that is because *think* hurts less than *feel*, so I found rational explanations for everything. During the early stage of my life I tried to make sense of physical ailments through a biomedical model, trying to accept that my body was like this: extremely sensitive and prone to anything (to get hurt), and the solution was to isolate myself and always take medication. I did not like this, it was very hard for years feeling the continuous exclusion and discrimination of almost all the environments in which someone of my age participated. Entering adulthood and already immersed in a career of psychology, there was a friend and a couple of teachers who began to crack my beliefs about the "weakness" of my health, and I began to wonder about the real causes of my discomfort.

It took a long time, a lot of tears and a lot of pain to realize that my primary environment was the main reason for my ailments. The violence and attacks in which I had grown up caused me to stop breathing and to unconsciously leave for a safer environment: hospital. I started thinking that it was not only asthma attacks, but panic and anguish attacks. There were nights when we had already emerged from emergencies and I was "stable", but after I would come back home with more fights and screams, I got sick again and we returned to emergencies. How could we not see it? The answer was always there. Going forward, along with various processes of recognition, emotional and physical healing and transformation through deep introspection, almost always through art and trips to my roots, my spiritual beliefs, and with much love from my friends (who never knew what I was going through), everything became more meaningful with my connections and my resistances, and I kept looking for the sunlight, as a sunflower.

The liberty of different hats

In 2017, the last year of my degree study, as part of my pre-professional experience, I had the opportunity to travel to other places to learn a little more about new ways of working that we could build in Peru with people with intellectual and psychosocial disabilities. That year, one year before the Civil Code Legislative Reform for the recognition of the legal capacity of people with disabilities,[1] we started the Pilot Project "Support networks for decision-making and community life" focused on people with intellectual and psychosocial disabilities. The main objective of this project was to promote support networks for the exercise of legal capacity (article 12 of the UN Convention on the Rights of Persons with Disabilities – CRPD) and community life of people with disabilities (article 19 of the CRPD). This proposal sought to generate empirical evidence to strengthen and continue the development of the Legislative Reform process.

The Reform process was quite complicated and took years of struggle from civil society groups of people with disabilities, even though Perú had ratified the United Nations Convention o+n the Rights of Persons with Disabilities (UN CRPD)[2] 10 years earlier as well as other international and national instruments based on the current human rights paradigm. It was a challenge to transform the existing vision rooted in centuries of discrimination and exclusion. For this reason, in parallel with this struggle at the legal and legislative level, our project began directly involving people with disabilities at the social and community level. This initiative was carried out by the NGO Society and Disability – SODIS,[3] with the support of the Inter-American Foundation.[4]

Almost at the end of the implementation of the project and in order to share the learning and the experiences, I travelled to the city of Santiago de Chile as the supporter of one of the participants with psychosocial disability. The gathering was called "The first Latin American Meeting of Mental Health and Social Movements"[5] organized by the Latin American Network of Mad Studies.[6] It brought together people from all over the region, including mental health professionals and people with experience of using mental health services. One of the programmed activities was to hold a separate meeting for mad people, users or ex-users, people with psychosocial disabilities, among other identities who had experiences in mental health services and/or of madness. That moment was a milestone that marked an important before and after in my life.

My role on that trip and at that time was strictly professional, I was there to support a participant of the project and that was part of my job. During all this time, in my mind there was no possibility of having a personal space for myself, because according to my professional training that would be unethical and could even harm the process of accompanying the other person. At that moment, I had to decide whether to leave or stay, and to stay I had to go through a quick introspection to identify where I belonged. I was quite nervous, laughing, and did not know what to do, so I dared to share my doubts with one of the organizers who was a survivor of psychiatry, and with Alberto Vásquez, president of the NGO SODIS (which I was a member of), and who identifies as a person with psychosocial disability (I did not know that). He taught me that we all have different "hats" and we can choose which one to wear each time. Neither did he seem surprised nor did he judge me at all, but told me that it was my decision, and what I decided would be fine. I was the person most surprised to stay, the one who was most shocked, conflicted, confused, and the one who had been probably judging myself the most. From that moment on, that trip became a revealing experience.

While having discussions with some of the people I was meeting in that space, I rediscovered more and more things about myself, my life and its meanings, and saw everything with new eyes. I remember having a conversation with Manuel Rodríguez and Victor Lizama, commenting that I did not feel like I fitted in because I had not gone through traumatic situations of internment or forced medicalization (psychiatric, because of another type I actually had). I did not feel as "survivor", because I had not overcome as many things as other people. Between self-stigma, confusion and guilt, I told myself that this was just a brief episode, one more experience on my journey.

As we talked, I realized that more than the consequences, what united us were our motives and characteristics of our diversity: our sensitivity. I remember having lots of insights. I remember referring to my sensitivity as a "superpower" that in my profession allowed me to easily connect with people, but that also for years it seemed to have been something that I should change or I should put away from me because from the outside it was seen as a sign of weakness … but I could not, I never could. I remember that everyone told their stories, experiences and anecdotes, and I had so much in common with them, my way of experiencing similar situations, despite people being from different countries and cultures. It seemed incredible to me (even up to now). Manuel called me "little sister" and he said that I already belonged. What people always told me was my weakness and I should change it of myself, that day it connected me with these wonderful people, and they made me feel that my way of being was always right, that I was not alone in the world and that we could change the system together. I began to accept and thank that day that changed my life.

As I write these lines, I just realized that exactly two years have passed since then. So many things have happened, my whole life has taken on a different meaning, it recovered an essence that I believed was lost – an essence that gives meaning, not only to the present, but to the past and the future. Being aware of and accepting my madness from self-love and appreciation of my neurodiversity, physically healed me and emotionally saved me. I realized that my way of being, thinking, feeling and perceiving the world crosses very human thresholds of sensitivity, so it is easy for me to connect with all nature (flora and fauna), all artistic expressions, all energies, and other people and their feelings (including to feel their pain easily).

Our body-mind-spirit speak: Listen and trust

Thanks to this international sharing between peers, I questioned in my personal life the medical-rehabilitative model in which I was professionally trained, and approached my experiences, finding new meanings. I realized that there was a pattern of violence prior to mental and physical discomfort – not only in me, but in everyone I knew – and ways in which the mind tried to get out of there, build and go to alternatives to the pain. Nothing is ever out of nowhere, all discomforts have a reason behind them, and the body (including our mind) wisely warns us with a signal (call it a symptom) that there is something we are not paying the attention, space, time and/or the love it deserves.

In some people these signs can be through psychosomatic discomfort, and/or in others through psychic discomfort. The first one is known as illnesses linking with unresolved repressed emotions and traumas. The second can lead us to experience intense expressions of pain, sadness, anger, fear – in mood, thought, through the senses and/or the personality. The ways of dealing with these discomforts can be very diverse. Some are socially accepted, while others are not and there is a consequence of exclusion for them (by prison or psychiatric system). Some accepted forms in Lima's middle-class society are repression, frequent consumption of legal drugs such as alcohol and cigarettes, anxiety feeding, therapy, medication, among others; while unacceptable forms are emotional crises that can be seen as anger, crying, anxiety and panic attacks, ruminating thoughts and various sensory experiences (voices, visions, etc.).

I realized that if no violence of any kind has been suffered personally – very unlikely in such an unequal society and with so much social injustice – the structural violence of the neoliberal capitalism, colonialist and patriarchal system is present, where machismo, racism, classism, capacitism, cuerdism and other forms of primary repression and discrimination operate, excluding human existence and interaction. I realized that the further away you are from this system, the more possibilities you have to build alternative ways of interaction and living from the most human, collective and ancestral knowledge.

I realized how different it would have been to go through my psychic discomforts in the capital city, Lima, then where I was, Trujillo, a city on the north coast of Peru. Despite being from Lima and living here now, I lived for several years in Trujillo, where the cosmologies of my Northern and Andean roots, La Libertad and Ancash, link well-being/discomfort with the natural and spiritual world, as was reflected in the beliefs and practices of my parents mixing ancestral knowledge, spiritual beliefs and elements of nature. When I or anyone in my family went through or mentioned certain experiences related to psychic discomforts (emotional or of the senses), these experiences were (are) validated immediately (nobody ever tells you "you are crazy") and the actions to follow were/are processes and rituals of cleansing and healing with elements of nature (stones, plants, animals), along with prayers and invocations to bring wellness. In contrast, the most frequent option in Lima is a psychiatrist or psychologist, who, from their knowledge and scope, would probably have given me psychiatric medication from an early age. This was corroborated later, already in Lima, when the psychologist referred me to psychiatry – after another traumatic process of mourning. Coming from very questioning parents and closely linked to the medical field (my mother for her profession and my father for his life experiences), I could not just accept the derivation. I did a lot of research about it, I consulted with several people (many who were already taking medication), I visited some psychiatrists and after being very disappointed, in the end I was only able to trust a female psychiatrist a little more (gender matters). This is where I received prescribed psychiatric medication, and after much resistance, I agreed to take it. She prescribed anxiolytics, antidepressants and antipsychotics – I did not take the first one because I was very afraid of generating dependence (I had researched and studied this in my career and my peers confirmed it). It seemed the most functional option to end my university classes at my very expensive and private university. I was accompanied not only by my psychologist, but it was vital to have the support of my family (my parents and my brother) and my friends who became my peers (as they also took medication). My peers told me how I could feel when taking the medication, which helped me not to get too scared, since some symptoms "disappeared" (turned off or repressed), but new ones appeared. It seemed that I was no longer myself. Some months later, I progressively interrupted the treatment, due to the terrible side effects – I could not feel anything: I did not want to die or similar any more, but I could not feel pleasure in anything either … I was dead alive. I think the most important thing was that I had consolidated a network of supports and wellness factors to accompany me during all this process, and they respected my decisions (even my psychologist).

I realized that my sensitivity was an essential part of my neurodiversity, now considered by me as a "superpower", which carries a great responsibility for self-knowledge and self-regulation, for me and for others. I realized that one of the main differences between my story and that of other survivors was my privileges, my interculturality and my supports. Due to having access to formal higher education and my particular career, I knew the "symptoms" very well, and could find the sequence of why they were there, so I could explain it; and I was surrounded by people among family, friends and teachers who supported me. No one ever judged me. No one ever tagged me or pointed at me with a diagnosis label, and no one told me that I was unable to do something. I had adjustments in my courses and my supports were with me at every step. Now, I am almost sure they had been in my position before, feeling like I felt at some point in their lives – so they were like peers with me in some way, and that was very important. Perhaps the one who judged me the hardest, for being "weak" again, and for having been internally broken in the process of professional training in a mental health career, with all my self-demands of strength and perfection, was *myself*. Now, I know that being sensitive is not an antonym of being strong, and that strength is not about never breaking internally or never feeling pain, but rather about being able to transform that pain, anger, sadness and fear into something else to help us resurface.

Knowing that things could be completely different for many people who go through discomforts and psychic pain if they had support in their lives, as I had and have, it only reinforced my complete conviction in the project in which we worked and in the legislative reform: how can I not believe and fight for something that I live every day? My support network is present in my life and I turn to them individually or as a group when I need it, not only to make decisions in complex moments, or seeking diverse information, opinions and perspectives, but as a source of emotional support, increasingly elaborating our action plans and accompaniment. I realized many other things and the insights have not stopped, even now I keep discovering things and giving new meanings to experiences from the past for my present and future.

With this sum of reflections, the term with which I most identify myself currently is "crazy person". Sometimes, as a joke, people close to me used to change "psicóloga" (which means psychologist) and used to call me "psico-loca": "psico" is like psycho for the first part of psycho-logist and "loca" means crazy, linked to the "Mad Pride" movements in Spain, Chile, Argentina, Mexico, and elsewhere. I am not a survivor, as I do not think I have gone through situations of abuse from the psychiatric system. Nor am I a person with a psychosocial disability, because although I have an evident neurodiversity of which I am now proud, I do not face barriers in accessing my rights because I know them, so I can demand their compliance, I can ask for an adjustment if I need it and I can use my support networks as one of them.

In Peru, although it can be used derogatorily – just like almost any similar word – the term "crazy" is used a lot colloquially, and you can hear the term in songs, poems, movies, and in every-day conversations alluding to someone who does "follies" (being in love) or is out of the norm (inventions, creations, new postures, etc.). If being crazy is having my level of human sensitivity and not adapting to the neoliberal capitalist, colonial and patriarchal system that does not work and constantly hurts and kills us, so, yes, I am quite proud of being crazy, and I would not want to stop being like that.

Mad warriors united

In May 2018, in that separatist meeting, an organized Latin American space was created that would later be called "Latin American Sphere Network of Psychosocial Diversity – Latin Madness". On December 2018, months later, we had the "First Regional Meeting of the Latin American Red Sphere of Psychosocial Diversity – Latin Madness" in the city of Lima (Perú), and our declaration[7] of that meeting set out the following:

1. We are a historically discriminated collective formed of users, ex-users and survivors of psychiatry, crazy people, people with psychosocial disabilities, among other identities of psychosocial diversity. We live common experiences in which we face torture, deprivation of liberty, isolation, trauma, violence, stigmatization, exclusion and violation of our rights.
2. We re-vindicate our dignity, freedom, autonomy and personal independence, including the freedom to make our own decisions, as well as the active and leading role we want to exercise in our lives. No one knows and will not know better than we do what our needs and demands are.
3. We demand absolute respect for our human rights and fundamental freedoms, particularly those recognized in the United Nations Convention on the Rights of Persons with Disabilities (UN CRPD), ratified by all the countries of the region.
4. We denounce the pathologisation and medicalization of our diversity, and all other forms of discrimination and abuse exercised by psychiatry, psychology and other specialties in the name of "mental health" and "normality". We demand the construction of a new paradigm of subjective discomfort, which accepts "psychosocial diversity" as a fact and principle derived from human diversity and recognizes us as people expert by experience.
5. We absolutely reject deprivation of liberty, electroshock, forced sterilization, forced treatment, involuntary medication, mechanical and chemical restraints, and other forms of torture and violation of rights in the name of "mental health". We demand that these practices be abolished and that their victims be recognised and compensated.
6. We adhere to the struggle of the feminist movement and condemn all types of violence that patriarchy and its institutions have and continue to exercise against women and groups in situations of bigger vulnerability, especially against those who do not adhere to the expectations of gender roles and "normality". We also adhere to the demands of the movements for the rights of children and indigenous people.

7. We warn the serious situation of poverty and social exclusion in which our collective lives in Latin America, particularly those people who belong to the most marginalized and discriminated against groups, which significantly reduces our access to educational, job, artistic, cultural, recreational and political opportunities and full participation.

8. We defend that no person should be pathologized or psychiatrized on the basis of their gender identity, sexual orientation, or any other expression of sexual diversity outside of what is established as "normal". We reject "corrective therapies" and other heteronormative practices that are practised with the aim of "correcting" people.

9. We commit ourselves to work for the construction of a regional associative movement; promote the exchange of experiences, knowledge and alternative good practices, including demedicalization; collaborate in the development and consolidation of mutual support groups; promote knowledge and fulfilment of our rights; promote mad pride and the right to madness; and participate and promote legislative and public policy reforms in the region, supporting the transformation of our communities and our environments towards inclusive societies that value and respect human diversity.

10. We want to be a democratic, participative, open and horizontal space for all psychosocially diverse people in Latin America, without distinction of sex, gender, age, sexual orientation, disability, colour, language, religion, origin or any other condition of diversity. We promote gender equality, the criterion of parity in participation and an intersectional perspective within and outside our community.

11. We are open and willing to form alliances and work with people and allied organizations that share our principles, within a framework of respect, equality and equity to advance the construction of just and inclusive societies.

This space has grown a lot since then and today it is strengthened by the presence of activists from 10 countries in Latin America.[8] All our actions are framed in terms of the rights recognized in the UN CRPD and all our countries have ratified their fulfilment of it. In 2019, one of the most outstanding works was the cycle of webinars[9] that touched on the following topics: mad pride, mutual support groups (GAMs), demedicalization, human rights, feminism and gender, and art and madness. In 2020, in the face of the global crisis of the COVID-19 pandemic, pronouncements[10] have been made and it is planned to continue influencing, at the national, regional and international levels, together with the following networks: Pan African Network of Persons with Psychosocial Disabilities, Transforming communities for Inclusion of persons with psychosocial disabilities – Asia Pacific (TCI Asia Pacific), European Network of Ex-Users and Survivors of Psychiatry (ENUSP), Center for the Human Rights of Users and Survivors of Psychiatry (CHRUSP) and World Network of Users and Survivors of Psychiatry (WNUSP). Currently, we continue to manage and articulate intersectional actions in various spaces.

Although some people find it contradictory in terms of my sensitivity, another of my main characteristics is my strength and my identity as a warrior – in a world that always seems to be at war, with or without weapons – a warrior against individualism, selfishness and colonial patriarchal neoliberal capitalism. It is a continual challenge but we are not alone: "We already know that sunflowers look for sunlight, but what few know is that on cloudy days they look at each other looking for energy in each one – Nature teaches us that if we do not have sun every day, we have each other".[11] One of the things that I learned in the experiences described above and that I try to keep in mind and do not forget is that we are not alone in these struggles. As we were feeling and building it in feminisms, many times feeling us fight against the current, with more certainties than fears, we are not alone and we have never been alone. We have always been everywhere, we are only dispersed, because the system has taken care of that and it wants us to stay the same way ... but not anymore. Now that we are raising our voices, accompanying and organizing ourselves, we know more than ever that we are not alone in these struggles and we go to fight together.

In 2019 in Peru, after the meeting of the Latin American Sphere Network of Psychosocial Diversity, the people from Lima organized to continue meeting in a peer support group (GAM), which worked weekly, for some months, until some difficulties in its functioning coincided with a combination of urgent situations for us. In April, a Mental Health Law Project was presented and approved by the Legislature and only required the President's signature to be published. This surprised and outraged different civil society groups, as none of them were consulted, apart from some psychiatrists.

For this reason, on 11 April 2019, an emergency meeting was convened for groups and associations of users and ex-users of mental health services, people with psychosocial disability, and people with diverse experiences of mental health, to debate the Mental Health Law Project. As a result, it was decided to create a workspace called "Coalition for Mental Health and Human Rights" with the aim of analysing the document and generating a joint document that communicated the points that should be adjusted, and respective proposals. This workspace also included family members, professionals, organizations, associations, and organized groups linked to and interested in a collective and intersectional contribution.

On 23 May, the Mental Health Law[12] was approved and, from now on, meetings focused on advocating for active participation in the elaboration of the Regulation of the Mental Health Law. The main arguments that were advanced on these regulations regarding rights, mental health and disability, were the following. First, the Draft Law was prepared without taking into account the central participation of those concerned, that is, users and people with psychosocial disabilities, although this was their (our) right, so the entire document required a thorough review. Second, carrying out this review, numerous contradictions and shortcomings became evident in the internal coherence of the text of the Law with some articles that defended rights and others that, contradictorily, violated them.

On 26 July, the Coalition for Mental Health and Human Rights meets at the National Mental Health Directorate (DSAME) of the Ministry of Health with the temporary Sector Commission, responsible for preparing the report containing the proposed regulation of Law No. 30947, Mental Health Law. In this working meeting, an attempt was made to collect comments and suggestions for the elaboration of the Regulation, and the points mentioned above were clarified, specifying the concerns and proposing joint alternatives. On 15 October, the Regulation of the Mental Health Law was pre-published, a stage at which civil society can make and send in comments, during 30 calendar days, to be incorporated prior to the final publication. The Coalition presented a sum of general and specific comments and contributions to the entire document, as adjustments in the approach used in consistence with the CRPD and the Legislative Reform No. 1384 that recognizes the legal capacity of persons with disability (2018).

On 5 March 2020, the Regulation of the Mental Health Law[13] was published, incorporating almost all (80% approx.) the contributions made by the Coalition. Some of the terms and definitions used were: deinstitutionalization, experts by experience, accessible informed consent, community empowerment, support for decision-making, among others. There are still actions to continue influencing, as well as monitoring for compliance; however, a State of National Emergency for the COVID-19 pandemic[14] was declared almost a week after this publication, so these measures have been put on hold for now.

One of the main sources of resistance to the incorporation and transformation of this rights-based approach, are the Administrators of Health Insurance Funds (IAFAS) and the Peruvian

Psychiatric Association presenting pronouncements and objections to certain articles of the Mental Health Law that directly concern them. On the other hand, the Peruvian College of Psychologists not only did not agree with the Law due to its non-incorporation in an article that indicates their power to carry out diagnoses, but also demanded its repeal, for which it carried out more than three marches, encouraging civil society to accompany them. Finally, the Single Union of Workers of the Larco Herrera Hospital ruled on the reform that it seeks to de-institutionalize, since they are against that and carried out pro-institutionalization activities. Recently, this last initiative has been joined by the staff of the Noguchi Institute, as well as gaining the adherence of the Valdizán Hospital, joining together the three psychiatric hospitals in the country.

In Peru, there are these three psychiatric hospitals,[15] all in the capital city of Lima – with almost a third of the national population. One having become the National Institute of Mental Health Honorio Delgado – Hideyo Noguchi has beds for 80 people, the Hermilio Valdizan Hospital has a capacity of 220 people, and the one that massively houses more than 480 people in deplorable conditions, the Víctor Larco Herrera Hospital, with people who have been there for more than 70 years. Regarding this, it is considered that there is a deficit of psychiatric hospitals and psychiatrists, since there are "only" three psychiatric hospitals in the whole country and they are in the capital Lima; while there is only 1 psychiatrist per 300,000 Peruvians.[16] The opinion of the majority of the population seems to follow this line of thought: Let's no longer stigmatize mental health, we need more psychiatrists and more psychotropic drugs! There is a huge absence regarding the human rights approach, questioning of the psychiatric system and alternatives to the psychiatrization of lives.

The Ministry of Health, through the National Directorate of Mental Health, many years ago tried to incorporate a Community Mental Health Care Reform (2012), however, it is a long process of transformation and it had some gaps in accordance with a Human Rights approach. More than 154 Community Mental Health Centers have been established throughout the country and 11 Protected Homes have been adapted,[17] which also follow the line of this Reform. With the new Mental Health Law, being a historical milestone to have regulations aimed at this subject, there is an opportunity to establish paradigm changes; however, the existing resistance to struggles of egos, powers and politics make it a long-term transformation challenge.

Meanwhile, the Coalition, a year after first being brought together, in a context of a lack of participation from people with lived experiences and in the midst of the global crisis due to the COVID-19 virus, has strengthened its efforts to organize internally. A logo and a page have been created to spread the message and a pronouncement on mental health and COVID-19 published. In these spaces, the Coalition for Mental Health and Human Rights[18] has been formally presented as a collective work space made up of activists who include people with experiences in mental health, neurodivergent people, users and ex-users of psychiatry, people with psychosocial disability, family, professionals, and members of allied organizations that seek to promote and defend the full exercise of the right to health and well-being of individuals, families and the community in Peru. It is worth mentioning that people with diverse experiences in mental health and madness play a leading role in this space, consistent with its main objective of guaranteeing their rights established in the UN CRPD. Currently, we are working to advocate again for urgent measures to be taken for people who live in psychiatric institutions, as well as health personnel at the Larco Herrera Hospital, because we know that for some time people had been infected with COVID-19 and on 11 May the first death occurred.[19]

Although we are now in a fairly complex context of crisis that has gone beyond health, to become a social, economic and political crisis as well, the deinstitutionalization of this population has been a task requiring completion since the CRPD was ratified and subsequently supported by the Mental Health Law and its regulation. Today more than ever it requires immediate actions, because these are areas and locations where more lives around the world are being lost. Beyond immediate measures such as the relocation of people to other settings where they would be cared for as required, in the long-term further steps have been discussed to support and respect their well-being and autonomy. From SODIS and the Coalition we have participated in a regional audience of the Inter-American Commission on Human Rights (IACHR)[20] as one of the countries most affected in the world by the COVID-19 pandemic, and with the demand to take urgent measures for people in a situation of institutionalization that are among the most affected populations, now more than ever.

From the Coalition for Mental Health and Human Rights, and the Feminist Madness Collective[21] – which was born from a feminist peer support (GAM) initiative – three strategies have been discussed. On the one hand, the promotion of GAMs or peer support is beneficial for those who face loneliness and other barriers in the midst of a complex process such as psychological distress. Then a feeling of understanding and belonging can have a direct effect on well-being as a protective factor, as well as offering its own transformative space for respect and confidentiality, open dialogue and active listening; and provide an opportunity to exchange ideas, advice, knowledge from your own experience, make decisions with support, among other things.

On the other hand, the Advance Directives of Will are the result of the Advance Planning of Decisions in Mental Health makes it possible to explore together with the person the elements of their processes of discomfort and well-being, crisis situations, barriers, support networks, and other resources that the person considers pertinent to add, such as the use of any medication, the acceptance/denial of particular interventions, etc.

Finally, the generation of collectives and community spaces can arise from any particular interest, concern, knowledge and/or experience; with a two-way welfare effect, not only on those who receive them as a target audience, but those who manage them constantly learning. In these ways, collective knowledge and actions are built, respecting the voice and autonomy of people with such experiences, exercising active citizenship and validating a multidisciplinary and intersectional equity of knowledge.

Personal is definitely political. For this reason, I have shared in this space, from the personal and intimate, to the social and political, to demonstrate how everything connects and has an impact on the development, well-being and exercise of rights of a person and their participation in the community. All the knowledge that we have as people expert by experience is lost in the middle of the system that absorbs, represses and divides us. Our resistance should be based on validating our own voices, raising them, sharing them among our peers, and organizing ourselves collectively. Precisely at this moment, Peru is going through exactly all this in the midst of a very strong political crisis – added to the sanitary, economic, social and systemic crisis – a historic moment that restores faith to our generation that resists this oppressive system; that does not accept more invisibility; whose members communicate, connect, and strengthen each other; who fight for what we think is fair, not just for one, but for all. This is a challenge for us to promote in capital cities as individualized as ours in Latin America; but we have amazing knowledge in non-capital cities that continue to function cooperatively – in tribes, in communities, in mutual support, where social responsibility is not relegated to particular acts of kindness and solidarity, but is a duty of all, and if there is no way out or solution to a problem, one is sought and created, since it is not an option that someone is left behind or excluded. It is quite difficult and we see it in other intersectional struggles that we encounter, however, every time it happens, it confirms the great power we have when we raise and unite our voices against the system. I am convinced that if everyone assumes their part in the social commitment that connects all of us, we can transform the system into one that truly includes us and represents us, respecting and valuing our human diversity. This fight is not exclusively for what we call "mental health", but for social justice.

Long live the madness that transforms the world!

Notes

1 Legislative decree 1384: https://busquedas.elperuano.pe/download/url/decreto-legislativo-que-reconoce-y-regula-la-capacidad-jurid-decreto-legislativo-n-1384-1687393-2
2 CRPD: https://www.un.org/esa/socdev/enable/documents/tccconvs.pdf
3 SODIS: https://sodisperu.org/
4 IAF: https://www.iaf.gov/
5 Images from event: https://www.facebook.com/sodisperu/posts/1269135723219378
6 Latin American Network of Mad Studies: https://www.facebook.com/Centrodeestudioslocos/
7 Declaration: http://www.rompiendolaetiqueta.com/blog/2019/5/8/declaracin-red-locura-latina?fbclid=IwAR1ccURmC_mG1WxVG6DgLl72E9j_2yXZXcyFW9c7ud0FuanCFfyNZ582ZsE
8 Sphere Network: https://www.facebook.com/laredesfera/
9 First six videos: https://www.youtube.com/channel/UC1DxblQVyo702z1isap3BYQ
10 Principal pronouncement: http://www.chrusp.org/home/covid19
11 Quote from unknown author
12 Mental Health Law: https://busquedas.elperuano.pe/download/url/ley-de-salud-mental-ley-n-30947-1772004-1
13 Regulation of the Mental Health Law: https://busquedas.elperuano.pe/normaslegales/decreto-supremo-que-aprueba-el-reglamento-de-la-ley-n-30947-decreto-supremo-n-007-2020-sa-1861796-1/
14 State of National Emergency for the COVID-19 pandemic: https://busquedas.elperuano.pe/normaslegales/decreto-supremo-que-declara-estado-de-emergencia-nacional-po-decreto-supremo-n-044-2020-pcm-1864948-2/
15 Official report of the ombudsman "Defensoría del Pueblo": https://www.defensoria.gob.pe/wp-content/uploads/2018/12/Informe-Defensorial-N%C2%BA-180-Derecho-a-la-Salud-Mental-con-RD.pdf
16 Approximate data: http://web2016.cmp.org.pe/i-jornada-peruano-espanola-de-psiquiatria-y-salud-mental/
17 Official data: http://www.minsa.gob.pe/salud-mental/
18 Coalition for Mental Health and Human Rights: https://www.facebook.com/coalicionporlasaludmentalperu/
19 News: https://www.sucesos.pe/nota/577-covid-19-silenciosa-muerte-pacientes-larco-herrera?fbclid=IwAR0diBIBZO9Mgs-UnReM0jmChXEU63KTYHrd0ak33SHUdzzkYRBw5AGrqUU#.XrrHu61oY6o.facebook
20 Audience IACHR: https://www.facebook.com/194263083953643/videos/341902073700564
21 Neuro-divergent Madness Collective: https://www.facebook.com/neurodivergentefeminista/

References

Declaration of Latin American Sphere Network of Psychosocial Diversity – Latin Madness. http://www.rompiendolaetiqueta.com/blog/2019/5/8/declaracin-red-locura-latina?fbclid=IwAR1ccURmC_mG1WxVG6DgLl72E9j_2yXZXcyFW9c7ud0FuanCFfyNZ582ZsE Accessed: 20 December 2020
Legislative Decree No. 1384 that recognizes and regulates the legal capacity of people with disabilities on equal terms. Official Gazette El Peruano (4 September 2018) https://busquedas.elperuano.pe/download/url/decreto-legislativo-que-reconoce-y-regula-la-capacidad-jurid-decreto-legislativo-n-1384-1687393-2 Accessed: 20 December 2020
Law No. 30947, Mental Health Law. Official Gazette El Peruano (23 May 2019) https://busquedas.elperuano.pe/download/url/ley-de-salud-mental-ley-n-30947-1772004-1 Accessed: 20 December 2020

Regulation of Law No. 30947, Mental Health Law. Official Gazette El Peruano (5 March 2020) https://busquedas.elperuano.pe/normaslegales/decreto-supremo-que-aprueba-el-reglamento-de-la-ley-n-30947-decreto-supremo-n-007-2020-sa-1861796-1/ Accessed: 20 December 2020

United Nations (2006) Convention on the Rights of Persons with Disabilities. Recovered from: https://www.un.org/esa/socdev/enable/documents/tccconvs.pdf Accessed: 20 December 2020

5

REFLECTIONS ON SURVIVOR KNOWLEDGE AND MAD STUDIES

Irit Shimrat

Survivor knowledge is more than just the accumulation and recounting of each of our stories of incarceration, torture, poisoning, electroshock, humiliation, etc., at the hands of psychiatry; the resultant terror, rage and angst; and how all of this can be used against us by "helping professionals" and hostile researchers. Our knowledge is essential beyond the importance of collecting, studying and exposing the evidence of psychiatry's fraudulence and dangerousness. Our critiques of psychiatry, psychology, and related pseudosciences, of "community mental health services," the effects of pharmaceutical marketing, etc., form the basis of innumerable ways in which survivors can assist, not only ourselves and each other, but also those people believed to be "sane." Our knowledge can help all of us relate to ourselves and to others. It can teach all of us, not just to cope with extremes of emotion and difference, but to learn from them – to find in them meaning, insight, and sometimes even joy – and consequently to live better, richer lives.

As for Mad Studies, my initial reaction to the very idea is a wincing distrust of academia, fed by unpleasant memories of trying to read documents written in "social science" jargon. Many psychiatric survivors are repelled, or at least mystified, by the academization of our suffering and of our ideas. For example, a blog I follow recently elicited this comment from a reader: "This is great, what I could understand. Part of my hope is that we can also write so that everyone can understand. Academic writing, I am not so good at. But these are very important ideas." Important ideas never require the use of jargon, and I have spent a portion of my editing life de-jargonizing academic writing. And I have written, in very plain language, essays, articles and even a book that have been used as texts in university courses.

Survivors who have been part of, or whose work has been used in, the area calling itself Mad Studies have made important contributions to the discovery and promotion of alternatives to psychiatry. Many have created wonderful organizations, publications, documents, websites, etc., that offer vital information, encouragement, advice, and interaction. Some are pushing to make the United Nations Convention on the Rights of Persons with Disabilities, and other pieces of legislation, work in our favour Some have dedicated themselves to Mad Studies (and related areas of study) as such, doing meaningful qualitative research, having their work published in respected journals, earning academic credentials, becoming professors, and so on. Mind you, not all the psychiatric survivors I know agree with the name "Mad Studies." Indeed, not all

DOI: 10.4324/9780429465444-7

like either the word "mad" or the term "psychiatric survivor." Nevertheless, I believe that all of this work has some potential to prevent our lives from being destroyed by the "mental health system."

Of course, many decades before Mad Studies became a thing, recipients of psychiatric "care" and the people who actually do care about us – including academics, dissident professionals, enlightened family members and others – began speaking out and writing about the dangers of, and alternatives to, psychiatry. And, despite all these efforts, more and more people have been, are being, and are in danger of being subjected to the expanding grip of psychiatry, whose practices just get more and more pernicious. (I think, for example, of the ubiquity of polypharmacy and multiple simultaneous diagnoses, the increasing use of electroshock "therapy," and the invention and promotion of implanted electronic devices.) At the same time, survivors are increasingly co-opted into the system, working in "partnership" with professionals in situations where they have no real power but serve as mere window-dressing, providing an illusion of co-operation and progress. This illusion is also at play when survivors are "trained" to become "peer" workers in situations where they may be able to comfort psychiatric inmates, but can never actually stop them from being held and drugged against their will.

Even outside of the mainstream "system," new therapeutic modalities have sprung up in which people who used to be patients make money off people who are trying to stop being patients. I imagine this sometimes works out well for both sides. But many psychiatric survivors are somewhat or very poor, and I know of situations in which people spend more than they can afford on "peer services," only to be abandoned, and end up back in hospital, when they get too upset or behave too strangely. I'm sorry to say that I also know of instances of serious emotional and even sexual abuse of survivors at the hands of "peer service providers" – an extreme example of how holders of survivor knowledge can perpetuate the power imbalance inherent in the "therapist/client relationship." And of course the sense of betrayal and resultant despair can be even more terrible than what is experienced within mainstream "services."

I see a profound problem with the exchange of money for "care." To me this is one of the nastiest aspects of the commodification of everything in a society driven by the profit motive; by market-driven ideology and greed and the delusion that infinite economic growth is possible or desirable, together with denial of the fact that the creation of extreme wealth requires the existence of extreme poverty. The Covid-19 pandemic has epitomized this: workers who make barely enough, or not enough, to live on are suddenly called "essential" and praised as "heroes," without any thought of more than (at most) a temporary wage increase. Meanwhile, gargantuan corporations are bailed out as a matter of course. CEOs are assumed to have special knowledge, skills and virtues, while those who actually do the work that keeps us all alive are seen as unskilled and, if they get sick and die, easily replaced. These and other, equally awful ideas are highlighted by increasingly vehement protests against all kinds of injustices, up to and including state-sanctioned murder, perpetrated on the poor, and especially on those not born with white skin; the darker the skin and the deeper the poverty, the more terrible the oppression. Race- and class-based oppression, like the oppression of women, elders, foster children, etc., plays out in psychiatry – and, indeed, in the psychiatric survivors' movement – just as it does in every other area of life.

We live in a world where citizens are seen as "consumers" of products and "targets" of advertising and marketing schemes, and non-citizens are too often viewed as people who do not deserve full rights, but who are needed to fill the kinds of jobs that citizens don't want. It's hardly surprising that those whose behaviour – or protest – causes discomfort or inconvenience can be molded into "consumers of mental health care services." Or that those who refuse such services can be forced into a life of psychiatric incarceration, outpatient committal, and perpetual "medication" with substances that silence us by brutally damaging our brains, bodies, minds and souls.

Where do survivor knowledge and Mad Studies come into all this? Psychiatry keeps expanding its markets (to children, to the elderly, to prisoners – to everyone who must be controlled and kept down in order for the status quo to be maintained), and the ways in which it captures people keep getting sneakier and being met with less and less resistance. That is why the need for education is more urgent than ever. Students of all ages, at all levels and in every area of study, as well as the general public (any of whom may fall victim to psychiatry), should learn to distinguish between "mental health" propaganda and what is really needed to improve relations between people. And those who have survived "care" need our voices heard and our views considered and – dare we hope? – understood. Such learning has huge potential to make the world a better place, for everybody.

Psychiatric treatment, to which I have been subjected many times both in youth and in middle age, has been, unequivocally, the worst thing that has ever happened to me. My utter rejection of it, however, has led to many of the best experiences of my life. And this would never have been the case, but for the psychiatric survivors' movement (or the Mad movement, as I named it in my book, mainly for the sake of brevity; again, there is no agreement on terminology). And some of the amazing experiences I've had certainly come under the umbrella of Mad Studies. Encounters and events at conferences attended partly or entirely by crazy people (including conferences and events arranged by academics and held at universities) have filled me with wonder and joy and hope. So has reading and hearing and seeing work created by other crazies, and sometimes by our allies. My own work in collecting, editing and publishing other survivors' stories has given purpose, structure and meaning to my life. Almost always, everyone involved, including me, ends up feeling less alone and more alive.

And of course it has been a delight, always, to write and present my own creations. I get so much joy and strength, and such a sense of "okayness" – of being allowed to be in the world, without fear that my difference might result in incarceration and brutality – through expressing my views and experiences and beliefs. And then there is the understanding and appreciation I get from friends and allies; from those who had never thought about any of this except from the mainstream perspective; and, best of all, from my fellow survivors.

I consider myself wildly fortunate to have been invited to address students of sociology, nursing, psychology, etc. Sometimes I have even been paid for it! It is sweet to see people who are working towards achieving positions of direct or indirect power over others swayed by accounts of the personal experiences of those who have been subjected to such power. And inevitably after class, and very occasionally during, at least one person will confess to having been psychiatrized themselves, and thus especially moved by my words. I think nothing but good can come of such confessions, and of all opportunities to bring survivor knowledge into the consciousness of as many people as possible.

Survivor knowledge has also been an important part of my life in ways that have nothing to do with words. One of my favorite of the many fabulous things that happened when I was working with the Ontario Psychiatric Survivors' Alliance occurred during a field trip to a "mental health clubhouse." These outings always involved my colleague and I kicking all staff out of the room (the things we got away with!); telling our own stories of coming into, and then out of, psychiatry, and then into activism; and encouraging "clubhouse" members to start their own unsupervised, autonomous groups. But this one time we somehow ended up in the kitchen, making rhythms together by banging on pots and pans, and all of us together entered a state of bliss, and in that moment it didn't matter one bit that some of us were still patients and some had graduated into activism.

Finally, on the topic of divisions and overcoming them, we must always keep in mind that anyone might become a mental patient, through circumstances beyond their control. And that the fear of other people's madness comes in large measure from fear of madness in oneself. So, exposing people to the idea that madness is not something outside of "normal" human experience, but rather part of a continuum of thought, emotion and perception, is good for everyone. Ultimately, survivor knowledge can bring all of us together, and liberate all of us, by toning down the fear of difference, and sense of isolation, at the root of so much of what's wrong in the world.

6

SPEAKING FOR OURSELVES

An early UK survivor activist's account

Peter Campbell

Peter has been described as a survivor who has "devoted his life and incredible talents to the pursuit of survivors' rights and justice".[1] He is one of the pioneers of the UK survivor movement. In an email interview with Peter Beresford for this book, this is what he had to say.

I first became involved in action by mental health system users/survivors in the UK in the mid-1980s. At that time the range of activity was extending considerably and would be actively involved until at least the end of the century. The three groups I was most involved in were Survivors Speak Out, founded in 1986; Survivors Poetry founded in 1991 and Survivors History Group founded in 2005.

Survivors Speak Out was my prime focus from 1986 to 1996, so much so that I limited my activity in Survivors Poetry within 18 months of being a founder member. There was not enough time for me to devote to the two groups and I felt Survivors Speak Out had my first loyalty. After 1996 I was not involved in a group but spent my energies as a freelance trainer of mental health workers. Then, in 2005, I became a founder member of Survivors History Group, a gathering of mental health system survivors interested in ensuring they should write and research their own histories. This is the only group I am still involved in.

Any discussion of what we call ourselves must start and end in the principle of self-definition. People must always be able to choose how they describe themselves and have that respected. This is important whether they want to call themselves consumers, service users, survivors, schizophrenics, anorexics or the mentally ill. We have been burdened for too long with alien names. We must not alienate others by calling them names they do not own. Having said that, I do have a clear preference of term – mental health system survivor. First of all, I feel that survivor (I am surviving not I have survived) is a positive term and points rightly to the obstacle course of the mental health system that I am endeavouring to survive. But equally important it is not a question of mental health services or psychiatry alone. These are important and can be oppressive but they are part of a wider system, a socio-political system that is founded on prejudices and misunderstandings of people diagnosed with so-called mental disorders. I feel most comfortable thinking of my life in relation to a mental health system. It points to the true nature of my dilemma in a way "psychiatric" survivor or mental health service survivor does not.

The main nature of my action has been in three areas. These have been, first the organisation and activities of the UK networking group Survivors Speak Out (1986 to 1996). Second,

DOI: 10.4324/9780429465444-8

freelance training with mental health workers – especially clinical psychologists, social workers and mental health nurses, with a particular focus on the lived experience of mental health system survivors; the reform of the 1983 Mental Health Act and work on the role and function of mental health nurses. Third and finally, the writing of numerous chapters, usually on the 'service user/survivor movement' and allied topics, in various mental health textbooks and including regular articles and book reviews in OpenMind, the bi-monthly and now much-missed magazine of MIND (formerly the National Association of Mental Health) which gave mental health system survivor activists an unparalleled voice for many years.

Much of this work was time consuming. Most of it was poorly paid if paid at all. I believe my last three years work at Survivors Speak Out led me to "burn out". Instead of planning new campaigns or publications like the very successful "Self Harm – From Personal Perspectives", I was addressing envelopes, dealing with membership fees, answering personal correspondence and other administrative tasks. The eventual arrival of paid workers brought many managerial challenges. Maintaining the infrastructure of action groups was often less enjoyable than action itself. A fact which may help explain why some groups found it to hard continue long term.

My areas of action included working with mental health system survivors and working with mental health workers. With both groups I emphasised the importance of self-advocacy – individuals and groups speaking and acting for change on their own terms. This made clear at the outset the possibilities of action, of people being the masters of their own destiny. It also encouraged diversity rather than agreed agendas and platforms. The aim was not to replace one dominant force (psychiatry) with another – a monocultural survivor movement.

Alongside self-advocacy speaking and acting for yourself – with particular relevance to services, was advocacy – an innovation of the 1980s. The survivor movement championed the right of service users to have another person support them in voicing their wants and needs or to speak up on their behalf completely. As a freelance trainer I promoted the understanding and practical application of both these concepts. Unfortunately, the very real gain in life choices that resulted, was mystified by the false rhetoric of "user empowerment" which suggested much more was going on than actually was. It is true that service users had more control over their lives, within and outside the system, but they certainly were not equal. People with a diagnosis of a so-called "mental disorder" remain, as ever, a disempowered rather than an empowered group.

The United Nations Convention for the Rights of People with Disabilities (UN CRPD) has not really played a part or been relevant to me and my work. I will be very surprised if the compulsion-free care and treatment the UN CRPD appears to envisage will be introduced in the UK in the foreseeable future. Developments seem to be going in the opposite direction with more, not less, compulsory detention and treatment. It has taken 37 years to outlaw the use of police station cells as places of safety under Section 136 of the 1983 Mental Health Act. If a minor but vital change of this kind is so long in coming, the sweeping changes the UN CPRD encourages seem unlikely to arrive any time soon.

In my view there are three main aspects of our first-hand knowledge. First, knowledge of living in, and receiving, mental health services. Secondly, living with mental distress in society. Finally, first-hand knowledge of the interior experience of distress (the "madness" experience). These are of varying interest to service providers. They are enthusiastic about service users as consumers, not particularly interested in the experience of living in society with mental distress and often uninterested or hostile to first-hand accounts and alternative accounts of distress.

The 1990s were the era of "user involvement" when activists were first invited to contribute their knowledge to community care plans. At the same time they told their life stories in training mental health workers.

By the end of the decade, the service user as conveyor of "consumer expertise" was widely accepted. At the same time another rather different development had been taking place. A number of groups emerged using their first-hand understandings of mental distress to put forward alternatives. The Hearing Voices Network (HVN) and the National Self Harm Network (NSHN) are good example of these. These groups were radical and their challenge to psychiatric orthodoxy was rooted in first-hand knowledge. Their work helped first hand understanding to gain a new value.

First-hand knowledge does now have a new respectability. But it is not entirely a rosy picture. Professionally derived knowledge is still regularly given a higher value than our first-hand knowledge. Survivor-led research is not respected in the way other research is. It would be good to see our knowledge existing on a level playing field with professional knowledge. It would also be good to see more emphasis on our first-hand knowledge of living with distress in society and see our experience being considered alongside that of other disabled people. Above all else, our first-hand knowledge of the interior experience of mental distress/madness deserves to hold a central place whenever psychiatry is taught.

I see psychiatry in the United Kingdom as a mechanism of social control. Individuals are controlled by being compulsorily detained and "treated" often for considerable periods. Psychiatry is at the heart of a system that creates a second class of citizens; people who can be treated differently even if they have retained the capacity to make decisions. It concentrates on the individual pathology of these people, suggesting that they are incompetent and "do not know what is in their best interests". Psychiatry acts conservatively, re-inforcing social prejudice and fitting its recipients into the status quo, rather than trying to change their social environment. While ostensibly looking only to help the distressed, psychiatry is in fact moulding them for roles as the disempowered.

The big question for the survivor movement is whether to try to improve psychiatry or to build alternatives to it. In the UK, the movement has by and large sought to improve psychiatry, while leaving the deeper problem virtually untouched. In this way they have achieved some important positive change without fundamentally challenging psychiatry as a potentially oppressive practice. In the 1980s there was a constant challenge to psychiatry as a form of social control, but that seems to have receded now. It could be claimed that the survivor movement has been co-opted into the mental health system and its challenge fundamentally blunted. The more radical demands of activists have been almost completely resisted. Whatever its history, by and large the survivor movement has become a reformist enterprise.

Unfortunately, the emergence of Mad Studies coincided with my stepping back from involvement in the survivor movement. In short, I know too little of Mad Studies to make meaningful comments. Having said that, any survivor-controlled initiative that provides a radical critique of psychiatry and seeks to build alternatives to it would have my support. Whether Mad Studies does those things will have to be for others to judge.

Note

1 This was said of Peter Campbell when he was awarded the title of Honorary Doctor of Education in 2010 by Anglia Ruskin University, see https://aru.ac.uk/graduation-and-alumni/honorary-award-holders2/peter-campbell

7

FOSTERING COMMUNITY RESPONSIBILITY

Perspectives from the Pan African network of people with psychosocial disabilities

Daniel Mwesigwa Iga

Introduction

I got involved in organizing people with psychosocial disabilities after being retired from paid work on the basis of my disability. I co-founded *Mental Health Uganda* (MHU) which later connected me to the *World Network of Users/Survivors of Psychiatry* (WNUSP). After being co-opted as WNUSP board member representing the African region I co-founded the *Pan African Network of Persons with Psychosocial Disabilities* (PANPPD) and was later chosen to represent Ugandan civil society in negotiating the United Nations Convention on the Rights of Persons with Disabilities (UN CRPD). I was also involved with the *International Disability Caucus* and the *International Disability Alliance*. In this chapter (based on conversation with Jasna Russo) I share my experiences and views on both Ugandan as well as international organizing of people with psychosocial disability – which is my preferred way to identify.

Broadening the action agenda in the African context: Working towards inclusion

We began under the name *Pan African Network of Users and Survivors of Psychiatry* as a branch of the *World Network of Users and Survivors of Psychiatry*. Later when we convened in Cape Town for another general assembly, we changed the name because people felt that the terms 'users' and 'survivors' are somehow stigmatizing and also present a bad image to our service providers – psychiatrists. We felt that 'people with psychosocial disabilities' is a more friendly and respectful way of referring to ourselves. I also use the term 'people with mental health challenges' to try and minimize stigma.

In Uganda we did have a national organization which was user-founded and user-led. But there was also a mental health organization founded by professionals where there was a lot of coercion and the user voice was not coming out. We then founded *My Story Initiative* in order to train what we call self-advocates. This is peer-founded and peer-led organization with peer support as its central value. The concept of raising awareness is very important because you cannot demand your rights if you do not know them. We train people about the CRPD and

DOI: 10.4324/9780429465444-9

about Sustainable Development Goals (SDGs), which is the United Nation's programme. We are using the latter because we want to be included in their Agenda 2030 – Leaving Nobody Behind. This is a more general agenda, it is much broader than just mental health. We realize that after a stay in a mental health institution or after a crisis a human being has all the same needs as any other person. For that reason, we need the broader inclusion agenda. The Global North can learn from this non-coercive approach. It is also cost effective to work with people in the community. It mitigates stigma and fosters community responsibility.

Community responsibility means that when a person living with mental health challenges is confused or having a problem they quickly come and say: 'Oh this is a son or daughter of so and so, we know him/her, (s)he is our person and we are responsible for helping him/her'. When a person is in a crisis, perhaps moving up and down and before they get into an accident or something difficult happens – people take responsibility and inform the parents or the next of kin and they see how best to address the situation. Or when a person comes back out of an institution – they are scared, they fear that person and think that maybe they are a danger to the community. Of course, there are communities with no awareness, but the communities that are sensitized, they actually know what to do and are being helpful. We see it as our responsibility and also the obligation of the government to sensitize the community – so that people with mental health challenges are also included and can have independent living within the society.

Awareness raising of course costs money and creates a need for finances which we think should be a government obligation, but we also know that the government may not see it as a priority. So civil society can address this; especially those of us who are passionate about it and who have gone through such experiences. People can then see the benefits that result. Because if I talk and explain that somebody can have challenges but nonetheless remain human and become a professional and do lot of things which are beautiful and when I give myself as an example, then people get the message.

For some of the difficulties I have – like anxiety and depression – you need to find out their cause. Instead of just medicating, you talk to that person, find out about the cause and try to address it. Now we have a programme, a mainstream initiative that we call peer support. We talk to our peers and encourage them that there is a life after crisis and encourage them to learn about themselves and seek help.

We are trying to advocate for community services but the Global North in contrast invests a lot of money in psychiatric facilities. When you arrive in a mental health institution in Uganda they are already thinking about using drugs on you – it is the fall-back position. For them it is about financial cost, but these drugs cause lot of side effects to our bodies. Such new developments could be useful, but the negatives are hidden and they are never told to people. In the long run we have discovered that a lot of damage has been done. Maybe some of these new drugs are even being tested on us and that's the problem. This is our fear. They may try drugs to find out whether they really work and our peers are treated as guinea pigs.

Challenges and potentials of international advocacy work

My experience with WNUSP is that it combines people from the northern and southern globe, with different levels of economic growth. Our members in the northern globe generally have welfare and services from the state. But for us in the southern globe, our service users have nobody to care for them apart from their core families. So that is the challenge that I've seen. And another challenge I have seen is that our friends in the North are being coerced into treatment. Yet in the Global South, there are virtually rudimentary mental health units so there are all together less conventional psychiatrically based services given to the people. So, our colleagues from the North are really negative about coercion because their situation is very different.

Those are the challenges I experienced in international advocacy because sometimes they don't understand why I talk about family. To us family is very important. I am also against coercion but to some extent we have to be realistic. Before we become stabilized we need psychiatric services. When they are not there someone's condition can become severe. My approach is holistic and pragmatic – combining the medical model with a social and human rights-based model. Then I believe we can come with good, hybrid solutions. At one point we need the medical model because sometimes natural remedies and alternatives might not help you as psychiatric medication can help you, but of course with informed consent. The medical treatment should always be with personal consent, not coercion. We are emphasizing the right to informed consent and doing away with guardianship and caging, which is not care but torture. We are advocating for community mental health services as opposed to institutionalization.

People from the Global North and Global South can work together because we face similar conditions: depression is depression, anxiety is anxiety. We can share the best practices: what has been done in the Global North and what has worked in the Global South. We can work together with mutual respect for one another's opinion. In the Global South building family networks is a very beautiful thing. In the Global South, families have worked well in caring for people with psychosocial disabilities. The North can buy this practice from the South. I believe we can share success stories. The North can also share some success stories. In both the Global North and Global South we need to amplify user voice, the voice of persons with psychosocial disabilities so that we are recognized as equal before the law and that we eradicate the use of phrases such as 'of unsound mind' which causes a legal death and which de-personalizes our humanity and our dignity.

8

USING SURVIVOR KNOWLEDGE TO INFLUENCE PUBLIC POLICY IN THE UNITED STATES

Darby Penney

Since the 1970s, people with psychiatric labels in the United States have organized to protest the inhumane treatment we have experienced from psychiatry; to critique the biomedical model of "mental illness"; to protect and expand our human and civil rights; to end forced treatment and other harmful practices; and to demand broadly available alternatives to psychiatric treatment for people experiencing emotional distress or extreme states.

Judi Chamberlin, a movement pioneer in the U.S., described the movement's rise in the early 1970s, with grassroots groups in different cities, each not knowing that other groups existed. She said it was:

> [l]ike a mushroom […] there was this big thing underground and then it popped up in a whole bunch of different places "[…] a lot of groups got started, not only in different parts of the United States, but different parts of the world.
>
> *(Chamberlin and Penney, 2002: 20)*

These groups initially focused on consciousness-raising, helping participants recognize that they were not broken or deficient, but that they and their peers had been harmed by the coercive psychiatric system.

These groups quickly moved from consciousness-raising to organizing. Judi Chamberlin recalled the early days in New York City:

> Oh, it was really exciting […] We were challenging this thing that was this horrible force in our lives and we're going to bring out the truth. We're going to expose it. We wrote up these flyers, and we used to distribute flyers in front of Bellevue Hospital so that people could take them into the people they were visiting, to let people know they're not alone. And we organized. We got invited to talk at college classes. And we got invited to talk on the radio. And "One Flew Over the Cuckoo's Nest" was playing Off Broadway, and we leafleted the audience to say it's not just the things on the stage, this is real.
>
> *(Chamberlin and Penney, 2002: 18)*

DOI: 10.4324/9780429465444-10

As the movement grew and spread across the country, local groups learned about each other's existence through word of mouth. Beginning in 1973, they organized an annual low-budget national Conference on Human Rights and Psychiatric Oppression, and developed a common agenda focused on opposition to involuntary commitment and all kinds of forced treatment. *Madness Network News* started as a San Francisco-area newsletter in 1972 and gradually evolved into a newspaper format covering the ex-patient movement in North America and worldwide. Movement groups worked to get a seat at policy-making tables at the local, state, and national levels, and made some headway in the 1980s.

By the mid-1980s, the movement had made inroads with the National Institute of Mental Health and survivor activists started to get invited to policy meetings. But in 1986, that agency began funding an annual "consumer" conference called Alternatives, which allowed them to censor and control the agenda. This was the start of the co-optation of some parts of the movement, as the government-funded conference soon supplanted the survivor organized Conference on Human Rights and Psychiatric Oppression. The more moderate "consumer" wing of the movement, which was not overtly anti-psychiatry, gained a foothold as they competed for limited government funding. The introduction of government funding began to highlight rifts between groups that opposed the medical model and forced treatment, and the more moderate groups who were generally in agreement with the philosophy of mainstream psychiatry and wanted to act in partnership with the system, rather than in opposition (Chamberlin, 1990; Chabasinski, 2012).

My own introduction to the movement came in 1989, when, as a staff member at the New York State Office of Mental Health, I worked on a planning project that required the agency to seek input, not just from mental health professionals, but from people who had used mental health services. Until then, I had not realized that my own negative experiences with the psychiatric system as a teenager and young adult had relevance to my work. On this project, I met activists in the consumer/survivor/ex-patient movement, and immediately recognized that I was one of them. Perhaps naively, I came out as a psychiatric survivor in a large meeting that included professionals. The ex-patients in the group seemed excited to learn that I was one of them; many of my colleagues seemed shocked, although my supervisor was supportive.

The consumer/survivor/ex-patient activists took me under their wing, gave me materials laying out the movement's critique of biological psychiatry, talked with me about movement history, and introduced me to activists around the country. Two years later, I was appointed special assistant to the state Office of Mental Health commissioner, charged with bringing the perspectives of current and former service users into policy-making. This was initially empowering; I hired several other psychiatric survivors as staff, we met regularly with movement activists to strategize on policy matters, and we ensured that service users were included in important policy discussions.

But official enthusiasm for our participation dimmed as the leadership slowly came to the realization that we were not interested in "reforming" the system or making it more "consumer-friendly," but that we took issue with the underlying premises of the psychiatric system and considered its coercive power a threat to human rights. This fundamental disagreement came to a head when the governor proposed, and OMH leadership supported, legislation to create what they called Assisted Outpatient Treatment and we called Involuntary Outpatient Commitment. This law allows forced treatment in the community, including forced drugging, of people who do not meet the criteria for inpatient commitment. The consumer/survivor/ex-patient movement rightly saw this as a serious deprivation of liberty. My staff and I helped the movement organize to oppose the legislation, while our employer worked to get it passed.

The law passed, I ultimately lost my job, and the agency leadership made sure my former position was filled by a "consumer" who shared the values and beliefs of the psychiatric establishment. At the same time, I watched as "peer specialists", a job title I helped create to bring genuine peer support to people within the mental health system, became increasingly co-opted, as the role became focused on supporting the treatment system. Peer specialists' roles changed; they now are required to do things like pressure people for medication "compliance" and report their behavior to clinicians. The use of "peer specialists", particularly in coercive settings, has exploded in recent years. Many mad movement activists are alarmed by this rampant co-optation and call for a moratorium on these roles, with a renewed focus on funding independent peer advocacy (Penney and Stastny, 2019).

In 2020, the situation of the psychiatric survivor movement in the U.S. feels somewhat discouraging. While the independent psychiatric survivor movement grew in the 1970s and 1980s, several factors, including the co-opting effects of government funding, resulted in the contraction of the independent movement in recent decades. There has been a corresponding rise of the so-called "peer movement" and "recovery movement", which have philosophies more in line with the beliefs of the mainstream mental health industry. As discussed earlier, in the 1970s and 1980s, organized survivors worked hard to get a seat at federal and state policy-making tables, demanding to present alternative views to the patriarchal medical model of psychiatry (Chamberlin, 1990). Currently, many ex-patients who work inside the system are not even aware of the history of the psychiatric survivor movement, which was rooted in opposition to the oppressive policies of the system. In the U.S, it feels as though survivor knowledge currently has no more influence on mental health public policy now than it did 40 years ago – and perhaps even less, as the pharmaceutical industry now has more power and the state has more authority to coerce people with psychiatric labels into "treatment".

I see the emergence and growth of Mad Studies in Canada and the U.K. as a very promising development that gives me hope. A field of academic study that focuses resources and attention on survivor's experiential knowledge and that supports research conceived of and led by survivors will hopefully provide increased opportunities to have our views taken seriously by policy-makers and practitioners. I would love to see this development take root in the U.S. While I'm aware of a handful of psychiatric survivors who are researchers or hold academic appointments, the term Mad Studies does not appear to be used in the U.S. In the 1990s, I was part of a national group called the Consumer/Survivor/Ex-Patient Research and Policy Workgroup; it would be wonderful to revive that group.

References

Chabasinski T (2012) The history and future of our psychiatric survivor movement. *Mad in America.* https://www.madinamerica.com/2012/08/the-history-and-future-of-our-psychiatric-survivor-movement/. Accessed: 12 June 2020

Chamberlin J (1990) The ex-patients' movement: Where we've been and where we're going. *Journal of Mind and Behavior*, 11 (3): 323–336.

Chamberlin J and Penney D (2002) Oral history interview of Judi Chamberlin by Darby Penney. *The Community Consortium.* http://www.community-consortium.org/projects/chamberlin-judy.pdf. Accessed:12 June 2020

Penney D and Stastny P (2019) Peer specialists in the mental health workforce: A critical reassessment. *Mad in America.* https://www.madinamerica.com/2019/10/peer-specialists-mental-health-workforce/. Accessed: 12 June 2020

9

THE SOCIAL MOVEMENT OF PEOPLE WITH PSYCHOSOCIAL DISABILITIES IN JAPAN

Strategies for taking the struggle to academia

Naoyuki Kirihara
Translated by Kasumi Ito

Origin and nature of movements

The first aim here is to set out the histories of social movements of people with psychosocial disabilities in Japan. These movements originated in the 1960s and gradually became more active. A national organization was first established in the 1970s.

A key reason why the movements became active was the existence of student movements developed by students in medical departments. Especially in western Japan, after medical students declared their support for anti-psychiatry and called for the reformation of psychiatry obtained their doctor's license and were subsequently assigned to a mental hospital, they organized self-governing groups of patients and supported patients' discharge. The Japanese government had promoted a policy to increase the number of beds in mental hospitals after World War II. Subsequently, long-term hospitalization and abuses in institutions became serious problems in the second half of the 1960s. The government, however, did not take any measures to address this and, finally, after 2000, budgetary measures for the reduction of the number of beds and community transition began to be taken. Thus, the discharge of long-term inpatients in western Japan from around 1969 continued uncertainly, without a systematic basis.

In Japan, over 90% of residences are located in the private market, and the custom is that renters' family members need to cosign lease contracts. However, most people with psychosocial disabilities who have no relatives are unlikely to have a cosigner. People who could not rent these residences because of such circumstances have had no other choice but to live in areas where residences do not have strict conditions for renting. Many people with psychosocial disabilities settled in these areas after their hospital discharge and naturally interacted with one another. For example, they visited one another's homes. Around 1969, people with psychosocial disabilities had very few social resources in their community. When they were

DOI: 10.4324/9780429465444-11

not feeling well, peers living nearby offered them lodging and cared for them. In this way, communities of persons with psychosocial disabilities helping one another were gradually created in these areas.

In one such area, a learning group for citizens called *Osaka kibo no kai* (group for hope in Osaka) was established mainly by student movements. Persons with psychosocial disabilities were influenced by the learning group and started their own unique activities. Shiro Nishiyama, who lived in the area, established an organization of people with psychosocial disabilities, called *Tomoshibi kai* (Group of Lamplight), based on his painful inpatient experiences. He also joined *Osaka kibo no kai*. He then rented an apartment in 1973 and started to host *Shabette tomaru kai* (Group to Talk and Stay Together) where people with psychosocial disabilities from eastern and western Japan could be together at weekends (Nishiyama, 1995).

Around this time, mental hospital inpatients started other unique activities that were different from the activities in communities. In 1970, some mental hospital inpatients who worked at companies out of the hospitals in rehabilitation schemes in daytime and slept in the hospitals at night, demanded wage increases for outside working, seeing it as a labor or employment issue. Reformist psychiatrists developed cooperative relationships with the labor unions of nurses and other mental hospital staff members. The labor union eventually came into contact with inpatients who demanded wage increases for outside working. Subsequently, people with psychosocial disabilities decided to set up their own organization to represent inpatients. The first self-governed group of inpatients in Japan was established in 1972. This group began to express opinions on the improvement of mental hospitals and legislation (Editorial Committee on the Histories of Iwakura Hospital, 1974). Such activities in and out of hospitals were also initiated in other areas of Japan and spread widely.

The Japanese government introduced an amendment to the Penal Code in May 1974. This included security measures that aimed to prevent crime among people with 'mental illness' who were recognized as not having criminal responsibility. It was the first government action to systemize the legislation of security measures, and it was met with an outcry from people with psychosocial disabilities, psychiatrists, lawyers, and labor unions. In 1973, shortly before the drafting of this bill was completed, an open letter titled "Let persons with psychosocial disabilities get together to protest against security measures" written by a person with psychosocial disabilities was published by a major newspaper company. People got together as a response to this call and established the *Tomo no kai* (Group of Friends) in the same year (Yamada, 1974). Since then, people with psychosocial disabilities have sought to form a national organization and develop a movement against such security measures. Finally, *Zenkoku "seishin-byo" sha shudan* (Japan National Group of Mentally Disabled People (JNGMDP), was established as the first national organization of people with psychosocial disabilities in May 1974 (Higashikawa, 1974). I write as a member of this organization.

Since its foundation, JNGMDP has argued against security measures, called for the abolition of the Mental Health Act, and protesting against damage from psychiatric practice. JNGMDP was less interested in making accusations against medical malpractices in individual hospitals, than in criticizing psychiatry itself. This objective is reflected in the name of JNGMDP, in which "*seishin-byo* (mental illness)" is enclosed in quotation marks to represent doubt in the very idea of "mental illness." The organization called for the participation of people who had histories of mental hospital admission based on the diagnosis of mental illness, without questioning whether the person actually had mental illness. In addition, the members of JNGMDP, who had had experiences of being excluded due to deviance from the regulated norms of organizations, thought that their group of people with psychosocial disabilities should not exclude others based on such organizational principles. Therefore, JNGMDP adopted a form of group that was different from both traditional communal societies and organizations; it did not have an instruction system, and did not establish bylaws nor elect representatives. The decision-making of JNGMDP as a group was not made by majority voting of the executive, but basically by mutual consent of members who gathered at the group's office. JNGMDP, however, was active not as an aggregation of individuals but as a group. JNGMDP intended to avoid the risk of their complaints being medicalized. This was because when concrete harm is experienced in mental health systems, allegations from individuals with psychosocial disabilities are often regarded as delusionary and dismissed as meaningless.

From its establishment, JNGMDP has been managed solely by people with psychosocial disabilities. To provide such mutual help, JNGMDP has relied on public assistance for individual members and the wages of leaders as their main financial resource. This has meant that they have had a vulnerable, but stable, financial basis because the amount of public assistance in Japan has been comparatively larger than that in other countries. Actually, many members had jobs. Therefore, the cost of mutual help could not be judged as fully covered only by public assistance in a wholesale manner. Members could cover at least their daily costs using public assistance and did not have to request financial assistance from patient groups. Their main activities included providing mutual help, in which people with psychosocial disabilities invited their peers to their own house and cared for them. Subsequently, some members found it necessary to have a place for getting together, and they would call for donations and get such places.

Thus, the groups of persons with psychosocial disabilities in Japan were not forced to demand financial assistance from the government and did not have to introduce relationships as providers and clients among members. Moreover, their activities were variable, without fixed service menus. Most of the activities were independent and voluntary and did not need to develop a well-organized service system.

Claims-making on security measures and the Mental Health Act

The government's plan to set up security measures in the Penal Code was decided on May 29, 1974. The provisional draft of the bill for revising the Penal Code, opened in April 1940, provided four types of security measures: labor measures to correct the work behavior of vagrants and people who were seen as averse to work, preventive measures to detain people who had committed serious crimes, custodial measures for people diagnosed with mental illness and with hearing and speech impairment, and corrective measures for people with addiction to alcohol and anesthetic drugs. In the discussion on the bill, some security measures had to be deleted or changed, and finally, only security measures to prevent recidivism among "persons who had caused serious cases under the condition of insanity" were adopted. Mass movements against the security measures were staged by well-known intellectuals, labor unions, and citizens. The Criminal Affairs Bureau of the Ministry of Justice summarized the movements as criticisms against the growth of state power (Criminal Affairs Bureau of the Ministry of Justice, 1974).

The Japanese Society of Psychiatry and Neurology, an organization of psychiatrists, argued that the security measures provided in the bill of the Penal Code were inapplicable to psychiatry, because it was impossible for health care to foresee offence and for treatment to prevent repeat offences. The Society also argued that health care exists for the benefit of patients, and giving priority to the public while excluding patients under medical treatment is contrary to the main principles of medicine (Japanese Society of Psychiatry and Neurology, 1972, 1974a, 1974b). The Japan Federation of Bar Associations, an organization of lawyers, argued that the establishment of the security measures represented the expansion of punishment rights by destroying the principle of no punishment without law, and that discussions were not enough, noting the lack of national participation despite the Bill's profound influence on the entire nation. In addition, the Federation stated that mental impairment is the reason for the repeat offences of specific persons with mental illness, and argued that enrichment of psychiatry was needed more than revision of the law because repeat offences could be prevented by the treatment of mental illness. They further argued that the enrichment of psychiatry would prevent the first offence, while revision of the Penal Code would only be able to prevent repeated offences. Based on these arguments, the Federation demanded that the Ministry of Health and Welfare revise the Mental Health Act (Japan Federation of Bar Associations, 1974, 1981a, 1981b, 1982).

In contrast, JNGMDP opposed the security measures and the Mental Health Act, on the grounds that they were discriminatory. They referred to their own humiliating experience of forced hospitalization under the Mental Health Act, and judged the security measures as having the same problem as the Mental Health Act in terms of the possibility of detention on the basis of "mental disorder." They also argued that the security measures were founded on discriminatory beliefs that looked upon people with mental disorders as people with criminal predispositions. Discriminatory belief is thus a belief that links mental disorders to offences, considers persons with mental disorders as offenders and other people as victims, and alienates persons with mental disorders, in spite of the possibility of any person becoming an offender and having mental impairment in the future. Such a belief undermines people's ability to consider the security measures as something that could affect them. People with psychosocial disabilities believed that each citizen could be persuaded that the security measures were their concern too by sharing their experiences of forced hospitalization under the existing Mental Health Act as a precedent for the security measures. They warned that anyone could become a person with mental disorder and be detained as a result (JNGMDP, 1977, 1981). In summary, the JNGMDP believed that perceptions of affinity and exclusion that draw boundaries between persons with mental disorders and other people privileged the security measures in the Penal Code and forced hospitalization in the Mental Health Act. Thus, they opposed both security measures in the Penal Code and forced hospitalization in the Mental Health Act because they saw these as promoting discrimination and exclusion.

Pioneer of international activities

Deliberations in the Japanese parliament, the Diet on the Bill on security measures in the Penal Code drafted by the government in 1974 were postponed because of opposition by psychiatrists, lawyers, labor unions, lawyers, and people with psychosocial disabilities. Discussions to legislate security measures restarted in 1980, triggered by a case of arson by a person who had a history of being hospitalized in a mental hospital. The main point of the discussion was the conflict between the Ministry of Justice, which sought to revise the Penal Code and establish security measures, and the Japan Federation of Bar Associations, which aimed to prevent persons with mental disorders from committing crimes by revising the Mental Health Act and enriching psychiatry. The Japan Federation of Bar Associations prepared a report of their visits to the United Kingdom, which has a system of high-security psychiatric hospitals in their Mental Health Act, and a suggestion to revise the Mental Health Act in Japan (Special Committee for Revision of the Penal Code and Committee for Protection of Human Rights of the Daini Tokyo Bar Association, 1982).

Discussions between the Ministry of Justice and Japan Federation of Bar Associations continued with an additional focus on whether legalization of the security measures should be achieved by the revision of the Penal Code, revision of the Mental Health Act, or establishment of independent law on social welfare. Suddenly, the discussions were halted in March 1984 after the incident known as the Utsunomiya Hospital Scandal became public. Reports revealed that nurses at Utsunomiya Hospital brutally beat and caused the death of two mental hospital inpatients. The scandal attracted wide attention as an issue of human rights in mental hospitals, later influencing the revision of the Mental Health Act (Yasui, 1984, 1986).

Meanwhile, political abuse in relation to psychiatry in the former Soviet Union was revealed as problematic by the World Psychiatric Association from the second half of the 1970s to 1983, when the Soviet Psychiatric Association withdrew from the World Psychiatric Association in a tumultuous manner. This incident shed light on the problems with human rights in psychiatric practice, not only in the former Soviet Union, but worldwide. Subsequently, the momentum to establish international principles on mental health increased. The Sub-Commission on the Prevention of Discrimination and Protection of Minorities within the UN Human Rights Committee nominated Erica-Irene Daes as special rapporteur. Principles in relation to mental health began to be drafted on September 10, 1980. The Principles, Guidelines and Guarantees for the Protection of Persons Detained on Grounds of Mental Ill-health or Suffering from Mental Disorder (UN Doc. E/CN.4/Sub.2/1983/17), drafted by the Sub-Commission and known as the Daes draft, were published on August 31, 1982. The Daes draft was designed to eliminate arbitrary decisions in psychiatry via due process and fair judgment. The International Commission of Jurists, an international organization of lawyers, was involved in drafting the Daes draft and took the initiative in promoting its legal model. The World Psychiatric Association, however, pointed out that the Daes draft would make it possible for the state to control the relationships between patients and medical staff by introducing due process, and criticized the Daes draft for opening a door to potential political abuses of psychiatry by the state. They recommended a medical model that gave discretion to medical professionals.

In response to the Utsunomiya Hospital Scandal, the International Commission of Jurists sent a letter to the Prime Minister of Japan in May 1984 to request that the government establish an independent committee to examine the treatment of persons with mental disorders and related legislation. The Japanese government did not reply to this letter. Then in September 1984, the International Commission of Jurists dispatched a joint investigation team to Japan, in cooperation with the World Health Professions Alliance. This team interviewed some organizations related to the hospital scandal, including the JNGMDP. The investigations were summarized in a report and published by the Sub-Commission on the Prevention of Discrimination and Protection of Minorities. The "Conclusion and recommendation" of the report included a request to revise the Mental Health Act immediately, stipulating the processes of hospitalization, and providing legal and judicial protections to inpatients. Hidesuke Kobayashi, chief of the Mental Health Division of the Ministry of Health and Welfare, in attending the 38th conference of the Sub-Commission on the Prevention of Discrimination and Protection of Minorities in Geneva on August 21, 1985, promised revision of the Mental Health Act by saying "We will revise the Mental Health Act with the aim of protecting the human rights of inpatients" (International Commission of Jurists, 1996). The series of actions of the International Commission of Jurists was carefully prepared by them to impress the legitimacy of the legal model in the drafting of the principles of mental health.

JNGMDP expressed their rejection of the principles through the Disabled People's International, established in 1981, at the Sub-Commission on the Prevention of Discrimination and Protection of Minorities. As there was no international organization of persons with psychosocial disabilities at the time, Disabled People's International was a suitable organization to express opinions internationally from the position of people with disabilities. JNGMDP expressed their opinions from the viewpoint of people with disabilities themselves and criticized adversely the way forced hospitalizations were made possible by due process or the judgment of a doctor. This report of the JNGMDP to the International Commission of Jurists attracted attention as the world's first opinion from persons with psychosocial disabilities themselves (JNGMDP, 1990). However, such opinions had little influence on the drafting of the principles because the conflicts between the International Commission of Jurists' legal model and the medical model of the World Psychiatric Association dominated the discourse.

A statement of Principles and Guarantees for the Protection of Mentally Ill Persons (UN Doc. E/CN.4/Sub.2/1984/19), known as the Palley draft, was submitted to the Sub-Commission on the Prevention of Discrimination and Protection of Minorities on September 2, 1988. The Palley draft put more emphasis on medical paternalism compared with the Daes draft. Subsequently, discussions were held and the draft was continually revised. The Principles for the Protection of Persons with Mental Illness and the Improvement of Mental Health Care (UN Doc. A/Res/46/119) were adopted at the UN General Assembly in December 1991. The adopted principles included some conditions that justified involuntary admission on the basis of mental disorders.

The World Federation of Psychiatric Users was established in 1991, and so the first international organization of people with psychosocial disabilities was born (World Federation of Psychiatric Users, 1991). The WFPU became a member of the monitoring committee of the Standard Rules on the Equalization of Opportunities for Persons with Disabilities (UN Doc. A/Res/48/96), and was then involved in the establishment of the International Disability Alliance. It changed its name to the World Network of Users and Survivors of Psychiatry (World Network of Users and Survivors of Psychiatry, no date), and subsequently played a large role in drafting the Convention on the Rights of Persons with Disabilities from the viewpoint of a social/human rights model. The Convention on the Rights of Persons with Disabilities (UN Doc. A/Res/61/106) recommends state parties to take measures to prohibit the deprivation of liberty and restriction of legal capacity on the basis of disability.

Blocking the revision of the Mental Health Act

In July 2016, a former staff member at an institution for persons with disabilities in Sagamihara City, Kanagawa Prefecture, killed 19 residents. The suspect, now a death-row inmate, was later revealed to have carried out the murder because of his belief that "the life of persons with disabilities has no use." The mass media, however, focused on his history of forced hospitalization in a mental hospital and consecutively aired many sensational reports.

I believe that the incident occurred because of policies that gathered and isolated people with disabilities in institutions and that the problems of institutions are similar to problems of forced hospitalization. Institutions make society one without persons with disabilities by placing people with disabilities in separate designated places. As a result, many people lose the chance to meet people with disabilities and tend to internalize the prejudice that people with disabilities are powerless. Likewise, forced hospitalization deprives people of the chance to meet persons with psychosocial disabilities and aggravates the prejudice that persons with psychosocial disabilities are dangerous. Such a chain of exclusion reinforces false beliefs about such offenders (see the incident in Sagamihara City). Strengthening forced hospitalization is only likely to prevent true resolution. However, revision of the forced hospitalization policy was strongly promoted, according to the intentions of the government. Subsequently, the government submitted a Bill for the amendment of the Mental Health Act, which included provisions to monitor persons with psychosocial disabilities by police after discharge from forced hospitalization (Kirihara, 2017).

When JNGMDP started its movement to oppose this Bill, no one had been protesting against it. Nonetheless, we in JNGMDP, decided to treat this situation as a good opportunity to showcase the power of persons with psychosocial disabilities, especially if such movements of people with psychosocial disabilities could lead to obstructing the passage of the Bill to revise the Mental Health Act. We carefully prepared and formulated detailed strategies. First, JNGMDP requested that the message, "Do not replace the issues relating to the incident with matters directed at forced hospitalization" was explicit in resolutions and programmes of events relating to the incident in Sagamihara City, undertaken in cooperation with organizations of people with disabilities. Second, JNGMDP continued to voice opinions to the Ministry of Health, Labor and Welfare, request action from organizations of mental health professionals and lawyers and, lobby against the Bill in the Diet. After the Bill was put on the agenda, JNGMDP was involved in activities in the Diet that aimed to make the position of opposition parties against the Bill at the examinations of bills at Policy Research Councils, send people with psychosocial disabilities as witnesses to the committee for the deliberation on the Bill, and demand circumspect deliberation while preparing to submit a supplementary resolution.

We concentrated our biggest efforts on developing theories to oppose the Bill. Consequently, most opposition parties took positions against the Bill, and JNGMDP succeeded in sending their member to the Diet as a witness. Deliberations on the Bill to revise the Mental Health Act were confusing, took a long time, carried over to the next session, and finally the Bill was abolished. The government intended to put out a Bill to revise the Mental Health Act again in the next session without changing the contents of the previous bill. JNGMDP, however, lobbied the ruling parties intensively against the Bill on a daily basis. As a result, the government gave up putting the Bill on the agenda. The Bill fell into a situation where it could not be put on the agenda without having its contents changed, though the situation was called a deferral state (Kirihara, 2020).

Joint, tense relations and conflicts between research and movements

In July 2017, the Japanese government released "Guidelines to ensure the provision of high-quality and appropriate medical care to persons with mental disorders" and formally institutionalized the role of peer supporters of persons with psychosocial disabilities. The preamble of the guidelines states as follows:

> The government promotes peer support, such as mutual supports by exchanges among persons with mental disorders, promotes developing independent relationships of persons with mental disorders and their families by supporting the families, who closely support persons with mental disorders, and pushes forward activities to prevent isolation from society.
>
> *(Ministry of Health, Labour and Welfare, 2014)*

I believe that the government's systemization of peer support has overall been positive, but the definition of peer support was changed after the systemization. Currently, peer supporters described by the government refer to persons with psychosocial disabilities who are employed by mental health and welfare offices. Therefore, mutual help in social movements of persons with psychosocial disabilities is being stripped from the meaning of peer support. The belief that only persons with psychosocial disabilities who are employed by mental health and welfare offices are accepted as peer supporters is problematic because it precludes as peer supporters those organizations of persons with psychosocial disabilities, which are involved in the domestic implementation of the Convention on the Rights of Persons with Disabilities and lobbying against the revision of the Mental Health Act. In addition, "recovery" is described as the adjustment of people to society, through treatment and rehabilitation and the goal of care in the field of care management.

There is no doubt that peer support and recovery were innovations that had their origins in the social movements of people with psychosocial disabilities. In Japan, however, the meanings of peer support and recovery have been increasingly undermined. They have been deconstructed to become concepts shaped by the medical models of medical professionals, as in many other countries. Meanwhile, movements of people with psychosocial disabilities have tended to explain abstractly the concepts of peer support and recovery. For example, recovery has been explained in terms of "self-definition," "having hopes," and "beliefs different from psychiatry." These explanations are unfortunately problematic as they leave room for arbitrary interpretation and distortion. Movements of people with psychosocial disabilities cannot progress with only passion. It is necessary to prove our uniqueness by putting into clear words the differences between our definitions and those of mental health professionals. Without such clarification and verbalization, we cannot differentiate our ideas from others', and the ideas will remain vulnerable to becoming distorted by professionals. I believe that the academics should help to put the ideas of movements into words and play a part in preventing the movement of persons with psychosocial disabilities from being distorted by professionals.

Ways forward

Movements of persons with psychosocial disabilities in Japan tend to be critical of academia. The criticism comes from misgivings that when they cooperate in research, it is the contribution and influence of researchers that increases, whereas their own circumstances do not improve. Such criticisms are often too passive for activists, because the main actors to change society should be social movements. Societal change should not be left to researchers. Activists need to have their own code on how they use academia and realize the desires of their movements. In particular, movements of people with psychosocial disabilities should pay the most careful attention to research to create evidence for national policy and this is a field where activists and academics should work together. Activists need to use academia effectively.

Activism and the academia are separate things. However, they are not necessarily caught in dualism, because the latter should involve the former in tackling issues of disability within its structures. Some academics promote a social/human rights model against the prevailing traditions of academia, in which the medical model is dominant and are involved in social movements to change academic society. Moreover, many academics who are involved in such social movements are persons with disabilities themselves.

I am involved in both social movements and research and comply with the criteria of the social/human rights model in both fields. Activities must be pushed forward, based on the achievements of histories of movements of persons with disabilities and in accordance with the social/human rights model.

Acknowledgment

I am grateful to Kasumi Ito, who translated my paper into English. She is a National Government Licensed Guide Interpreter and supports organizations of persons with disabilities in her capacity as an academic. For more information about her work please see http://www.arsvi.com/w/ik17e.htm.

References

Criminal Affairs Bureau of the Ministry of Justice (1974) *Keiho kaisei wo do kangaeru ka: Hosei shingikai no kaisei keiho soan wo kore ni taisuru hihan wo megutte (What should we think about revisions of the Penal Code?: About the draft revision of the Penal Code by Legislative Council of the Ministry of Justice and criticisms against it).*

Editorial Committee on the Histories of Iwakura Hospital (1974) *Iwakura byoin shi: Sono 1* (Histories of Iwakura Hospital: No. 1). *Seishin iryo dai 1 ki (Psychiatry: The first period).* 4: 57–62.

Higashikawa G (1974) *Dai 1 kai zenkoku kanja shukai wo owatte* (After the first patients' national assembly). *Seishin iryo dai 1 ki (Psychiatry: The first period).* 4(1): 98–99.

International Commission of Jurists (1996) *Seishin shogai-sha no jinken: Kokusai horitsu-ka iinkai repoto (Human rights of people with psychosocial disabilities: Report of the International Commission of Jurists).* Akashi shoten.

Japan Federation of Bar Associations (1974) *Keiho zenmen "kaisei" ni-kansuru seimei* (Statement on complete "revision" of the Penal Code).

Japan Federation of Bar Associations (1981a) *Seishin iryo no bappon-teki kaizen ni-tsuite: Yoko an* (About a drastic improvement of psychiatry: Draft outline).

Japan Federation of Bar Associations (1981b) *Seishin iryo no kaizen hosaku ni-tsuite: Kosshi* (About measures to improve psychiatry: Summary).

Japan Federation of Bar Associations (1982) *Seishin iryo no kaizen hosaku ni-tsuite: Ikensho* (About measures to improve psychiatry: Written opinion).

Japanese Society of Psychiatry and Neurology (1972) *Hoan shobun ni hantai-suru iinkai hokoku* (Report of commission to oppose security measures). *Seishin shinkei-gaku zasshi (Psychiatria et Neurologia Japonica).* 75(11): 831–833.

Japanese Society of Psychiatry and Neurology (1974a) *Hoan shobun ni-tsuite no riji-cho danwa* (Comment of chairperson on security measures). *Seishin shinkei-gaku zasshi (Psychiatria et Neurologia Japonica).* 76(6): 453.

Japanese Society of Psychiatry and Neurology (1974b) *Seimei* (Statement). *Seishin shinkei-gaku zasshi (Psychiatria et Neurologia Japonica).* 77(3): 218.

Japan National Group of Mentally Disabled People (JNGMDP) (1977) *11.13 dai 3 kai "seishin shogai-sha" zeikoku sou kekki shukai* (The third whole national rally of "people with psychosocial disabilities" on November 13). JNGMDP.

Japan National Group of Mentally Disabled People (JNGMDP) (1981) *Kizuna* (Bond) No. 7. JNGMDP.

Japan National Group of Mentally Disabled People (JNGMDP) (1990) *Zenkoku "Seishin-byo" sha shudan nyusu 2 gatu-go* (Newsletter of the Japan National Group of Mentally Disabled People: February). JNGMDP.

Kirihara N (2017) Sagamiha jiken kara seishin hoken fukusi ho kaisei made: Teiko no kiseki (From the incident in Sagamihara City to the revision of the Mental Health Act: Track of resistance). Hori T (ed.) *Watashi-tachi no Tsukui-yamayuri En jiken: Shogai-sha to-tomoni <kyosei shakai> no asu he (Our incident of the Tsukui-yamayuri En: Toward 'convivial society' with people with disabilities).* Shakai hyoron sha.

Kirihara N (2017) Sagamiha jiken kara seishin hoken fukusi ho kaisei made: Teiko no kiseki (From the incident in Sagamihara City to the revision of the Mental Health Act: Track of resistance). In Hori T (ed.) (2017) Watashi-tachi ha Tsukui-yamayuri En jiken no "nani" wo sabaku bekika: Miho-san Tomoko-san to Ko-Z-san wo yo no hikari ni!("What" should we punish regarding the incident of the Tsukui-yamayuriEn?:Miho, Tomoko, and Ko-Z would be the light of the world!). Shakai hyoronsha.

Ministry of Health, Labour and Welfare (2014) Ryoshitsu katsu tekisetu na seishin-shogai-sha ni-taisuru iryo no teikyo wo kakuho-suru tameno shishin (Guidelines to ensure the provision of high-quality and appropriate medical care providing good quality and suitable medicine to persons with mental disorders) https://www.mhlw.go.jp/file/05-Shingikai-12201000-Shakaiengokyokushougaihokenfukushibu-Kikakuka/0000032568.pdf. Accessed June 19, 2021.

Nishiyama S (1995) *Chi wo hau tomoshibi-kai* (Group of Lamplight crawls on the ground). In *"Byo"-sha no hon shuppan iinkai* (Publication committee of books by people with "mental illness") *Tenjou-tenge "byo"-sha hangeki: Chi wo hau "seishin-byo"-sha undo (People with "mental illness" counterattack in the whole universe: Movements of people with "mental illness" crawling on the ground).* Shakai hyoron sha, 118–127.

Special Committee for Revision of the Penal Code and Committee for Protection of Human Rights of the Daini Tokyo Bar Association (1982) *Kiro ni tatsu yoroppa no hoan shobun: Oshu jinken saiban-sho hanketsu to eikoku no hoan shobun shisetsu no jittai* (Security Measures in Europe, standing at a turning-point in: Judgement of the European Court of Human Rights and actual situations of institutions for security measures in the United Kingdom). Daini Tokyo Bar Association.

World Federation of Psychiatric Users (1991) WFPU first committee meeting, Mexico City. *World Network of Users and Survivors of Psychiatry*. http://wnusp.rafus.dk/wfpu-first-committee-meeting-mexico-city. html. Accessed: November 13, 2020.

World Network of Users and Survivors of Psychiatry (no date) History of the World Network of Users and Survivors of Psychiatry. *World Network of Users and Survivors of Psychiatry*. http://wnusp.net/index. php/history-of-the-world-network-of-users-and-survivors-of-psychiatry.html. Accessed: November 13, 2020.

Yamada K (1974) *Tachiagaru kanja-tachi* (Patients standing up). *Tomo no kai* (Group of Friends) (ed) *Tetsu-goshi no naka kara: Seishin Iryo ha korede iinoka (From grated space: Should we leave psychiatry the way it is?)*. Kai cho sha, 118–127.

Yasui T (1984) *Utsunomiya byoin no jittai* (Actual situations of Utsunomiya Hospital). *Seishin iryo dai 2 ki (Psychiatry: The second period)*.13(2): 12–19.

Yasui T (1986) *Akuma no seishin byoin: Hotoku-kai Utsunomiya Byoin (Devilish mental hospital: Hotoku-kai Utsunomiya Hospital)*. San-ichi shobo.

10

RE-WRITING THE MASTER NARRATIVE

A Prerequisite for Mad Liberation

Wilda L. White

Introduction

In the United States, we have the highest rates of unemployment (Henry et al., 2016), the highest rates of disproportionate incarceration (Human Rights Watch, 2006; James and Glaze, 2006), are most likely to be killed by police (Fuller et al., 2015), and die 20 to 25 years prematurely (Walker et al., 2015; Hayes et al., 2015; Siddiqi et al., 2017).

Sixty-eight percent of Americans do not want someone with a mental illness marrying into their family and 58 percent do not want people with mental illness in their workplaces (Martin et al., 2000). While most of us are able and willing to work, surveys of U.S. employers reveal that 50 percent are reluctant to hire someone with a past psychiatric history, approximately 70 percent are reluctant to hire someone currently taking antipsychotic medications, and 25 percent say they would fire someone who had not disclosed a mental illness (Stuart, 2006).

We are the butt of jokes on late night television, scapegoated for gun violence[1] (Obama, 2015; Trump, 2019) and routinely demeaned in the media. *The New York Times*, America's newspaper of record, frequently carries headlines such as "Who's the Real American Psycho?" (Dowd, 2018) or "Is Mr. Trump Nuts?" (The New York Times, 2018).

During his tenure, former President Barack Obama referred to his adversaries as "the crazies," (Fabian, 2015) and his wife, Michelle Obama (2018:352) who has a reputation for taking the high road, characterized Donald Trump's birther campaign against her husband as "crazy," and designed to stir up the "wingnuts and kooks." For his part, Trump, Barack Obama's successor, frequently refers to his detractors as "psycho" or "crazy," and the mainstream media reprint these epithets without a murmur of critique (Johnson, 2017).

Despite this persistent and pervasive marginalization and discrimination, our advocacy focuses almost exclusively on the mental health system and/or critiques of psychiatry. Most advocacy efforts are aimed at increasing "peer" participation in the development of mental health policies, persuading policymakers of the value of a recovery-based, mental health system, and spearheading alternatives to the mainstream mental health system.

Even the burgeoning discipline of Mad Studies delimits its scope as a "critique and transcendence of psy-centered ways of thinking, behaving, relating and being." (LeFrançois et al., 2013:13).

DOI: 10.4324/9780429465444-12

This hyper-focus on psychiatry and the mental health system has left the many sites of our oppression uncontested. And even in the arena that we do contest – the mental health system – our advocacy typically neither acknowledges nor challenges the root cause of the oppression and discrimination that effectively results in our erasure from society.

Against the backdrop of a psychiatric medical malpractice trial, this chapter introduces the concept of epistemic injustice to illustrate how the failure to focus our advocacy beyond psychiatry and the mental health system facilitates the denial of our basic rights such as the right to redress harm done to us.

The chapter argues that unless and until we, including the discipline of Mad Studies, expand our gaze beyond psychiatry and the mental health system, we will fail in our efforts to liberate ourselves because our oppression is largely rooted in epistemic injustice, an injustice which we much directly confront if we are ever to overcome our oppression both within and beyond the mental health system.

Until we achieve epistemic justice – that is, until society considers us credible witnesses to our own experiences and until we are able to render intelligible to ourselves and others our experiences of oppression – the discrimination and oppression that we experience in all realms of our lives will endure.

Epistemic injustice

In 2007, philosopher Miranda Fricker coined the term epistemic injustice to describe the harm that results when, because of prejudice, a person is deprived of her capacity as a "knower" or "interpreter" of her own experience.

Fricker termed the deprivation a person suffers in her capacity as a "knower," testimonial injustice, and the deprivation a person suffers in her capacity as an "interpreter," hermeneutical injustice.

Testimonial injustice occurs whenever prejudice causes the hearer to "give a deflated level of credibility to the speaker's word" (Fricker, 2007:1). A classic example of testimonial injustice is the disbelief with which women are often met when they say they have been raped or sexually harassed. Black people also often find themselves on the receiving end of testimonial injustice during encounters with police or when testifying before juries.

Testimonial injustice is not limited to instances of formal, witness testimony. As conceived by Fricker, testimonial injustice encompasses the full range of speech acts, including asking relevant questions, sharing an opinion, or suggesting a hypothesis. Testimonial injustice arises whenever the relevant statement, question, opinion or hypothesis is disbelieved, ignored, deflected or ridiculed because of prejudice.

Fricker (2007) employed the term "hermeneutical injustice," to describe what happens when prejudice denies a social group the opportunity to contribute to the pool of knowledge that allows human beings to make sense of and explain their experiences to themselves and others. When a social group has an experience that is unique to that social group, and the group because of prejudice has been denied the opportunity to participate in the creation of the concepts, vocabulary and interpretative tropes necessary to understand, articulate and share that experience, the group is said to be hermeneutically marginalized.

In Fricker's (2007) conception, hermeneutical marginalization is a prerequisite for a situation to count as a case of hermeneutical injustice. If an experience or condition is not well understood merely because the knowledge has yet to be created, this would not count as a case of hermeneutical injustice, unless the gap in understanding arises from a prejudice that has precluded knowledge creation or knowledge sharing.

Psychiatric patients and survivors have been traditionally excluded from creating knowledge about issues that affect us (Wallcraft, 2009:133), although this is not widely known and is itself an example of hermeneutical injustice. Fricker, for example, during a presentation to a group of doctors, once said of people with psychiatric histories:

> … if you think they count as a member of a group which is hermeneutically marginalized, I don't really know how we should think about that, but certainly I've had some people say to me who themselves have a history of mental ill health, say we count as such a group. One is hermeneutically marginalized when one has mental illness.
>
> *(Fricker, 2015: 00:35:01)*

Fricker's uncertainty aside, there is ample evidence, such as that recounted at the outset of this chapter, that people labeled with mental illnesses are, in fact, hermeneutically marginalized.

When Fricker (2007:149–152) first introduced the concept of hermeneutical injustice, she used as an example the experience of women victimized by sexual harassment before the term "sexual harassment" was coined. Before sexual harassment was given a name, women did not have the language and concepts to grasp and explain their experiences of being sexually pressured in the workplace. Historically, women, owing to prejudice, were excluded from the business of knowledge-creation. As a group, then, women were hermeneutically marginalized. This hermeneutical marginalization created a gap in women's and society's shared tools of understanding the experiences of women in the workplace. This lack of shared tools of understanding owing to hermeneutical marginalization is an example of hermeneutical injustice.

Another example of hermeneutical injustice comes from the black feminist movement. In the mid-1970s, five black women sued General Motors alleging discrimination against them as black women.[2] At the time, General Motors hired black men, and it hired white women. It did not hire black women. Because General Motors hired women and it hired men, the court dismissed the lawsuit, reasoning that the law did not contemplate that black women could be discriminated against as "black women." While black women understood that they suffered discrimination as black women, because they were hermeneutically marginalized, their group understanding was not shared across the social space, including within American jurisprudence.

In 1989, Kimberlé Crenshaw, a UCLA law school professor, re-visited the General Motors case in a law review article and coined the term "intersectionality" to describe the entwined form of oppression black women experience both because of their race and also their sex (1989:139–142). Today, the concept of "intersectionality," is widely understood across social groups.

Hermeneutical injustice exists both when a marginalized group itself lacks the interpretative tools necessary to understand its own experience, as was the case with women experiencing sexual harassment in the workplace, and also when the marginalized group understands its experience but cannot explain it to those outside the group because of a lack of shared tools of understanding, as was the case with the black women suing General Motors for discrimination against them as black women.

As the foregoing examples illustrate, the harm from epistemic injustice can be significant, depriving people of equal access to employment or a workplace free of harassment. In addition, the capacity to know, reason and inquire is essential to human value. When people are not believed because of prejudice or people cannot themselves understand their experiences or convey them to others because of a dearth of concepts from which to do so, Fricker (2007: 55) argues that the harm is so great it actually prevents people from becoming who they are.

A case study

In 2012, a San Francisco psychiatrist diagnosed me with Attention Deficit Hyperactivity Disorder (ADHD) and prescribed dextroamphetamine, a stimulant, to treat it. At the time, I was 54 years old, held a senior level position at UC Berkeley School of Law, my alma mater, where I earned a six-figure salary. I was also licensed to practice law in three states and was an honors graduate of Harvard Business School. I was debt-free, lived on Telegraph Hill in San Francisco, was in a loving relationship, and was a member of San Francisco's vibrant squash community.

At the time the psychiatrist prescribed the stimulant, he told me a potential side effect was "mania"[3] and/or "psychosis," and after I asked what were the signs and symptoms of "mania" and "psychosis," he referred me to the Diagnostic and Statistical Manual of Mental Disorders (DSM). While I personally take issue with the DSM's nosology, I had put myself into the country of Western psychiatry where the DSM was the lingua franca. If I wanted to be understood by my psychiatrist, I felt I had to use his language. Thus, in the language of the DSM, within weeks of starting the dextroamphetamine, I was "manic" and "psychotic," and did not want to be, and less than a year later, I was also homeless, jobless, penniless, single, and deeply in debt.

According to the DSM, the rulebook to which psychiatry purports to abide, a "manic" episode is a distinct period during which a person's mood is abnormally and persistently elevated, expansive or irritable with at least three additional symptoms from a list that includes: (a) inflated self-esteem or grandiosity; (b) decreased need for sleep; (c) pressure of speech; (d) flight of ideas; (e) distractibility; (f) increased involvement in goal-directed activities or psychomotor agitation; and (g) excessive involvement in pleasurable activities with a high potential for painful consequences. "Psychotic" features such as "hallucinations" (perceiving things through the senses that are outside the consensus reality) and "delusions" (believing things that are outside the consensus reality) can also be present. The expansiveness, unwarranted optimism, grandiosity and poor judgment that are characteristic of "mania" often lead to an imprudent involvement in pleasurable activities such as buying sprees and foolish business investments (American Psychiatric Association, 2013:123–129).

Over the course of a year, I told my psychiatrist repeatedly that I was "manic" and later "psychotic." While I was aware of my behavior and activities, I had no power to control them. In fact, I felt somewhat possessed.

I told the psychiatrist I was not sleeping, felt more creative, and was spending more money than I wanted to spend, including buying a brand-new car for a niece. Overnight, I adopted a new goal to raise millions of dollars for the law school. I told him about plans to start a business to end racism and shortly thereafter, I told him I was placed on administrative leave at the law school after delivering a speech at a Gala during which I warned prospective students, who were visiting campus to decide whether to attend the law school, not to attend because the law school was racist. I told him colleagues had begun to call me "crazy."

The psychiatrist wrote:

> Pt. appears to be exercising sound judgment in making decisions; seems to understand risks/benefits/consequences of her actions/behaviors; … able to articulate her thoughts in a way that makes sense and is in keeping with her passion/experiences in life; noted to pt. that many people who have experienced racism may just stay quiet about it or not take action, but that she's different in a way because it is her calling to take action to address it.

I also told him that I took out a $20,000 line of credit to launch my business to end racism, which my friends felt was an expression of "mania," particularly in the way I was going about it.

The psychiatrist wrote:

> Her friend thinks that pt. starting the [business to end racism] represents mania; however, given pt's lifelong interest in ending racism and fighting for justice, it's difficult to glean whether this behavior represents grandiosity or bold entrepreneurial vision/ normal risk taking.

Friends also directly contacted the psychiatrist to report their observations. One reported that I had "lost a lot of weight, my apartment was a mess, I was not thinking clearly, and was clearly not myself." The psychiatrist wrote:

> I don't see any clinical evidence of hypomania or mania. … For the most part, when I ask her about the risks, consequences and benefits of the decisions she's making, she seems to be exercising good reasoning and is able to articulate her thoughts clearly.

A second friend wrote in an email:

> Changes that I have witnessed in her attitude and behavior include a shift from risk-avoidant to risk-embracing behavior in relation to her finances and work-life, elevated mood, a sense of greater openness and expansion of possibilities, and a development of a personal relationship to God.

The psychiatrist wrote:

> In my opinion, pt may have some degree of hypomania, but even that is not clear to me; she appears to understand the risks that she's taking and is sound in her thinking about it.

I told him I was communicating with my dead parents and at their instruction I flew cross country to purchase a half-a-million-dollar home for my niece.

The psychiatrist wrote:

> Unclear to me if pt is having true manic episode or speaking metaphorically or having more of a spiritual experience.

After I was fired for the remarks I made at the Gala, I applied for private disability insurance. The disability insurer's psychiatrist, relying solely on the psychiatrist's medical records found me disabled due to "mania" and "psychosis." Thereafter, my psychiatrist retroactively diagnosed me with "mania" and "psychosis." The psychiatrist wrote:

> Things that I saw that I now consider to be features of mania in her are: (1) increased confidence; (2) acting more aggressively; (3) decreased social inhibition, e.g., saying things in contexts where she would have previously exercised greater personal reserve; (4) increased spending; (5) feeling more religious/spiritual than she normally is. … I'm on my toes trying to pick up these clues/symptoms now (I still feel lousy for having missed them the first go around).

In other words, the psychiatrist acknowledged seeing for himself the same signs that I and my friends reported when we told him that I was "manic."

When I asked him how he could have failed to recognize the "mania" and "psychosis," which my friends and I pointed out repeatedly, he wrote that because I did not exhibit during sessions with him "racing thoughts, flight of ideas, pressured speech, grandiosity, sense of invincibility, and social disinhibition," it was difficult for him "to discern the characteristic mental status changes of a manic episode."

I would go on to learn that I did not meet the DSM criteria for ADHD and the unnecessary prescription of dextroamphetamine had most likely triggered the "mania" and "psychosis," which abated after I stopped taking the drug. By this time, my savings were gone, and with the loss of my job, so was my $2 million pension and net future earnings. A few months later, I was homeless.

For his part, my psychiatrist inserted a secret, five-page "updated diagnostic formulation note" in my medical records, which purported to diagnose me with narcissistic and paranoid personality disorder based, among other things, on my history of rape, my brother's diagnosis of schizophrenia, and the following:

> She reported to me that she refused to show identification to the police officer because she was concerned that, being black, there was a higher chance that the male officer would mistake her for taking out a weapon instead of her identification – and consequently that a firearm would be discharged against her preemptively.

The psychiatrist hid the updated note from me. I learned about the note months later from records the psychiatrist sent to my disability insurer.

Given the enormity of my loss, I decided to pursue a medical malpractice action. I contacted dozens of lawyers. None was willing to take on a case on behalf of a client with a psychiatric history. I eventually found one lawyer who was willing to meet with me. However, after helping me file the initial lawsuit, he decided not to follow through and in the end, I reluctantly served as my own lawyer.

Once I got to trial, the judge, who was white, was hostile to me and my case at the outset. When I proposed using a written, jury questionnaire to tease out issues of bias based on race, sexuality, gender or psychiatric history, she announced that no such biases existed in San Francisco. During jury selection, she refused to allow me to ask prospective jurors about their own psychiatric histories or experiences with psychiatrists because in her words that was too embarrassing and shameful. Of course, if the case had involved medical malpractice based on a physical ailment, I would have been permitted to ask jurors about their familiarity with the physical ailment and their experiences with medical doctors.

During conferences with the judge, whenever I reported the facts of the case in support of an argument, the judge would turn to opposing counsel and ask, "is that true?" She never asked me whether what my opposing counsel reported was true. She simply accepted it as true even though many times, it was not.

The jury was permitted to ask questions of witnesses during the trial and at one point a juror asked my former psychiatrist what was my diet. He replied without missing a beat that I was a lifelong vegan, which I was not.

Although my psychiatrist had admitted several times in his medical records that he believed the dextroamphetamine had triggered the "psychotic manic" episode, he changed his position at trial and maintained that the episode was an organic process caused by bipolar disorder.

Medical malpractice trials require expert witnesses. My expert witness testified that the psychiatrist's treatment fell below the standard care because he failed to conduct an assessment to justify the ADHD diagnosis; he unnecessarily prescribed dextroamphetamine for a presumed diagnosis of ADHD; and he failed to recognize and treat the "manic psychosis" that was triggered by the dextroamphetamine.

In the end, the jury sided with my former psychiatrist's expert witness who testified that amphetamines do not cause "psychosis" and that it was a shame that I had been told that the episode was iatrogenic, when in fact I had the severe and chronic mental illness of bipolar disorder.

Discussion

Distributive and Discriminatory Epistemic Injustice

Epistemic injustice can take on both distributive and discriminatory forms. The distributive form encompasses whether people have fair access to epistemic goods such as education, information, good advice, legal services, and similar resources. The discriminatory form, of course, involves unequal treatment owing to prejudice.

My inability to find a lawyer willing to represent me exemplifies the distributive form of epistemic injustice and also the discriminatory form because my inability was due to my psychiatric history. Discrimination against people with psychiatric histories is so normalized that lawyers freely admit to it. For instance, in a continuing legal education seminar on medical malpractice available on the internet, a New York trial attorney (Oginski, 2014:00:00:25) advises attendees "you should run as fast as possible away" from potential clients with psychiatric histories even where there is a valid basis for a claim, adding that this was the considered opinion of many experienced trial attorneys.

As an attorney, I was technically able to represent myself. However, I was severely disadvantaged as a self-represented litigant. The psychiatrist was represented by three lawyers whose fees and expenses were paid by an insurance company. My psychiatrist's insurance company even paid him to attend trial. In contrast, I worked alone with no support and the expenses of my under-funded lawsuit were paid by a GoFundMe campaign. And although the law permits a self-represented litigant to testify in narrative form, the judge would not allow me to do so. I was made to ask myself questions and answer them. The irony of a person with a history of "psychosis" effectively talking to herself on the witness stand was not lost on me and likely left a negative impression on the jury.

Testimonial Injustice

The psychiatrist not believing me when I reported that I was "manic" and "psychotic" is an obvious case of testimonial injustice. When I reported the symptoms that were concerning to me, he appointed himself the epistemic authority of my irreducibly subjective experiences of elevated mood, decreased need for sleep, and increased energy.

Not only did he disbelieve my subjective experiences, but also he substituted his judgment for my own. For example, where I said I exercised poor judgment in speaking at the Gala, he wrote that I "appeared to be exercising sound judgment in making decisions." When I told him I was concerned about the grandiose idea of starting a business to end racism, he not only dismissed my concerns, he enabled the idea, suggesting that I turn to Kickstarter to help finance the endeavor.

The jury's asking my psychiatrist, rather than me, about my diet also exemplifies a form of testimonial injustice which Fricker calls preemptive testimonial injustice. Preemptive testimonial injustice happens where prejudice on the part of inquirers causes them not even to bother asking your view. The juror's question signaled that I was not viewed as an attorney or an individual with agency from whom information was solicited. Rather, I was a specimen from which data was extracted. In other words, I was epistemically objectified.

In reality, the psychiatrist knew nothing about my diet. Perhaps believing that he was expected to know, he simply invented a response which received no credibility deflation notwithstanding how unlikely it was that a 60-year-old, American woman had been a vegan since infancy. In this instance, the psychiatrist received an inflation of credibility, which is yet another example of testimonial injustice because it arises out of the jury's epistemic objectification of me.

The judge's practice of asking the opposing attorney whether what I reported was true is another example of testimonial injustice. In fact, the judge's question reveals her deep-seated prejudice against me. As an attorney in the American legal system I am considered an officer of the court and as such entitled to the presumption of truthfulness. In my decades of practicing law, a judge had never questioned my veracity. In turning to my opposing counsel as the arbiter of my credibility, she revealed that she herself had no legitimate basis to disbelieve me. She made no credibility judgment. She simply found me inherently untrustworthy based on my status as a self-represented, black woman with a psychiatric history.

The psychiatrist's expert witness also did not believe my reports of symptoms. This is yet another example of testimonial injustice. Fricker's conception of prejudice is fairly broad and is defined as a motivated resistance to counter-evidence owing to close-mindedness. Here, I was ultimately vindicated by the disability insurer's determination that I was experiencing a manic episode, by my psychiatrist's retroactive diagnosis of the same, and by the catastrophe that befell my life as a result of activities I engaged in while "manic." However, the psychiatrist's expert witness resisted this evidence without any rational basis.

The jury's decision to side with the psychiatrist's expert witness is also an example of testimonial injustice when you consider that the evidence was far more compelling that the dextroamphetamine triggered the episode. First, "mania" and "psychosis" are recognized side effects of dextroamphetamine. Second, the episode began within weeks of taking the drug and abated on its own when I stopped. Third, I had never before experienced a spontaneous "manic" episode. Fourth, at the time of trial, I had not seen a mental health practitioner in three years, had received no medical interventions, and showed no psychiatric symptoms, which according to the testimony would be an atypical course for chronic, lifelong bipolar disorder. Fifth, my psychiatrist had admitted in writing on numerous occasions that he believed the dextroamphetamine triggered the episode.

Unlike my expert, the psychiatrist's expert witness had never examined me. He nevertheless testified that I had chronic, lifelong bipolar disorder and that the "manic" episode was triggered by the loss of my job even though my employer testified that I lost my job because of behavior I engaged in while "manic" and even though both my friends and I reported our concerns to my psychiatrist many months before I lost my job.

The expert witness for the psychiatrist also testified that amphetamines do not cause "psychosis." On cross-examination I confronted him with the following passage from a report he wrote a few years before trial:

> In the 1950s, amphetamines began to be widely distributed for weight loss and the 1960s saw a peak in amphetamine use. However, this widespread consumption also

led to increased recognition of amphetamine's negative health consequences including amphetamine psychosis.

(Urman-Yotam and Ostacher, 2014:2)

And when I asked him on cross-examination if he warned his patients to whom he prescribed amphetamines that they can cause "psychosis," he said that he did because it was standard of care to do so.

I ultimately do not know precisely why the jury sided with the psychiatrist. Trials are complicated and there are many factors at play. I was not only a former psychiatric patient, I was also the only black person in the courtroom. As a self-represented litigant, I was also out-lawyered and out-resourced. However, none of that should affect the power of the evidence, which is why I offer this as an example of testimonial injustice. In the final analysis, the power of prejudice appears to have trumped the power of the evidence.

Hermeneutical injustice

The manner in which the psychiatrist's secret personality disorder diagnosis played out is an example of hermeneutical injustice.

For strategic reasons, I attempted to include as part of my lawsuit the harm I suffered upon discovering the secret personality disorder diagnosis. Essentially, I argued it was a fraudulent diagnosis. In pre-trial proceedings, the psychiatrist's lawyers opposed this attempt. The judge ultimately sided with the psychiatrist, asking why would a psychiatrist make a fraudulent diagnosis. The judge simply could not imagine a scenario under which a psychiatrist would offer a diagnosis that was motivated by anything other than helping a patient.

Although the judge could not imagine such a scenario, I was well aware through my contacts with other psychiatric survivors that a personality disorder diagnosis is the most charged psychiatric diagnosis of all. "You know you've really pissed off a psychiatrist when they diagnose you with a personality disorder," a fellow psychiatric survivor once told me.

Other psychiatrists also had no difficulty recognizing the secret diagnosis for what it was. The psychiatrist who interviewed me for eight hours and reviewed my records on behalf of my disability insurance company wrote in his report to the disability insurer:

> I am skeptical of the fact that … only just before their final session when Ms. White angrily confronted [the psychiatrist] over his failure to note her manic psychosis and treat her appropriately and terminated treatment with him, telling him that she no longer trusted his judgment, did he diagnose her with a personality disorder.

And the psychiatrist who prepared a rebuttal to the personality disorder diagnosis, wrote:

> It is worth observing, in my opinion, that there is a conflict of interest here for [the psychiatrist]. In making this diagnosis, he provides an alternative explanation for the suffering that she experienced during her manic episode, one that shifts responsibility for this suffering predominantly to her, thereby mitigating the moral responsibility he might otherwise feel for prescribing her a stimulant medication which, in all likelihood, triggered her mania.

However, owing to the hermeneutical marginalization of psychiatric survivors, I did not have available to me shared concepts, background information, and interpretive tropes to help the judge understand why a psychiatrist would make a fraudulent diagnosis. As a result, I was unable to hold the psychiatrist accountable.

My psychiatrist not believing me when I reported that I was "manic" and "psychotic" is also an example of hermeneutical injustice, based both on my race and my status as a psychiatric patient.

The psychiatrist rationalized my behavior at the Gala through the lens of race, reasoning that I made the inappropriate comments that led to the loss of my employment based on a "calling to take action to address [racism]."

First, I cannot resist noting the irony of the psychiatrist characterizing the remarks that led to my employment termination as consistent with my passion and life experiences and thereafter pathologizing as indicative of a personality disorder my refusal to comply with a police officer's unlawful demand to see my identification.

Second, no black psychiatrist or perhaps any psychiatrist with any knowledge of how black people negotiate their professional lives would have reached this conclusion. How could I both work at the law school and tell students not to attend and expect to have my job at the end of the day? In this sense, I was harmed by the psychiatrist's ignorance about how black professionals navigate white professional spaces. While this information is known among black people, owing to hermeneutical marginalization, it was not within society's common pool of knowledge sufficient to reach the awareness of this psychiatrist.

This example also counts as hermeneutical injustice based on my status as a psychiatric patient. However, to understand this as such requires background information that is simply not within the common pool of societal knowledge, owing ironically to hermeneutical injustice. It was not even within my own ken at the time I attempted to get my psychiatrist to take the reports of my symptoms seriously.

What I have come to understand is that the term "mental illness" connotes not just a state of mental ill health. The term is also deeply ideological and includes a set of beliefs, values and assumptions that shape public opinion, drive mental health policy, and influence treatment decisions. The ideology of mental illness conceptualizes mental illness as extreme, aberrant, often deviant behavior, which makes others uncomfortable and is so simple to recognize that everybody knows.

Thus, while there are 35 unique combinations of symptoms all of which meet the DSM definition of a "manic" episode, practitioners learn to recognize and act upon a single, stereotypical portrayal of "mania."

A witness for the psychiatrist testified, as follows, about how he was trained to recognize "mania" and "psychosis":

> What I recall from my days in graduate school … is that one of the cardinal signs for manic diagnosis, at least the way that it was taught to me, is that the therapist actually feels the – an oddity, an exaggeration in the way that the client is expressing themselves or a rapidity in their speech, a pressure in their speech; there is sometimes such a fluidity between one idea to another idea to another idea that it starts to feel uncomfortable to the therapist, and that experience is something that we were taught we should pay close attention to as a way of hypothesizing that perhaps we have someone that is having a break with reality.

After the disability insurer's doctor stepped in, my former psychiatrist readily acknowledged that he had indeed observed the signs of "mania" all along. However, he disregarded them because I did not manifest stereotypical signs such as racing thoughts, pressured speech, distractibility, and flight of ideas. There is also an unsubstantiated, but dominant clinical and research view that people experiencing "psychosis" have pervasive cognitive, reasoning deficits (Sanati and Kyratsous, 2015), which I also did not exhibit.

Thus, because of the ideology of mental illness and its focus on behavior that is disconcerting to others, my psychiatrist's recognition of my condition depended on a complex chain of circumstances in which my symptoms were not paramount. How I felt about my symptoms was much less important than how others felt about me. The effect I had on a clinician, the stereotypical manifestation of "mania" and "psychosis," and an unawareness of my mental state were all more important to a diagnosis of "mania" and "psychosis" than whether my symptoms met DSM criteria or whether I was bothered by them.

In fact, my awareness of my symptoms worked against me because psychiatrists have been incorrectly taught that individuals who are "psychotic" do not typically recognize that they are. To say you are "psychotic" is to prove you are not. The combination of this classic Catch-22 and my ignorance about the ideology of mental illness deprived me of the conceptual tools to convince my psychiatrist that I was, according to his own nosology, "psychotic," and did not want to be.

Importance of epistemic equality

What I have set out to demonstrate through the example of my trial is that (1) the oppression we experience in the mental health system is not confined to the mental health system but infiltrates every aspect of our lives; and (2) the root cause of that oppression is epistemic injustice.

Fricker (2014) has suggested that social epistemic contribution – the contribution of concepts, meanings, interpretations, beliefs, and knowledge to the pool of shared knowledge – is so crucial to political freedom, freedom of speech, and non-domination, that it is worthy for inclusion on philosopher Martha Nussbaum's list of central human capabilities. Nussbaum (2000) conceived the list as a description of basic things considered necessary for survival and to avoid or escape poverty or other serious deprivations.

I agree with Fricker. Epistemic justice is fundamental to political freedom and in my estimation, epistemic injustice underlies, among other things, the barbaric practice of psychiatric forced drugging, a separate and inherently unequal mental health system, our underemployment and overincarceration, and the grip of biomedical psychiatry despite its largely conjectural nature.

Epistemic injustice led to the destruction of my health, and the loss of my home, my livelihood, and my savings. And owing to epistemic injustice, I could hold no one to account. I could not retain an attorney to represent me. I could not make the judge and jury understand the harm I suffered or my psychiatrist's improper motives. I could not even serve as a credible witness to my own experience and witnesses who testified on my behalf were painted with the same broad brush of testimonial injustice.

Trials are ultimately about storytelling through shared tropes, shared concepts and common knowledge. Those who are excluded from the creation and dissemination of interpretive tropes, concepts and knowledge are seriously disadvantaged in such a process, a process that is essential to American democracy and its promise of freedom.

A fundamental tenet of American jurisprudence is due process, meaning notice and an opportunity to be heard. However, the concept of epistemic injustice teaches that it is not enough simply to be heard. One also needs to be believed and understood.

Thus, epistemic justice is foundational. Without epistemic justice – both distributive and non-discriminatory – there can be no other justice. It is impossible to contest the many sites of our oppression if we are not believed and if we cannot render intelligible to ourselves and others the harm that has been done to us sufficient to redress those harms.

Epistemic justice: How do we get there?

Overcoming epistemic injustice necessarily begins with an awareness of its existence. And just as voting rights were for black Americans, epistemic rights for us must be central to our advocacy and scholarship. While we cannot simply demand that people find us credible, there are ways of being in the world and actions we can take that confront hermeneutical injustice, and in the process, transform the social attitudes that perpetuate discrimination and oppression against us.

The rallying cry of consumers/ex-patients/psychiatric survivors – "Nothing about us, without us" – has led some of us to fight solely for the right to be present when decisions are made about us and to require only our lived experience as the price of admission. However, epistemic justice requires more than merely the presence of our lived experience during discussions about us. We must have something useful to say and we must be heard, believed, and understood.

To that end, we must ask more of ourselves and each other. Each of us must offer more than our lived experience or stories of recovery in the venues where our advocacy takes form. We must strive to create theories, concepts, meanings, interpretations, beliefs and knowledge that combine our lived experience with thought, reason, and creativity. And we must disseminate this new knowledge through mainstream media, including social media. We need more letters to the editor, more blogs, more magazine articles, more TED Talks, more YouTube videos, more tweets and more Op-Ed pieces directed to a mainstream audience that challenge the dominant conception of who we are. We must not allow our challenges to be reduced simply to recovery from illness. Rather, we must interrogate the ideology of mental illness, which keeps us underemployed, overincarcerated, prematurely deceased and ghettoized and mistreated in a doctrinaire mental health system.

The burgeoning discipline of Mad Studies has a critical role to play in this regard. However, for the field to contribute to Mad liberation, it must aim higher than transforming the mental health system or adopting alternatives to biomedical psychiatry or replicating other social justice movements and critical studies disciplines that have found a place in society by fitting neatly within society's tax-paying, law-abiding, we-are-just-like-you-and-want-what-you-want Master Narrative. Invariably, these movements have replicated and perpetuated the oppression of the dominant culture and have left many members of those movements behind.

For true liberation, Mad scholars and activists must re-write the Master Narrative in its entirety, and that narrative must be grounded in difference not sameness, humanity not sanity, and the inherent value of people not the transactional value of money.

Notes

1 Following the October 2015 shooting in Oregon, President Barack Obama said: "And it's fair to say that anybody who does this has a sickness in their minds, regardless of what they think their motivations may be." Following the August 2019 mass shootings in Texas and Ohio, President Donald Trump said: "Mental illness and hatred pulls the trigger, not the gun."
2 *DeGraffenreid v. General Motors*, 413 F. Supp. 142 (ED Mo 1976).
3 Throughout this chapter, except when quoting others, terms of art from Western psychiatry will be enclosed in quotation marks in an attempt to mitigate their violence and underscore that I do not endorse these terms. I used these terms in relation to myself only in the context of trying to be understood by my psychiatrist and others whose mother tongue is the DSM.

References

American Psychiatric Association (2013) *Diagnostic and Statistical Manual of Mental Disorders* (5th ed.). Washington, DC: Author.

Crenshaw K (1989) Demarginalizing the intersection of race and sex: A Black feminist critique of antidiscrimination doctrine, feminist theory and antiracist politics. *The University of Chicago Legal Forum* 139.

Dowd M (2018) Who's the real American psycho. *The New York Times* 10 November. https://www.nytimes.com/2018/11/10/opinion/sunday/dick-cheney-donald-trump-vice-movie.html. Accessed: 20 February 2020.

Fabian J (2015) White House: Obama 'flip' in referring to 'crazies'. *The Hill.* 25 August. https://thehill.com/homenews/administration/251926-white-house-obama-flip-in-referring-to-crazies. Accessed: 20 February 2020.

Fricker M (2007) *Epistemic Injustice: Power and Ethics of Knowing.* Oxford: Oxford University Press.

Fricker M (2014) *Epistemic Equality?* [Lecture] Social Equity Conference, University of Cape Town Philosophy, Cape Town. August. https://www.youtube.com/watch?v=u8zoN6GghXk. Accessed: 31 October 2019.

Fricker M (2015) *Epistemic Justice and the Medical Expert.* [Lecture] University of Sheffield. 25 February. https://www.youtube.com/watch?v=duNAXfOAvK0. Accessed: 31 October 2019.

Fuller D A, Lamb H R, Biasotti M, and Snook J (2015) *Overlooked in the Undercounted: The Role of Mental Illness in Fatal Law Enforcement Encounters.* Arlington: Treatment Advocacy Center.

Hayes J F, Miles J, Walters K, King M and Osborn D P J (2015) A systematic review and meta-analysis of premature mortality in bipolar affective disorder. *Acta Psychiatrica Scandinavica* 131(6): 417–425.

Henry A D, Barkoff A, Mathis J, Lilly B and Fishman J (2016) *Policy Opportunities for Promoting Employment for People with Psychiatric Disabilities.* Shrewsbury: University of Massachusetts Medical School and the Bazelon Center for Mental Health Law.

Human Rights Watch. (2006) U.S.: Number of mentally ill in prisons quadrupled. *Human Rights Watch* 5 September. . Accessed: 20 February 2020.

James D and Glaze L (2006) *Mental Health Problems of Prison and Jail Inmates.* Washington, DC: United States Department of Justice Bureau of Justice Statistics.

Johnson J (2017) President Trump angrily lashes out at 'Morning Joe' hosts on Twitter. *Washington Post* 29 June. https://www.washingtonpost.com/news/post-politics/wp/2017/06/29/trump-angrily-lashes-out-at-morning-joe-hosts-on-twitter/. Accessed: 20 February 2020.

LeFrançois B, Menzies R and Reaume G (eds) (2013) *Mad Matters: A Critical Reader in Canadian Mad Studies.* Toronto: Canadian Scholars' Press.

Martin J, Pescosolido B and Tuch S (2000) Of fear and loathing: The role of 'disturbing behavior', labels, and causal attributions in shaping public attitudes toward people with mental illness. *Journal of Health and Social Behavior* 41(2): 208–223.

Nussbaum M (2000) *Women and Human Development: The Capabilities Approach.* Cambridge: Cambridge University Press.

Obama B (2015) *President Obama's Statement on the Shooting in Oregon.* Washington, DC: President Barack Obama White House Archives 2 October. https://obamawhitehouse.archives.gov/blog/2015/10/01/watch-president-obamas-statement-shooting-oregon. Accessed: 20 February 2020.

Obama M (2018) *Becoming.* New York: Crown.

Oginski G (2014) New York medical malpractice - psychiatric injuries & emotional trauma: Are they good cases? [Lecture] Bridge-the-Gap: New York City Bar Association Lecture – New York Medical Malpractice Law for the Non-Medical Malpractice Attorney, Part 11. 4 January. https://www.youtube.com/watch?v=M4o2awgOFOM. Accessed: 20 February 2020.

Sanati A and Kyratsous M (2015) Epistemic injustice in delusions. *Journal of Evaluation in Clinical Practice* 21: 479–485.

Siddiqi N, Doran T, Prady S L and Taylor J (2017) Closing the mortality gap for severe mental illness: are we going in the right direction? *The British Journal of Psychiatry* 211: 1–2.

Stuart H (2006) Mental Illness and Employment Discrimination. *Current Opinion in Psychiatry* 19(5): 522–526.

The New York Times (2018) Is Mr. Trump nuts? *The New York Times.* 10 January. https://www.nytimes.com/2018/01/10/opinion/is-mr-trump-nuts.html. Accessed: 20 February 2020.

Trump D J (2019) *Remarks by President Trump on the Mass Shootings in Texas and Ohio*. Washington, DC: President Donald J Trump White House Briefings 5 August. https://www.whitehouse.gov/briefings-statements/remarks-president-trump-mass-shootings-texas-ohio/ Accessed: 20 February 2020.

Urman-Yotam M and Ostacher M (2014) Stimulants: amphetamine, cocaine, and synthetic cathinones. In M Caplan (ed) *Reference Module in Biomedical Research* (3d ed.). Amsterdam: Elsevier BV.

Walker E R, McGee R E and Druss B G (2015) Mortality in Mental Disorders and Global Disease Burden Implications: A Systematic Review and Meta-analysis. *JAMA Psychiatry* 72(4): 334–341.

Wallcraft J (2009) From activist to researcher and part-way back. In A Sweeney, P Beresford, A Faulkner, M Nettle, and D Rose (eds) *This is Survivor Research*. Ross-on-Wye: PCCS Books, 132–139.

PART 2

Situating Mad Studies

11

A GENEALOGY OF THE CONCEPT OF "MAD STUDIES"

Richard A. Ingram

On May 3, 2008, I gave a presentation at an academic conference at Syracuse University on what I termed an "in/discipline," Mad Studies (Ingram, 2008). Alongside me, Jijian Voronka presented on Britney Spears, a paper that was an example of doing Mad Studies. My presentation was mostly impromptu, in spite of the large amount of writing that I had done in the first four months of 2008 on Mad Studies.

In addition to launching the concept of Mad Studies at an academic conference, I shared ideas on the Mad Students Society listserv. My thinking was that Mad Studies was a concept that had emerged from Mad movement groups and communities, and it was important to ensure that Mad Studies was understood as an invitation and an opportunity shared as widely as possible.

In this chapter I want to trace the concept back to the first time it entered my consciousness in the academic year 2000–1, and to trace how my thoughts about the concept have evolved since 2008. I want to describe some of the events, collaborations, and groups that provided a context for the concept of Mad Studies to emerge in 2001, and to be launched in 2008.

Having completed my comprehensive examinations, I was working in 2000 on a chapter plan for my doctoral dissertation. In addition to this task, I had to declare the subject areas of my dissertation. During this period, I heard what Michel Foucault termed "the thought from outside" (1990). Indeed, it was at once a voice and a vision. What I heard, and what I foresaw, was that a day would come when Mad Studies was an important concept, and formed as a field of knowledge.

In 1997, Irit Shimrat's book, *Call Me Crazy: Stories from the Mad Movement*, had established the concept of a Mad movement. "Mad movement activists in this country," Shimrat writes, "have started self-help, political and creative groups that have made a real difference" (1997:152). When I read this book, I realized that I was far from alone in my intuition that psychiatrization as a process was doing me far more harm than good. Shimrat's inclusion of writings by many Mad activists demonstrated that there was a Mad movement across Canada. The book also showed the overlaps between LGBTQ+ movements and the Mad movement.

On the one hand, the concept of Mad Studies seemed like an obvious step from a knowledgeable Mad movement to a body of knowledge with its own name. On the other hand, it was not inevitable that a field of knowledge called Mad Studies would emerge. In a sense,

DOI: 10.4324/9780429465444-14

thinking the concept of Mad Studies involved losing touch with reality. It was not the only time I would have the experience of losing touch with reality in order to imagine Mad Studies.

In March 2001, a demonstration took place outside of the Vancouver Convention Centre, where the World Assembly for Mental Health was being held. It was at this demonstration that I first met leading activists including Irit Shimrat and David Oaks. It was also during this time that the World Network of Users and Survivors of Psychiatry held its first General Assembly, though this event was not one I attended in person.

In the wake of this momentous demonstration, a series of events called "Madness 101" were held at the Humanities Storefront, which was situated in Vancouver's downtown Eastside. Like other events at this location, Madness 101 was intended to bring educational opportunities to people for whom such opportunities were scarce. Madness 101 was an example of what I thought of as Mad Studies in a formal dimension. Meanwhile, a satirical online website, Mad Nation, was an example of Mad Studies in a more informal dimension.

By the time I was ready to defend my dissertation in April 2005, I felt that its subject matter fell under the heading of Mad Studies. However, I had not declared Mad Studies as one of my subject areas. The reason for this decision was that I had become interested in the principle of "copyleft," which is an invitational approach that opens up ideas for use by others. I was concerned that declaring my dissertation as belonging to the field of Mad Studies would make the term "Mad Studies," like the dissertation itself, copyright of the University of British Columbia.

In taking a copyleft approach, I was inspired by a collective with the name, Critical Theory Ensemble. Personally, I had been involved in a collective called ETC, or Ephemeral Theory Collective.[1] The four members of this collective had given papers at a conference at the State University of New York, Buffalo in the fall of 2001. Together we had read Gilles Deleuze and Felix Guattari's magnum opus, *A Thousand Plateaus* (1987). Writing and presenting as collectives de-emphasizes the role of the individual, highlighting how our ideas are developed through conversation.

In the spring of 2006, I was invited to be an organizer of Vancouver's Mad Pride events, which are coordinated by Gallery Gachet and take place each July. Being involved in Mad Pride gave me a better understanding of the Mad community in Vancouver. Meanwhile I was interviewed for a post in the School of Disability Studies at Ryerson University in Toronto. Although I was not offered the advertised position, I was offered a one-year position as a Senior Research Fellow for 2007, which I was pleased to accept.

Being located in Toronto enabled me to collaborate with Ephemeral Theory Collective member, James Overboe, on a series of workshops with the title, PsychoCrips. The concept of psychocrips was intended to draw attention to the commonalities between psychiatrized and disabled communities in the Toronto region; for example, by highlighting the disabling effects of psychiatric treatment and the traumatizing effects of medicalizing disability. In these workshops there was an emphasis on envisioning futures which was intended to balance research into eugenics, the bleakness of which often seems to suggest that disabled people have no future. These workshops covered a variety of issues, including intersections between dis/ability, race, and gender.

My position at Ryerson finished at the end of December 2007. In January 2008, I found myself with time to reflect upon the concept of "Mad Studies." One of the highlights of my year at Ryerson had been guest lecturing in David Reville's class, Mad People's History. I had known about Reville since reading Shimrat's *Call Me Crazy* (1997), to which he is a contributor. What I began to wonder was whether the kind of course that Reville had crafted in Disability Studies might be the basis for a new discipline of Mad Studies.

In my writings, my goal was to prepare material for the conference organized by Robert Menzies: Madness, Citizenship and Social Justice. I thought that the upcoming conference was a clear sign of a field of knowledge beginning to coalesce, and that this entity needed a name. To bestow a name, however, would have complicated effects that were worthy of careful consideration. To this end, I returned to Deleuze and Guattari's *A Thousand Plateaus* (1987) to think about the two sides of Mad Studies: Mad Studies as discipline, and Mad Studies as indiscipline.

The articulation of "Mad" to "Studies" produces a phrase that appears paradoxical. Is it even possible to establish a field of knowledge when the subject and object is Mad? There is, in short, something senseless about Mad Studies. This indiscipline is subversive in relation to existing disciplines, and therefore in relation to academia. In Deleuze and Guattari's terminology, this knowledge is rhizomatic and nomadic, as opposed to arboreal and settled (1987). To the extent that Mad Studies unfolds as sense, it becomes another discipline alongside existing disciplines. What I foresaw in 2008 was that Mad Studies would have sense and senselessness, and would therefore become an in/discipline.

In preparing for my presentation at Syracuse in May 2008, I drew on the study of linguistics that had formed part of my MA in Ideology and Discourse Analysis in the Department of Government at the University of Essex. As with Women's Studies, Disability Studies, and Deaf Studies, Mad Studies would act as a nodal point (Laclau and Mouffe, 1985); that is, as a point of condensation of meanings supplied to its position at the centre of a growing discourse. There would be two sides to Mad Studies. On the one side, it would bring together writings from the perspectives of Mad subjects; on the other side, it would enable Mad subjects to write about any topic in which madness was prominently mentioned, so as to deconstruct rationalist logics by showing the extent of their dependence on the signifiers "mad" and "madness."

As the date of my Syracuse presentation approached, my mind unravelled. By the day of the presentation, I was no longer able to coordinate my thoughts as intended. Instead, I took Antonin Artaud as an example of someone performing in spite of, or rather, inspired by, madness. I had to trust that a stream of consciousness presentation would produce a valuable talk. I began by reading out a brief manifesto:

We hold these truths to be self-evident…

We crazies can heal ourselves of the destructive side of madness. We need others to understand that we are the primary victims of this destructive side, while acknowledging that others are too often subjected to its effects.

We can heal ourselves when we have space and time to learn how to bring forth the creative side of madness. Individually and collectively, we are working to acquire the skills required to shift from destruction to creation. Yet under the current regime of state-run and for-profit management of madness, the conditions for acquiring these skills arise all too rarely.

We hope that societies will recover their lost wisdom by coming to recognize once again the tremendous potential that resides in our unorthodox imaginations. We remark that this potential is already recognized in a select few; among whom privileged individuals are often business leaders and entertainment stars. We long for the gap between the select few and the abandoned multitudes to be bridged.

We await the time when our epiphanies are no longer misrecognized as mania or psychosis; when our dry spells are no longer misrecognized as depression; when our frenetic energies are no longer misrecognized as ADHD or borderline personality disorder; and when our search for an inner place of refuge is no longer recognized as autism.

> A time will come when our "bodyminds" are no longer declared incompetent, and
> are no longer regarded as accidents waiting to happen. A time will come when we can
> laugh and cry, love and hide, freely, and without fear. A time will come when there
> will be no punishment for allowing your imagination to run wild.

As the presentation proceeded I decided to end by talking about Franz Fanon, champion of "The Wretched of the Earth" (1963). The result was an impassioned plea at the intersection of madness and anti-colonialism on the part of the emerging in/discipline of Mad Studies. It is my view that I needed to be at least in part "out of my mind" in order to call for an in/discipline that only came into existence through speculative articulation.

I want to emphasize, though, that Mad Studies did not begin only in an academic environment. During my visit to Toronto in the summer of 2006 I had attended a meeting of the group formed by Lucy Costa, the Mad Students Society. On the day I attended, the guest speaker was long-time local activist, Don Weitz. I introduced the term Mad Studies to the Mad Students Society listserv in the spring of 2008, showing how Mad Studies might be done by sharing ideas on which I was working for my presentation at Syracuse. Given that this listserv reached Mad activists in the community, this act of sharing ideas meant that Mad Studies was an invitation and an opportunity available not only to academics, but also to grassroots activists. It was my hope that Mad Studies as a in/discipline would also thrive beyond the bounds of academia.

In 2011, Margaret Price's book, *Mad at School*, was published. The title and content were, in my view, consistent with the concept of Mad Studies as in/discipline: *Mad at School* announced a new discipline, and proclaimed indiscipline as valid knowledge. At the time I was working at Simon Fraser University, thanks to a two-year Canadian Institutes of Health Research postdoctoral fellowship, for which Marina Morrow was the principal investigator. In the course of my research, I came across an article by Rebecca Birnbaum, the daughter of Morton Birnbaum, the doctor and lawyer who coined the term "sanism."

In May 2011 I presented the paper, "Sanism in Theory and Practice" at the 2nd Annual Critical Inquiries Workshop, which was organized by Marina Morrow's Centre for the Study of Gender, Social Inequities and Mental Health at Simon Fraser University. In this paper I showed that the concept of sanism emerged at the intersection of race, gender, and madness-as-disability. The concept of sanism has been further developed by lawyer and legal scholar, Michael Perlin, in *The Hidden Prejudice* (2000). Naming the ideology that is resistant to madness and Mad Studies is itself an important step forward. The speech act of giving a name to a phenomenon brings into being, as J.L. Austin posited, entities that did not exist previously as such.

Since July 2012, I have not been able to sustain regular employment due to fibromyalgia and chronic fatigue, as well as ongoing mind problems. In particular, pain has corroded my ability to think. I was invited to write the Introduction to the book, *Mad Matters: A Critical Reader in Canadian Mad Studies* (LeFrançois et al, 2013), which was not possible due to these health problems. It is this book that is commonly seen as putting Mad Studies on the map in the English-speaking world and beyond.

In 2015, I was invited to give a keynote presentation at the conference, Making Sense of Mad Studies at Durham University. As part of this presentation, I asked for a show of hands to indicate who supported and opposed Mad Studies becoming an academic discipline. The results were roughly even between those who preferred Mad Studies to remain outside academia and those who saw its future within academia. The other purpose of this poll was to decentre myself, so as once again to underscore that Mad Studies is an invitation and an opportunity for others.

During my stay in Durham, I was interviewed by Victoria McGowan for Mentally Sound Show 9. I mentioned that "not everyone […] is happy with Mad Studies in the way that it's taking shape. That's important, it's important to acknowledge the differences that exist, and to give room for dissent." Introducing a new concept is not only a reason for acknowledging a contribution, but is also a reason for assigning responsibility for shortcomings. There is plenty of scope, for example, for intersectional work to expand the diversity of Mad Studies.

In this overview of the genealogy of Mad Studies, I have sought to describe the context in which different ideas about the meaning of Mad Studies emerged. I am delighted that what began as a crazy idea in my head has become an idea that is inspiring an increasing number of people to contribute to Mad Studies as an in/discipline.

Note

1 Members of the ETC were: Joy James, Charles Barbour, James Overboe, and myself.

References

Deleuze, G. and Guattari, F. (1987) *A Thousand Plateaus: Capitalism and Schizophrenia.* Translated by Brian Massumi. Minneapolis: University of Minnesota.

Fanon, F. (1963) *The Wretched of the Earth.* Translated by Constance Farrington. New York: Grove Press.

Foucault, M. (1990) *Maurice Blanchot: The Thought from Outside.* Translated by Brian Massumi. New York: Zone Books.

Ingram, R. (2008) *Mapping 'Mad Studies': The Birth of an In/discipline.* First Regional Graduate/Undergraduate Disability Studies Symposium. Syracuse University.

Laclau, E. and Mouffe, C. (1985) *Hegemony and Socialist Strategy: Towards a Radical Democratic Politics.* London: Verso.

LeFrançois, B., Menzies, R. and Reaume, G. (2013) *Mad Matters: A Critical Reader in Canadian Mad Studies.* Toronto: Canadian Scholars.

Perlin, M. (2000) *The Hidden Prejudice: Mental Disability on Trial.* Washington DC: American Psychological Association.

Price, M. (2011) *Mad at School: Rhetorics of Mental Disability and Academic Life.* Ann Arbor: University of Michigan.

Shimrat, I. (1997) *Call Me Crazy: Stories from the Mad Movement.* Vancouver: Press Gang.

12

HOW IS MAD STUDIES DIFFERENT FROM ANTI-PSYCHIATRY AND CRITICAL PSYCHIATRY?

Geoffrey Reaume

What are the differences between anti-psychiatry, critical psychiatry and mad studies? This question matters because by describing the distinctions behind each of these approaches their underlying impetus reveals the extent to which mad people have reclaimed knowledge that was more often *about* rather than *by* us. When distinguishing between anti-psychiatry, critical psychiatry and mad studies, it is important to point out from the start that these areas are significantly diverse within their own schools of thought to the point of being difficult to pin down as having a specific set of overarching doctrines. Part of this is due to the diffuse nature of the writers and activists in this area and the absence of one central person as an ideological leader to follow as the ultimate source of original reference. In many ways this is a positive aspect of this field of criticism since it does not require that anyone must meet a particular ideological litmus test measured against one esteemed person's beliefs. There are, nevertheless, a set of beliefs that do underline what it means to identify as being in one, or more, of these critical camps. When discussing these developments, it helps to point out in regard to many of the references cited herein that this chapter is written from a Canadian perspective, while also taking account of views beyond this country. Keeping in mind the above point about the immense diversity of views within the topics to be discussed helps to provide some awareness of the plurality of views as to what each of these fields represent, beginning with the oldest of these three areas.

The term "anti-psychiatry", coined in 1967 by radical psychiatrist David Cooper, has been used to categorize hugely diverging critiques of institutional psychiatry's history and contemporary practices (Cooper, 1967). This has ranged from using this term to describe critics from within the mental health profession such as Thomas Szasz, Cooper and RD Laing as well as academic theorists such as sociologist Erving Goffman and philosopher Michel Foucault (Szasz, 1961; Cooper, 1967; Laing, 1960, 1961; Goffman, 1961; Foucault, 1965; Shorter, 1997). Anti-psychiatry has also been used to describe a writer critiquing aspects of her own personal experiences within the psychiatric system, such as Kate Millett (Millett, 1991; Murray, 2014). It has also been used to refer to well-known activists engaged in the mad and psychiatric survivor communities, such as Judi Chamberlin, and still other activists who commemorate the histories of asylum inmate labourers from the past (Chamberlin, 1978; Dain, 1994; Flis and Wright, 2011). It is worth noting that ascribing someone, or a group of people, as "anti-psychiatry"

DOI: 10.4324/9780429465444-15

does not mean those so described agree with this identification. Szasz, for instance, being one of the most well-known figures in this category and who was also a psychiatrist, repeatedly rejected the use of this externally imposed descriptor for most of the last fifty years of his life, instead referring to himself as "anti-coercion, not anti-psychiatry" (Szasz, 2010: 230).

Given the vast differences in outlook and motivations behind what is a diffuse group of people described as anti-psychiatry, it should be no surprise that this term ends up in many cases to be confusing at best or meaningless at worst. It has been used as an easy way of slapping a convenient, intellectually inconsistent, and even unexplained label on critics of psychiatry in a way that is intended to diminish the seriousness of such criticisms (Dain, 1994, Shorter, 1997; Flis and Wright, 2011). Perhaps the most egregious example of this is when critics of those who have been described as anti-psychiatry, are equated as being in league with members of the Church of Scientology, a sort of 'reds under the bed' form of medical McCarthyism (Brean, 2010). Szasz did at one point in his career support Scientology in its efforts to attack psychiatry, though he was never a member of the organization itself; nevertheless this association with a cult-like group cost him significant credibility (Carey, 2012). It is worth observing that individuals in the mad movement whom this writer has met who have described themselves as being anti-psychiatry have mentioned at different times that they are not and have no interest in being Scientologists. If we put aside the misinformation about, and distancing from, this imposed descriptor by some of the supposed initiators of anti-psychiatry, as well as their significant overall ideological differences – Szasz being a libertarian free marketeer, Cooper being a Marxist revolutionary, for example – there remains the point of needing to figure out just what is meant by the term "anti-psychiatry".

At its most basic, anti-psychiatry in its most radical form advocates for the abolition of psychiatry (Burstow, 2005, 2015a). In this sense, it is distinct from mad studies which has no such unequivocal agenda, though there are similarities in regard to both camp's opposition to the medical model of mental illness and abolishing forced treatment, though even here there is room for differences. One of the basic critiques of the diverse group of people defined as anti-psychiatry is that psychiatric treatment should not be forced, though some, such as Laing would argue for exceptions to this argument (Double, 2006). Laing argued that madness was not biologically based but should be humanely treated and, like Szasz, rejected the notion of there being such a thing as mental illness as pathology. Szasz, however, differs from anti-psychiatrists like Cooper in that he regards madness as being due to problems in daily living on an individual basis, not a social level, a significant point of departure from critics who took a broader societal view of causation linking madness, poverty and marginalization (Laing, 1960; Szasz, 1961; Cooper, 1967; Double, 2006). Others who identify as being anti-psychiatry, such as Bonnie Burstow, clearly argue for the abolition of psychiatry and the creation of community supports run by mad people and allies who reject coercion in working with people in psychic crisis (Burstow, 2015b). An overarching critique by all of the above is in regard to the connection between legal systems, medicine, coercion and the impact of the pharmaceutical industry on contemporary treatments of people in psychiatric facilities or under psychiatric jurisdiction in the community. This is a common position of those who are identified as being anti-psychiatry regardless of whether or not this term is accepted by those so regarded (Szasz, [1965] 1988; Double, 2006).

More recently the development of critical psychiatry since the 1980s has sought to distance itself from the either/or debate about whether one is pro-psychiatry or anti-psychiatry (Ingleby, 1980). Instead, critical psychiatry attempts to remain respectable within the mental health profession, in a way that anti-psychiatry has never sought from mainstream psychiatrists. Critical psychiatry argues for a place within a hospital setting, while critiquing aspects of the mental health system, ranging from opposition to forced treatment, excessive use of medications particularly in regard to children, and systematically challenging the western orientation and racism in the mental health profession. This latter focus in particular reflects the influence of psychiatrist Suman Fernando whose anti-racist and ethno-psychiatric work has been of major importance in the field (Fernando, 1991, 2003, 2017; Moodley and Ocampo, 2014). Unlike some of the more radical activists who identify as anti-psychiatry, there are no advocates for the abolition of psychiatry among proponents of critical psychiatry; they are reformists from within the system. Like the group of people identified as anti-psychiatry, however, both groups started among academicians and mental health professionals and only later sought out mad people as direct participants in their line of inquiry. This in turn leads to the most significant distinction between anti-psychiatry, critical psychiatry and mad studies – the initiators and sustaining momentum behind the existence of each field.

In the first two fields discussed thus far, it is clear that while some activists who identify as psychiatric survivors have had engagement with anti-psychiatry, the main impetus for anti-psychiatry and critical psychiatry have been people who have not themselves been psychiatric patients, survivors, users or mad people. Mad studies does not claim to originate "solely" amongst mad people, particularly given the ongoing contributions from people who have never identified as mad (Menzies et al, 2013: 2). It is essential to point out, however, that the main premise of mad studies *from the start* has been and remains the centrality of empowering and engaging individuals who have had direct experience of the psychiatric system in the development of this area of study and fostering its practical application beyond the academy. It is this distinguishing feature at the source of mad studies that sets the field apart from what were professionally initiated concepts based within the mental health profession. Anti-psychiatry and critical psychiatry are initiatives that were originally externally developed concepts by people who later saw themselves as allies of mad people who critiqued the psychiatric system. This is unlike mad studies which has evolved from the activist histories and thinking of mad people ourselves in conjunction with allies. In other words, anti-psychiatry and critical psychiatry equals professionals first as central facilitators; mad studies equals mad people first as central facilitators in harmony with allies. As will become evident, this is not the only distinction but it is one of the most significant distinctions since all that follows is influenced by this difference in which an identifiable group has been central to developing and inspiring the field.

There are, of course, allies who have worked in mad studies to advance the field who do not themselves identify as mad – Robert Menzies, who was the primary initiator of the co-edited 2013 book, *Mad Matters*, is one example (LeFrançois et al, 2013). Mad studies, however, from its pre-history in the late twentieth century to its conscious inception in the early 2000s has always been based on the thoughts, theories and activism of mad people first. As such, the focus, while drawing intellectual support from aspects of anti-psychiatry in particular, is nevertheless distinct from it and critical psychiatry by placing mad people's interpretations at the centre of inquiry. It is therefore necessary to briefly note how these distinctions have evolved.

When considering how these critiques of psychiatry first self-consciously developed in each of their specific historical contexts – anti-psychiatry during the 1960s, critical psychiatry during the late 20th century and mad studies in the early 21st century – it is essential to point out that all of them were preceded by a long history of mad people expressing public critiques about their contemporary treatment dating at least to the 18th century. This is particularly evident as first, mad houses, and then, during the 19th century, the establishment of public insane asylums, raised concerns about the nature of madness, who decides, and how people so defined were treated by the developing profession of psychiatry, the state and legal systems which became intertwined in establishing this apparatus (Peterson, 1982; Porter, 2002; Reaume, 2017). By the second half of the twentieth century, then, public criticisms by ex-inmates, by some family members, and by some civil libertarians about the mistreatment and abuse of mad people, had a long history well before the existence of anti-psychiatry, critical psychiatry or mad studies. The radicals of the 1960s counter-cultural movement were not the first to attack institutional psychiatry by any means. They were, however, caught up in a political environment that was particularly advantageous to the wider reception and spread of the ideas they propagated. The social milieu in which these ideas evolved is important to underline. Anti-psychiatry caught on during the 1960s wider spirit of anti-establishment rebellion and civil rights protest, even though writers like Goffman, Laing, Foucault and Szasz had all been writing before the decade of the 1960s came to be a romanticized symbol for radical revolt against the existing order. Their initial publications by the early 1960s were not written at a time when the term "the sixties" had the rebellious connotations it did by the end of that decade and thereafter. It was only later on, as the tumultuous decade unfolded for all to reflect upon that their ideas came to be seen as reflecting the spirit of this period (Dain, 1994; Jones, 1998).

Yet, for all of their radicalism, this professional-led revolt against psychiatry had a degree of elitism. People in positions of power who did not experience madness themselves were telling the mad masses what was, or was not, good for them. Is this any different from mad studies? Time will tell, and those who will do the telling should be mad people outside of the academy rather than those of us inside for it to have any meaning beyond self-justification. In one most important comparative respect, mad studies has been advocated by academics and activists, some of whom are also "inside" the mad community and who have experiences of madness ourselves. Thus the connection between our subject of research and our own experience is not as distant as it was among the early anti-psychiatry theorists. This factor has the potential to lessen top-down preaching. Yet, as plenty of experienced activists can relate, elitism can take place within communities when individuals achieve higher socio-economic status than their peers with whom they have worked. It is this mad community activist history, in its more recent incarnation from the 1970s especially, that bears the most importance in possibly checking elitism when considering how this past continues to transform and challenge our work today.

Mad studies grew out of a later 20th century and early 21st century evolution of decades-long activism among mad people whose self-identity as mad sought to reclaim knowledge from professional outsiders of all persuasions (Menzies et al, 2013; LeFrançois et al, 2016). This was even though some mad studies activists/writers became, or were already, insiders within the academy and other places of power and privilege. On the other hand, the power and privilege which anti-psychiatry proponents enjoyed from the outset of their rebellion was related to their largely being a collection of white, European and North American males. Anti-psychiatry was very much "a guy thing" as far as who made the most publicized pronouncements which came to define the field in its heyday of the 1960s and early 1970s (Jones, 1998: 290). This makes it distinct from critical psychiatry and mad studies in which addressing race and gender have been at the forefront of analysis from the beginning of the development of these fields, undoubtedly because both of these fields' originators were not comprised solely of white males. Sexual orientation has also been a major part of the analytic approach of mad studies from its earliest inception, something which only later came to be the case for anti-psychiatry due to the activism of people in the lesbian, gay, bisexual, transgender and queer (LGBTQ) communities whose history of pathologization is as old as psychiatry (Burstow, 1990). Mad studies is particularly distinct in this regard since women, members of the LGBTQ community and racialized people who experience madness have been part of the foundational process in a way that eschews the domination of one privileged group from determining the field's ideas, as happened with anti-psychiatry. Yet, mad studies, like disability studies, continues to be predominantly white and focused on northern theories and concerns, though this too is changing from within (Lee, 2013; Gorman, 2013; Tam, 2013; Mills, 2014; Joseph, 2015; King, 2016; Stefan, 2018).

Given the prominent role of women in defining mad studies from the beginning, something which took longer among anti-psychiatry proponents, there has been a far greater focus from the outset on gendered and racial issues at the core of the field's critique than originally existed within anti-psychiatry. This later changed with contributions by Phyllis Chesler, along with other feminist critics of psychiatry (Chesler, 1972). Anti-psychiatry, critical psychiatry and mad studies have all had a significant analysis of class issues, particularly with writers like Cooper (anti-psychiatry) and Menzies (mad studies), reflecting Marxist influences in aspects of each field (Cooper, 1967; Menzies et al, 2013). While criticisms of the western medical model-oriented psychiatric system are a primary feature of mad studies there is no overarching call to abolish the entire psychiatric system as there has been among some anti-psychiatry activists. The most important distinguishing difference between anti-psychiatry and critical psychiatry, on the one hand, and mad studies, on the other hand, is the essential importance of prioritizing from the start of this field of inquiry, the first person critical analysis of mad people in all aspects of understanding our past and present contexts. This includes both individual and collective critiques. (e.g., Chamberlin, 1978; Farber, 1993; LeFrançois et al, 2013; Psychiatric Disabilities Anti-violence Coalition, 2015). In both anti-psychiatry and critical psychiatry, the focus is on a professionally based critique of the mental health system in its medical model orientation. Mad studies, by contrast, focuses on the experiences of mad people both as interpreters of our past and present and as active agents in bringing about change. There has been an effort in mad studies to open the doors to as wide a constituency of critics of psychiatry as possible, so long as the experiences and perspectives of mad people are at the centre of critiques. Burstow's description is appropriate to compare in this regard: "…what distinguishes antipsychiatry from other critical positions is the conviction that critiques of psychiatry are sufficiently conclusive, compelling, foundational, and damning to render psychiatry as an institution inherently undesirable and irredeemable" (Burstow, 2015a: 36). Thus, psychiatry cannot be reformed. Burstow also notes that, as a movement, anti-psychiatry is "floundering" in part due to past lack of respectful engagement with other members of the community, which, she argues, has changed, along with the entrenched power of psychiatry and the absence of an anti-psychiatry model to "guide its action" (Burstow, 2015a: 35). At the same time, it would be inaccurate to portray anti-psychiatry as a perpetually ineffective, marginalized influence wherever its proponents are engaged.

Given that mad studies is "steadfastly arrayed against biomedical psychiatry" its close connection in this respect to anti-psychiatry is evident (Menzies et al, 2013: 13). Critical psychiatry, on the other hand, while strongly critical of the predominance of the western medical model, continues to remain a willing part of the mental health system, seeking to change from within (Ingleby, 1980; Double, 2006; Moodley and Ocampo, 2014). At the same time, anti-psychiatry, as described above, provides a more definitive determination about what to do with psychiatry – get rid of it – than does mad studies, at least so far. Mad studies, amidst denouncing the power of psychiatry to medicate, control and confine people, calls for the

> radical restructuring of the 'mental health' industry […] [and thus] continues to be very much a project of abolition and transformation.
>
> *(Menzies et al, 2013: 17)*

At the same time, mad studies provides no single answer about what to do about psychiatry. Instead, it subsumes a loose assemblage of perspectives that resist compression into an irreducible dogma or singular approach to theory or practice.

(Menzies et al, 2013: 13)

Thus, while inclusive of anti-psychiatry theories, mad studies resists focusing solely on tearing down the mental health system as the principal aim of the movement, an objective that has come to characterize the most well-known feature of anti-psychiatry. Though mad studies as a field is relatively new, its close inter-disciplinary relation with other critically oriented fields in the humanities and social sciences from which it springs has been central to its development within the academy and beyond (Menzies et al, 2013; LeFrançois et al, 2016). It is this "beyond" that is particularly important to mad studies that sets it apart from the other two fields discussed here. Anti-psychiatry, particularly as practiced by RD Laing at Kingsley Hall, London, England, from 1965–70 did make a concerted effort to have theory match practice, and thus be a part of the local community (Miller, 2004; O'Hagan, 2012). There were also grassroots activist groups which identified as anti-psychiatry which also sought to organize amongst mad people (Shimrat, 1997; Dunst, 2016). Overall, however, anti-psychiatry was an academic pursuit without extensive, sustained involvement in the community of mad people, perhaps reflecting its origins from within the "psy" professions in the academy by academicians who did not themselves identify as mad. By contrast, mad studies from its earliest days began as an outgrowth of the broader mix of ex-patient activism within the psychiatric survivor community during the late 20th century, many of whom did not categorically subscribe to the call for the abolition of the psychiatric system, partly due to avoiding a stance that sounded all-encompassing and authoritarian (Campbell, 2011).

Related to this, the development of mad studies in the early 21st century coincided with the rise of mad pride, which originated as psychiatric survivor pride day in 1993 and had, by the early 2000s, spread to different places as mad pride. While mad pride as an organized movement may have had its day at the time of this writing, it nevertheless was an important catalyst within the wider mad community in several large cities in Canada, the United States, United Kingdom, Brazil, New Zealand, and elsewhere, for providing mad people, or users of psychiatry, with an idea of the potential for celebrating the abilities of mad people in ways that other movements up to then had not done (Finkler, 1997; Dellar et al, 2001; Abraham, 2016). It was not just about being "anti" but also "for" – an essential point in regard to mad people's inclusion and recognition in wider society. Depending on the locale, mad pride was, for over twenty years, a regular feature of efforts to fight discrimination in local communities, like Toronto, while also celebrating the place of mad people wherever we live. Mad pride's influence and legacy in mad studies is reflected in regard to efforts to ensure that mad people's perspectives, histories and critiques become part of the wider discussion around mental health and madness in the academy and beyond. This also happened at a time when alternatives to psychiatry were being promoted among psychiatric survivors and users (Farber, 1993; Stastny and Lehmann, 2007). Where anti-psychiatry places an overriding emphasis on critiquing the power of psychiatry and how it needs to be dismantled, mad studies, while also contributing to these ideas, goes further by having as pride of place, as it were, the experiences and perspectives of self-identified mad people. It is this "pride" in ensuring that mad perspectives are the primary inspiration for this field of studies that links mad pride with mad studies in a way that was not engaged by either anti-psychiatry nor critical psychiatry. This has ensured from the outset that the wider community of mad people are part of this endeavour.

Yet no matter how much the wider mad community is invoked, it is obvious that, so far, the main forum for published debate is where most of the money is for this purpose: the academy. Here, mad studies has become broadly based in a relatively short period of time. While anti-psychiatry and critical psychiatry have both been interdisciplinary, including academics from a range of fields, it is apparent how the foundational ideas emanating from both critiques have been initiated and largely sustained by mental health professionals. This is unlike in mad studies where mental health professionals, while welcome to contribute are not in leading positions as activists and writers in the field. Of course, mental health professionals can identify as mad people too, and indeed the increasing number of peer support workers underlines a further topic of analysis in regard to how mad people work within the psychiatric system as employees (Voronka, 2019). Generally speaking, however, when referring to mental health professionals, this usually identifies the person as a psychiatrist, psychologist or nurse who works within the system, a few of whom have contributed to mad studies already (Warme, 2013; Adam, 2015). Unlike the leading figures identified with anti-psychiatry during its earliest phases, no psychiatrist or psychologist has anywhere near the prominence or domination of Szasz or Laing, for example. Instead, the field includes people ranging from mad students and people who work in areas as varied as social work, sociology, law, the performing and visual arts, political science, literary studies, health policy analysts, cultural studies, women and gender studies, queer studies, disability studies, nursing and history. Thus it is a broad tent, intentionally so. These broad perspectives are also a sign that the reach of mad studies is intended to move far beyond the western academic tradition in a way that anti-psychiatry has not done.

This leads to another important point of distinction which is that anti-psychiatry in theory and practice has historically been focused on mental health diagnoses in a western context in the northern industrialized world. In contrast, mad studies, like disability studies more recently, seeks to incorporate a global approach, with a critical analyses of how madness is experienced and interpreted outside of a western oriented medical model approach in both the north and south (Nabbali, 2013; Mills, 2014). This leads to asking: Will mad studies appeal to more people than has anti-psychiatry in both the north and the south who have experienced and live with madness? Of course, this is impossible to answer without a much longer duration of time to reflect upon mad studies which, in name at least, is barely a decade old (Ingram, 2008). Given the wider demographic and geographic base of people who are participating in debates around what is now called mad studies, there is a potential for much broader interest in different parts of the world by a more diverse representation of mad people than have been attracted to anti-psychiatry, based as it is in the industrialized north. Mad studies, at present, may also be seen to be more current than anti-psychiatry with its reputation based on 1960s counter-culture, a context which, while of much historical interest, will be less and less relevant to the daily lives of more and more mad people as time goes on.

There needs to be some caution with this last point, however, and some humbleness. History has much to teach us about the need to be humble when thinking about our current place in the world in comparison to those who have gone before. It is worth observing that mad studies is more current with contemporary issues across the field – gender, race, sexual orientation, trans-national and global south approaches, for example, in large part because more recent activists and writers can reflect on what and who was left out of major consideration from earlier activist and theoretical efforts. Those of us involved in mad studies therefore should avoid a morally superior attitude towards anti-psychiatry or other critiques of institutional psychiatry. We have benefited from earlier generations' criticisms of psychiatry, while also seeking to correct and improve upon earlier omissions so that the field is more broadly relevant than before. Activists in decades to come may very well take a new critical approach by improving upon what mad studies proponents are doing now during a future we can only vaguely imagine. This is another reason for humbleness when reflecting upon our collective efforts to improve our world for ourselves and future generations of mad people when we distinguish mad studies from antipsychiatry and critical psychiatry – none of us can predict whether or not mad studies will appeal to mad people in future decades. We cannot even predict if mad studies will appeal to many mad people today beyond its current advocates. By distinguishing between these three fields, however, we can see from the past how we have arrived at this present juncture in the hope that mad studies will become relevant for mad people in a practical way that goes far beyond what it is at the beginning of the 2020s.

References

Abraham A (2016) Remembering Mad Pride, The Movement that Celebrated Mental Illness. *Vice.* https://www.vice.com/en_uk/article/7bxqxa/mad-pride-remembering-the-uks-mental-health-pride-movement. Accessed: 22 February 2019.

Adam S (2015) From subservience to resistance: Nursing versus psychiatry. In B Burstow, B LeFrançois and S Diamond (eds) *Psychiatry Disrupted: Theorizing Resistance and Crafting the (R)evolution*. Montreal & Kingston: McGill-Queen's University Press, 65–76.

Brean J (2010) Delusional: Movement to depose psychiatry emerges from the shadows. *National Post* 8 May.

Burstow B (1990) A history of psychiatric homophobia. *Phoenix Rising: The Voice of the Psychiatrized* 8(3&4): 38–39.

Burstow B (2005) Feminist antipsychiatry praxis: Women and the movement(s). In W Chan, D Chun and R Menzies (eds) *Women, Madness, and the Law: A Feminist Reader*. London: Glasshouse, 245–258.

Burstow B (2015a) The withering away of psychiatry: An attritional model for antipsychiatry. In B Burstow, B LeFrançois and S Diamond (eds) *Psychiatry Disrupted: Theorizing Resistance and Crafting the (R)evolution*. Montreal & Kingston: McGill-Queen's University Press, 34–51.

Burstow B (2015b) *Psychiatry and the Business of Madness: An Ethical and Epistemological Accounting*. New York: Palgrave Macmillan.

Campbell D (2011) *Unsettled: Discourse, Practice, Context and Collective Identity Among Mad People in the United States, 1970–1999*.Unpublished PhD thesis. Faculty of Environmental Studies, York University.

Carey B (2012) Dr Thomas Szasz, Psychiatrist who led movement against his field, dies at 92. *New York Times*. https://www.nytimes.com/2012/09/12/health/dr-thomas-szasz-psychiatrist-who-led-movement-against-his-field-dies-at-92.html. Accessed: 22 February 2019.

Chamberlin J (1978) *On Our Own: Patient Controlled Alternatives to the Mental Health System*. New York: Hawthorn.

Chesler P (1972) *Women and Madness*. Garden City, New York: Doubleday.

Cooper D (1967) *Psychiatry and Anti-psychiatry*. London: Tavistock.

Dain N (1994) Psychiatry and anti-psychiatry in the United States. In M Micale and R Porter (eds) *Discovering the History of Psychiatry*. Oxford: Oxford University Press, 415–444.

Dellar R, Leslie E and Watson B (eds) (2001) *Mad Pride: A Celebration of Mad Culture*. London: Spare Change Books.

Double D (2006) Historical perspectives on anti-psychiatry. In D Double (ed) *Critical Psychiatry: The Limits of Madness*. New York: Palgrave Macmillan, 19–39.

Dunst A (2016) 'All the fits that's news to print': Deinstitutionalisation and anti-psychiatric movement magazines in the United States, 1970–1986. In D Kritsotaki, V Long and M Smith (eds) *Deinstitutionalisation and After: Post-War Psychiatry in the Western World*. Cham, Switzerland: Palgrave Macmillan, 57–74.

Farber S (1993) *Madness, Heresy, and the Rumor of Angels: The Revolt Against the Mental Health System*. Chicago: Open Court.

Fernando S (1991) *Mental Health, Race and Culture*. Houndmills, UK: Macmillan.

Fernando S (2003) *Cultural Diversity, Mental Health and Psychiatry: The Struggle Against Racism*. New York: Brunner-Routledge.

Fernando S (2017) *Institutional Racism in Psychiatry and Clinical Psychology: Race Matters in Mental Health*. Cham, Switzerland: Springer.

Finkler L (1997) Psychiatric survivor pride day: Community organizing with psychiatric survivors. *Osgoode Hall Law Journal* 35(3/4 Fall/Winter): 763–772.

Flis N and Wright D (2011) 'A grave injustice': The mental hospital and shifting sites of memory. In C Coleborne and D MacKinnon (eds) *Exhibiting Madness in Museums: Remembering Psychiatry through Collections and Display*. London: Routledge, 101–115.

Foucault M (1965) *Madness and Civilization: A History of Insanity in the Age of Reason*. New York: Pantheon.

Goffman E (1961) *Asylums: Essays on the Social Situation of Mental Patients and Other Inmates*. Garden City, New York: Doubleday.

Gorman R (2013) Mad nation? Thinking through race, class and identity politics. In B François, R Menzies and G Reaume (eds) *Mad Matters: A Critical Reader in Canadian Mad Studies*. Toronto: Canadian Scholars' Press, 269–280.

Ingleby D (ed) (1980) *Critical Psychiatry: The Politics of Mental Health*. New York: Pantheon.

Ingram R (2008) Mapping 'Mad Studies': The birth of an in/discipline. Paper presented at Disability Studies Student conference, Syracuse University.

Jones C (1998) Raising the anti: Jan Foudraine, Ronald Laing and anti-psychiatry. In M Gijswijt-Hofstra and R Porter (eds) *Cultures of Psychiatry and Mental Health Care in Postwar Britain and the Netherlands*. Amsterdam & Atlanta: Rodopi, 283–294.

Joseph A (2015) *Deportation and the Confluence of Violence Within Forensic Mental Health and Immigration Systems*. New York: Palgrave Macmillan.

King C (2016) Whiteness in psychiatry: The madness of European misdiagnoses. In J Russo and A Sweeney (eds) *Searching for a Rose Garden: Challenging Psychiatry, Fostering Mad Studies*. Monmouth, UK: PCCS Books, 69–76.

Laing R (1960) *The Divided Self*. London: Tavistock.

Laing R (1961) *The Self and Others*. London: Tavistock.

Lee J (2013) Mad as hell: The objectifying experience of symbolic violence. In B LeFrançois, R Menzies and G Reaume (eds) *Mad Matters: A Critical Reader in Canadian Mad Studies*. Toronto: Canadian Scholars' Press, 105–121.

LeFrançois B, Menzies R and Reaume G (eds) (2013) *Mad Matters: A Critical Reader in Canadian Mad Studies*. Toronto: Canadian Scholars' Press.

LeFrançois B, Beresford P and Russo J (2016) Editorial: Destination mad studies. *Intersectionalities* 5 (3): 1–10.

Menzies R, LeFrançois B and Reaume G (2013) Introducing mad studies. In B LeFrançois, R Menzies and G Reaume (eds) *Mad Matters: A Critical Reader in Canadian Mad Studies*. Toronto: Canadian Scholars' Press, 1–22.

Miller G (2004) *R.D. Laing*. Edinburgh: Edinburgh University Press.

Millett K (1991) *The Loony-Bin Trip*. New York: Touchstone.

Mills C (2014) *Decolonizing Global Mental Health: The Psychiatrization of the Majority World*. London: Routledge.

Moodley R and Ocampo M (eds) (2014) *Critical Psychiatry and Mental Health: Exploring the Work of Suman Fernando in Clinical Practice*. London: Routledge.

Murray H (2014) 'My place was set at the terrible feast': The meanings of the 'anti-psychiatry' movement and responses in the United States, 1970s–1990s. *Journal of American Culture* 37(1): 37–51.

Naballi E (2013) 'Mad' activism and its (Ghanaian?) future: A prolegomena to debate. *Trans-Scripts* 3: 178–201.

O'Hagan S (2012) Kingsley Hall: RD Laing's Experiment in Anti-Psychiatry. *The Guardian*. https://www.theguardian.com/books/2012/sep/02/rd-laing-mental-health-sanity. Accessed 25 February 2019.

Peterson D (ed) (1982) *A Mad People's History of Madness*. Pittsburgh: University of Pittsburgh Press.

Porter R (2002) *Madness: A Brief History*. Oxford: Oxford University Press.

Psychiatric Disabilities Anti-violence Coalition (2015) Clearing a path: A psychiatric survivor anti-violence framework. https://torontoantiviolencecoalition.files.wordpress.com/2016/02/clearing-a-path-dec-2015.pdf. Accessed: 7 May 2019.

Reaume G (2017) From the perspectives of mad people. In G Eghigian (ed) *The Routledge History of Madness and Mental Health*. London: Routledge, 277–296.

Shimrat I (1997) *Call Me Crazy: Stories from the Mad Movement*. Vancouver: Press Gang Publishers.

Shorter E (1997) *A History of Psychiatry: From the Era of the Asylum to the Age of Prozac*. New York: John Wiley & Sons.

Stastny P and Lehmann P (eds) (2007) *Alternatives Beyond Psychiatry*. Berlin: Peter Lehmann Books.

Stefan H (2018) A (Head) Case for Mad Humanities: *Sula*'s Shadrack and Black Madness. *Disability Studies Quarterly* 38(4): 1. http://dsq-sds.org/article/view/6378/5123. Accessed 25 February 2019.

Szasz T (1961) *The Myth of Mental Illness: Foundations of a Theory of Mental Illness*. New York: Hoeber Harper.

Szasz T ([1965] 1988). *Psychiatric Justice*. Syracuse: Syracuse University Press.

Szasz T (2010) Psychiatry, anti-psychiatry, critical psychiatry: What do these terms mean? *Philosophy, Psychiatry, & Psychology* 17(3): 229–232.

Tam L (2013) Whither indigenizing the mad movement? Theorizing the social relations of race and madness through conviviality. In B LeFrançois, R Menzies and G Reaume (eds) *Mad Matters: A Critical Reader in Canadian Mad Studies*. Toronto: Canadian Scholars' Press, 281–297.

Voronka J (2019) The mental health peer worker as informant: Performing authenticity and the paradoxes of passing. *Disability & Society* 34(4): 564–582.

Warme G (2013) Removing Civil Rights: How Dare We? In B LeFrançois, R Menzies and G Reaume (eds) *Mad Matters: A Critical Reader in Canadian Mad Studies*. Toronto: Canadian Scholars' Press, 210–220.

13

MAD STUDIES AND DISABILITY STUDIES

Hannah Morgan

Introduction

Mad Studies has developed from within, alongside and, at times, in dispute with Disability Studies. Disability Studies, although still relatively new as an academic discipline, is older and more developed in terms of scope, size and global reach. As such, it has accrued some of the benefits of a more established position in the academy and in policy and practice arenas, while Mad Studies is at a much more formative and potentially precarious stage in its evolution, albeit with deep roots in critical approaches to mental distress. Both fields are part of wider political projects, grounded in the communities from which they emerged, that seek to resist oppressive forms of knowledge and practice through the creation of new forms of knowledge embedded in lived experience and committed to creating and promoting inclusive and enabling practices.

People who experience mental distress and their perspectives have been present within Disability Studies and the disabled people's movement since their formation, although they have often been overlooked or silent (Plumb, 1994). There have been deliberate attempts to broaden the focus of Disability Studies from its initial concern with the experiences of those with physical impairments and 'public' and environmental barriers, to better include all disabled people and their experiences. Survivors and their allies have made significant contributions to the field, helping to expand the focus of the social model of disability to better incorporate their perspectives, especially in relation to psycho-emotional disablism (Reeve, 2015), participatory and inclusive research (Beresford and Wallcraft, 1997; Beresford and Carr, 2018) and practices of dissent (Plumb, 1994) and resistance (Hunt, 2019).

Peter Beresford (2000; 2004; 2012) has made a particular contribution to promoting a positive, respectful and purposeful dialogue about the relationship between Disability Studies and psychiatric system survivors and madness which pre-dates the emergence of Mad Studies as a distinct project 'devoted to the critique and transcendence of psy-centred ways of thinking, behaving, relating and being' (LeFrancois et al, 2013:13). Thus, Mad Studies is both a continuation and a fresh intervention in the tradition of critical approaches to mental health. It maintains a sharp focus on experiential knowledge and brings to the fore a reconceptualization of mental distress as 'madness' as 'a reference to political categories of critique and exclusion' (Spandler and Poursanidou, 2019:1).

DOI: 10.4324/9780429465444-16

Perhaps most importantly for Disability Studies the project of forming the field of Mad Studies as an in/discipline (Ingram, 2016) provides an opportunity revisit its core operating tenets. Ingram's starting point in crafting Mad Studies (which he distinguishes from earlier work he describes as *mad studies*) was to consider the limitations of Disability Studies 'as a space within which to do research focusing on madness and Mad people' (2016:11). For him, thinking about madness was constrained by the 'overarching, or governing, concept of "disability"' which raises questions for Disability Studies itself that I will return to. The *in*discipline of Mad Studies, echoes discussions from the formative days of Disability Studies, by raising questions about whether it is a 'positive development if Mad Studies were to become an established academic discipline in universities' as well as outside the academy (Ingram, 2016:13). These are debates that have remained live and at times fractious within Disability Studies when considering the place and role of non-disabled people, the in/formal relationship between Disability Studies and the disabled people's movement and the extent to which Disability Studies realises its promise to effect transformation in understandings of disability and in naming and eradicating disablism.

Disability Studies

Disability Studies emerged in the 1980s in response to, and in dialogue with, the development of the disabled people's movement in Northern Europe and America. This relationship with the disabled people's movement is a defining characteristic of Disability Studies. It signifies a distinction between academic practices that start from the experiences of disabled people, seeing them as creators (and contesters) of knowledge than where they are the passive subjects of professional concern. Initially located in sociology, social policy and education, it has permeated the social sciences, humanities, health and professional education as well as other fields like design and engineering and become a global field of academic inquiry (Watson et al, 2012). While Disability Studies remains a broad church, inclusive of a wide range of disciplinary perspectives and areas of concern, what distinguishes Disability Studies from research and other scholarship 'on' disability is its foundation in the transformational work of the Union of the Physically Impaired Against Segregation (UPIAS). In their groundbreaking *Fundamental Principles of Disability* (1976) UPIAS rejected traditional notions that the disadvantage experienced by disabled people was the natural and inevitable result of their impairments arguing instead that it is society that disables physically impaired people. Disability is something imposed on top of our impairments, by the way we are unnecessarily isolated and excluded from full participation in society. Disabled people are therefore an oppressed group in society.

Thus, disablement is the outcome of a range of structural, social, cultural and political forces which are disabling, rather than the inevitable consequence of individual impairment. Sociologist Michael Oliver built on this analysis to articulate a *social model of disability* as a practical tool to help the social work students he was teaching understand the role of disablist economic, environmental and attitudinal barriers experienced by people with impairments (Oliver 1996). For Oliver (2004), the model was to be a 'hammer' to challenge the dominance of individual model understandings of disability (which views disability as a personal tragedy caused by impairment) and to identify and break down the barriers experienced by disabled people. As such, it has been extremely effectively wielded by the disabled people's movement, as the basis for a collective political identity and to effect legal, policy and societal change.

As the disabled people's movement and Disability Studies have grown in size and scope, so too has the social model and linked theoretical work evolved and expanded in response to a range of developments and concerns. A number of these have particular relevance and implications for the place of mental distress and psychiatric system survivors in Disability Studies. An underpinning question or consideration is whether Disability Studies should seek to be more inclusive of the experiences and perspectives of survivors, and at the same time, what should perhaps remain outside of the scope (although certainly not of the interest) of Disability Studies and be the concern of Mad Studies.

The place and continued significance of the social model of disability remains an ongoing debate at the heart of Disability Studies with strong defences of its continued relevance and fundamental nature (Barnes, 2012) while others view it as one element of a 'matrix of theories, pedagogies and practices' (Garland-Thomson 2002 in Goodley, 2017:11) and suggest Disability Studies is now in a 'post-social model' era (Goodley, 2017:11). These debates have raised questions about the (continuing) adequacy or contribution of the social model of disability to Disability Studies and what is gained and lost by its continued centrality? (Watson and Vehmas, 2020). A linked debate is concerned with whether questions about madness and the experiences of mad people can adequately be considered or explained solely from a social model of disability perspective and, if so, how does the social model need to further develop to become more inclusive of these experiences?

If not, the alternatives are specific models of mental distress or madness that may or may not align themselves with Disability Studies. For my part, I favour a middle way that sees Disability Studies as a practice that is 'in the wake of the social model' which necessitates a 'strong imperative to hold on to, return to and revisit its central texts and tenets' (Morgan, 2018:13) as well as exploring and engaging with new concepts and approaches. Beckett and Campbell (2015) make a helpful distinction between the social model (lower case) which refers to UPIAS' (1976) original work and Oliver's (1990, 2004) formal articulation of the Social Model (capitalised), a more fruitful way of exploring these ideas than the somewhat sterile debate that has crystallised around what is criticised by many as dogmatic Social Model. In this spirit I suggest it is probably impossible for the development of Mad Studies to be other than *in the wake* of the social model and Disability Studies. Thus, the focus should be on what can be gained, learned and shared by those of us in this wake, whether our primary focus is on disability, madness or the space(s) in between.

Disability, impairment and madness

That impairment has 'a unique, ubiquitous, and constantly troublesome position within disability studies' (Sherry, 2016:729) cannot be understated. The simplicity of the distinction between impairment and disability delineated by UPIAS is one of the most powerful elements of the social model. It is easy to grasp, resonates with the experiences of disabled people and provides the liberatory message that as Liz Crow put it 'gave me an understanding of my life, shared with thousands, even millions, of other people around the world …[that] It wasn't my body that was responsible for all of my difficulties' (1996:55). This creates a disability identity constituted through three components: the presence of impairment, the experience of disablism and self-identification as a disabled person (Oliver, 1996). This collective politicised disability identity has been a great strength of the disabled people's movement, however, there are a number of issues in relation to the place of impairment and identification as a disabled person that are pertinent to this discussion.

An early criticism was that the movement and Disability Studies were based on the experiences of a particular group of disabled people, the 'physically impaired' named in UPIAS and thus failed to adequately include or address the experiences of those with different impairments, especially people with learning disabilities and survivors, and the intersection with other forms of diversity like gender, race, sexuality and class (Oliver, 2004). I will return to this criticism in relation to mental distress and madness in the next section.

A second, and more enduring area of debate has been about the role of impairment. For many the distinction between impairment and disability appeared to signal a silencing of the experience of impairment, creating a significant gap in Disability Studies' ability to engage with the totality of disabled people's lived experience. Impairments are embodied, they have 'effects' (Thomas, 1999) which can be restrictive, painful and unpleasant. The experience of impairment is not neutral, it is mediated through social relations and structures that frequently don't prioritise or value this experience with the result impairment effects and consequences can be exacerbated or prolonged.

There have been sustained, and successful, calls for a greater empirical and theoretical work within Disability Studies, not least from some who locate themselves centrally in the social model tradition like Paul Abberley (1987) and Carol Thomas (1999). Indeed Oliver (1990) called for a sociology of impairment to be developed alongside and in dialogue with a sociology of disability. A useful example of this work came from empirical work with people living with Motor Neurone Disease (also known as ALS), a degenerative condition with very limited treatment options and generally a short prognosis after diagnosis. Ferrie and Watson (2015) highlighted the emotional trauma and uncertainty generated by living with the condition and anticipating its progress. They identified the ways in which people living with MND experienced impairment effects in relation to personal relationships and in private spaces. Thus, these impairment effects also caused psycho-emotional disablism, in terms of 'barriers to being', as Thomas (2007) puts it. This has the potential to resonate with the experience of some with mental distress where the impairment effects of their condition may be a barrier to creating and maintaining personal relationships.

For others, the conception of impairment as 'lacking part or all of a limb, or having a defective limb, organ or mechanism of the body' (UPIAS, 1976:14) was problematic because impairment remains a deficit or deviation from the norm. As Goodley suggests the word impairment 'symbolises social death, inertia, lack, deficit and tragedy' (2017:35). It is hardly surprising then that some disabled people reject the notion (and particularly the phrasing) of impairment. This has sometimes been based on a shared label of a particular impairment or condition. For example, Deaf people viewing themselves as a cultural or linguistic minority who are oppressed on that basis rather than in response to bodily deficit in relation to hearing norms (Scott-Hill, 2003). Similarly, some reject the notion of impairment because their experience of it is not as 'impairing' or restrictive of activity (particularly in inclusive contexts).

For others, it is the negativity of the phrasing and its failure to capture the diversity of the experience of impairment, which for some has benefits or is to be celebrated. For both reasons, impairment has been considered problematic in relation to madness. Many reject the notion of 'mental impairment' or the pathologisation of mental distress and highlight the difficulty of navigating a disability identity that requires professional classification and recognition of an impairment label for example as the basis for welfare benefits or to access treatment or other forms of support.

An interesting example that melds impairment and disability identities comes from discussions amongst people who identify as having 'psychosocial disabilities' in Asia (Davar, 2015). At a *Trans-Asia Initiative* event in 2013 in the light of the United Nations Convention on the Rights of Persons with Disabilities (UNCRPD), there was recognition of an 'identity crises'. 'Mentally ill patient' was a medicalised and legal(ly controlling) term, 'user and survivor' carried western baggage in a context where for many a lack of services meant 'there was no question of 'using' or 'surviving' a service' although it was the preferred term for some, while others found 'disability' useful in emphasising discrimination (225). As Davar suggests there remained questions about how, and perhaps more importantly, whether these differences could or should be reconciled. She argues that the newly formed identity of being 'psychosocially disabled', as framed in the UNCRPD 'comes with the promise of human rights and empowerment' has greater potential particularly for greater inclusion in the disabled people's movement and enabling those with this 'emerging disability identity' to organise collectively.

A helpful concept that has been developed in Deaf Studies and that could usefully be deployed more widely in relation to disability, is that of 'deaf gain' where the focus is on what is gained from being Deaf by the individual, the Deaf community and society more broadly (Bauman and Murray, 2014). Deaf gain is 'a form of human diversity capable of making vital contributions to the greater good of society ... without recourse to "normalization"' (Bauman and Murray, 2010:210) A simple example is teaching babies sign language to enable greater communication before spoken language is acquired. By extension this approach can identify what is lost to society by having a narrow definition of what is normal or deficient (Bauman and Murray, 2010). There are parallels here with the *affirmation model of disability* (Swain and French, 2000) which builds on the social model to present a non-tragic view of impairment and disability (as a direct challenge to personal tragedy theory which Oliver (1990) describes as the grand theory underpinning traditional individual and medicalised understandings of disability). The model enables disabled people to assert positive identities of disability *and* impairment and as such is 'an assertion of the value and validity of life as a person with impairment' (Swain and French, 2000:578).

There has been some resistance or caution to this approach within Disability Studies, as there has been to impairment-specific organisations or research. As Crow suggests the 'silence' on impairment in early Disability Studies work was often motivated by a concern that discussing impairment might bring an individualised and medicalised focus back and therefore 'impairment is safer not mentioned at all' (1996:58). Reflecting on 30 years of the social model, Mike Oliver (2013:2026) argued that 'emphasising impairment and difference was a strategy that was impotent in protecting disabled people' and insufficient in these neoliberal austere times when many of the gains won by disabled people are being eroded.

What is clear is that Disability and Mad Studies will both continue to grapple with these tensions and the inherently 'troublesomeness' of impairment: its biological yet socially mediated nature, that it can be (sometimes simultaneously) a positive or a negative experience, and that it can be appropriate to prevent the creation of impairment while also accepting and embracing impairment in all its human diversity. Here there is opportunity for dialogue and collective learning that can enhance both fields.

Social models of disability and madness

There has been such protracted debate about the place and continued relevance of the social model of disability in Disability Studies that Mike Oliver demanded that 'the talking has to stop' (2013:1026). Despite this there is no doubt that the conceptual shift the model demands – from an individual personal tragedy to the collective experience of oppression – remains the fundament of Disability Studies. It is a threshold concept (Meyer and Land, 2003) that is, once understood, is transformative and irreversible (Morgan, 2012), As such it is impossible for Disability Studies to be otherwise than in its wake (Morgan, 2018), whether writers seek to extend or break with it. In either circumstance their thinking and practicing of Disability Studies is inevitably influenced. The same is true for social models of mental distress or madness, whether writers choose to locate themselves in Disability Studies or out with its scope/boundaries, the social model of disability remains both a starting and inevitable reference point for these models.

It is useful to remind ourselves why, given the seemingly endless debate about the relevance of the social model, models matter. Why not simply consign the model (and models modelled on it) to history as a useful starting point for a new social movement and academic discipline but now a relic to which homage may be due but whose relevance has passed? I contend models continue to have useful work to do in disciplines that seek to transform understandings and effect social change. As Finkelstein asserts

> A good model can enable us to see something which we do not understand because in the model it can be seen from different viewpoints … that can trigger insights that we might not otherwise develop' (2001:3).

Indeed, Finkelstein (2001) developed a number of models to describe different processes of disablement. Like Oliver, he saw such models as a helpful first stage in identifying and challenging dominant, seemingly common sense, ways of explaining and understanding social processes and relationships. Their potential to effect change in lay and activist contexts cannot be understated. While it is necessary for them to be underpinned by more theoretical and conceptual work, their transformatory nature and utility as 'a hammer' (Oliver, 2004) is essential for political movements agitating for change.

At the heart of both Disability and Mad Studies is a responsibility to hear the concerns of those with lived experience as well as producing knowledge that is useful in challenging the discrimination and oppression they endure and promoting their rights and aspirations. As praxis disciplines which are defined by their commitment to practical action through and alongside more theoretical thinking, our work needs to speak to and be accessible to a variety of audiences. Therefore, Disability and Mad Studies must utilise concepts, approaches and ideas that can be readily understood and applied by 'lay' people as well as being robust enough for academic debate and defence.

If the purpose and benefits of such models is accepted as such, then the first question here is whether the social model of disability is or can be sufficiently expansive to include the experience of those who experience mental distress and/or identify as mad. While the second is whether a social model of distress or madness is constituted within the auspices of the social model of disability as an extension that builds on social model foundations in a similar way to the affirmation model or whether it should be articulated as a separate and distinct model.

Building social model insights and concerns, two linked reports (Beresford et al, 2010; Beresford et al, 2016) highlighted a reluctance amongst survivors to identify as disabled or find the social model of disability helpful as well a number of recommendations for action in response to this (Beresford et al, 2010). These included encouraging Disability Studies writers exploring how the model could be more accessible to and inclusive of survivors, for survivors themselves to spend time considering how this could take place and for discussions between disabled people and survivors to enable learning about and with each other. The second report (Beresford et al, 2016) describes the findings of this work, which took place as 'madness' was becoming a reclaimed and organising concept within parts of the survivor movement. They found that 'madness' like the social model of disability received a mixed reception amongst 'lay' survivors. The report concluded that survivors valued social models (particularly as a rejection of medical models) but found the social model of disability too narrow in focus to fully incorporate their experiences. Similarly, madness and Mad Studies was viewed with some hesitancy.

Therefore, the answer to the questions posed above, remain in flux, and perhaps appropriately so. Models of disability, distress and madness must be accessible to those whose experiences they seek to represent. They inevitably create 'troublesome knowledge' that unsettles, which for some is transformatory while at the same time remaining alien to the experiences and explanations of others (Meyer and Land, 2003 in Morgan, 2012). In this context, I disagree with Oliver, the talking between disabled people and survivors about the social model must not stop but be actively encouraged and supported and these discussions must inform academic thinking even if this is 'troublesome' for us. Moreover, both disciplines must remain vigilant in acknowledging the dominance of privileged perspectives and knowledge within as well as without. It is vital models and theoretical thinking are accessible, and learn from disabled and mad people globally, with particular recognition of the need to listen – and hear – indigenous and other marginalised voices, especially from the global south.

Doing Disability and Mad Studies: enabling and inclusive practices

As well as being fields of study Disability and Mad Studies are also practices or ways of being in the world, praxis disciplines (as I describe them earlier) that demand the practical utility of the knowledge we produce as well as practical application and action. We cannot interrogate ableism and disablism without a continuing reflexive examination of the ways in which we 'do' Disability and Mad Studies. As Beresford and Russo put it 'the 'how' of Mad Studies is as important as its whys and whats' (2016:273). That is, how we seek to teach, to research, to collaborate with and to serve disabled and mad people, colleagues, allies, activists, students and practitioners is as significant as the intellectual project underpinning both fields.

These were concerns that were more to the fore in the earlier days of Disability Studies, for example, debates in *Disability & Society* about the place of non-disabled people (Drake, 1997; Branfield, 1998; Oliver and Barnes, 1997) or on disability research more generally (Barnes and Mercer, 1997). Does this suggest that this a necessary stage or process in the formation of a newer field, that it is through this thrashing out of a set of values, etiquette and practices that a field is formed? Certainly, this appears to be the case in fields of study which are linked to identity and shared experiences of oppression and marginalisation. Developing these practices are a form of resistance against the traditional exclusions in established fields and opportunities for opening up more inclusive and attentive space for discussion. Disability Studies has rehearsed, although perhaps not resolved, many of the issues Mad Studies is grappling with. The questions raised by Spandler and Poursanidou in their recent article 'Who is included in the Mad Studies project?' (2019) echo earlier discussions in Disability Studies and benefit repeating. They suggest a necessary stage in any new project is establishing its boundaries and how permeable or malleable they should be asking 'who is inside and outside, included and excluded' (2019:1) Spandler and Poursanidou acknowledge there are inherent tensions in this questioning but that this is a necessity because it is in these borderlands and liminal spaces (Meyer and Land, 2003) that 'new and important areas of inquiry and critique' are opened up with the potential for the creation of 'alternative counter-cultures of critical inquiry, support and solidarity' (Spandler and Poursanidou, 2019:15).

However, as a field becomes more established and coalesces around particular values and practices, these values and practices can be taken for granted or assumed to remain relevant and inclusive. Recent interventions, frequently from early career academics, have questioned the accessibility of the academy for disabled scholars (Brown and Leigh, 2018), the inclusive nature of our practices like conferences and other events and of our discipline and debates about and for groups more recently brought under the umbrella term disability, for example those living with chronic illness (Scambler, 2012) or trans (disabled) people (Slater and Liddiard, 2018).

What can Disability Studies and Mad Studies learn from this and from each other? This, I believe, is one of the most helpful parts of the relationship, as the disciplines evolve at different paces and are engaging with different and difficult thorny issues or troublesome knowledge at different points, from which much can be learned and shared. They also draw on different literatures, traditions and experiences which provides opportunities for connection, provocation and challenge. This, of course, assumes that the disciplines are listening and actively engaging with each other, this happens when we contribute to each other's spaces but also create spaces for this to happen.

The recent dialogue between Mad Studies and neurodiversity is an example. It was 'framed within the field of disability studies' (McWade et al, 2015) at an event hosted at the Centre for Disability Research at Lancaster University, deliberately brought together participants from all three groups and from a variety of positions, academics, more established and early career, activists and those with lived experience (McWade and Beresford, 2015). The event led to a current issues piece in the journal *Disability & Society* written by three academics who would locate themselves within disability studies but also in Mad Studies (McWade and Beresford) and neurodiversity/critical autism studies (Milton). They build on Graby's earlier (2015) work that suggested neurodiversity 'bridge conceptual gaps between the disabled people's and survivor movements' (in McWade et al, 2015:306) and end with a concern about the wider current context of these discussions acknowledging that many activist concepts, from both Disability and Mad Studies, have been 'co-opted, appropriated and politically neutralised' (McWade et al, 2015:307). They end with the rallying 'let us build upon the rich histories of activism and bring our shared experiences of oppression and marginalisation together' (McWade et al, 2015:308).

Concluding thoughts: more in common

As I suggested in the section on models, one of the most significant challenges for Disability Studies, and perhaps even more so for the disabled people's movement has been the adoption and co-option of its ideas and languages by politicians, policy makers and providers. The pre-eminence of the model led Oliver, to contend 'it is tempting to suggest that we are all social modellists now!' (2004:18). While initially welcomed as an indication of the impact and power of the approach, the formal adoption of the social model of disability by professionals, service providers and policy makers has resulted in a set of unforeseen difficulties (Roulstone and Morgan, 2009). As Oliver and Barnes foresaw 'the assimilation of disability into mainstream political agendas will undermine the more radical aims and political struggles by disabled people and their organisations for social justice' (2012:169). Indeed, as Sheldon had suggested earlier 'perhaps the disabled people's movement is floundering on the shores of its own success' (2006:3). The implementation of anti-discrimination legislation like the Disability Discrimination Act 2005 (replaced by the Equality Act 2010) in the UK and the increased visibility of disabled people as the result of reforms to care and support can give the impression disabled people's rights have been won and are assured.

The 'common sense' understanding of disability is starting to turn full circle, if disability is created by barriers and those barriers are removed, then what remains can again by explained by individualising the problem. There are, of course, many counters to this simplified neoliberal reconceptualising of disability. For certain, many (although very definitely not all) of the most visible environmental barriers have been removed and there are reams of official policies concerned with preventing discrimination and promoting independent living and human rights. However, this masks a number of enduring problems. Barriers are increasing those to 'being' rather than to 'doing', while the psycho-emotional impact of living in an increasingly hostile environment becomes intensified when the problem is returned to one of individual agency and resilience (Ryan, 2019). There is also insufficient recognition of the legacy of the cumulative impact of historic barriers and attitudes that remain engrained in public attitudes and practices. Identifying and challenging this usurpation while continuing to amplify the voices of disabled people and (re)generate progressive knowledge has become the moral imperative for Disability Studies.

Similar challenges face the nascent field of Mad Studies with key writers Beresford and Russo asking whether Mad Studies can be 'protected from being undermined and subverted' in the ways the key ideas of Disability Studies and earlier formations of critical approaches to mental health have been (2016:271). However, there is considerable scope for solidarity and collegiately here particularly if both fields coalesce around Plumb's (1994) assertion that what unites them is a 'non-conformist' approach. The development of knowledges and practices that celebrate the non-conformism of the concepts of disability and madness retain great strength in challenging deficit thinking and provide a way to move on from the cul-de-sac of debate about impairment and sits more comfortably alongside the activism and identity of pride. Rather than focusing on differences and areas of discomfort (although they should continue to be areas of discussion and debate) we should take our lead from McWade, Milton and Beresford who argue we should seek dialogic alliances that move beyond the limitations of identity politics where 'the aim is to stop thinking about how we are the same and begin to work with our differences collectively' (2015:307). It is in this spirit that the vital and vibrant relationship between Disability Studies and Mad Studies can endure, respecting our differences and diversity, but remaining committed to that central claim 'there must be nothing about us without us'.

References

Abberley, P (1987) The Concept of Oppression and the Development of a Social Theory of Disability. *Disability, Handicap and Society* 2(1), 5–19. https://doi.org/10.1080/02674648766780021

Barnes, C (2012) Understanding the Social Model of Disability: Past, Present and Future. In N Watson, A Roulstone and C Thomas (eds). *Routledge Handbook of Disability Studies*. Abingdon: Routledge.

Barnes, C and Mercer, G (eds) (1997) *Doing Disability Research*. Leeds: The Disability Press.

Bauman, H and Murray J (2010) Deaf Studies in the 21st Century: "Deaf-gain" and the Future of Human Diversity. In M Marchark and P E Spencer (eds). *The Oxford Handbook of Deaf Studies, Language and Education* 2.

Bauman, H and Murray, J J (eds) (2014) *Deaf Gain: Raising the Stakes for Human Diversity*. Minneapolis, MN: University of Minnesota Press.

Beckett, A E and Campbell, T (2015) The Social Model of Disability as an Oppositional Device. *Disability & Society* 30(2), 270–283. https://doi.org/10.1080/09687599.2014.999912

Beresford, P (2000) What Have Madness and Psychiatric System Survivors Got to Do with Disability and Disability Studies? *Disability & Society* 20(4), 469–477.

Beresford, P (2004) Madness, Distress, Research and a Social Model. In C Barnes and G Mercer (eds). *Implement The Social Model of Disability: Theory and Research*. Leeds: The Disability Press. https://disability-studies.leeds.ac.uk/wp-content/uploads/sites/40/library/Barnes-implementing-the-social-model-chapter-13.pdf Accessed: 29 June 2020.

Beresford, P. (2012) Psychiatric System Survivors: An Emerging Movement. In N. Watson, A Roulstone and C. Thomas (eds) *The Routledge Handbook of Disability Studies*. Abingdon: Routledge.

Beresford, P and Carr, S (2018) *Social Policy First Hand: An International Introduction to Participative Social Welfare*. Bristol: Policy Press.

Beresford, P and Russo, J (2016) Supporting the Sustainability of Mad Studies and Preventing its Co-option. *Disability & Society* 31(2), 270–274. https://doi.org/10.1080/09687599.2016.1145380

Beresford, P and Wallcraft, J (1997) Psychiatric System Survivors and Emancipatory Research: Issues, Overlaps and Differences. In C. Barnes and G. Mercer (eds) *Doing Disability Research*. Leeds: Disability Press, 67–87. https://disability-studies.leeds.ac.uk/wp-content/uploads/sites/40/library/Barnes-Chapter-5.pdf Accessed: 29 June 2020.

Beresford, P, Nettle, M and Perring, R (2010) *Towards a Social Model of Madness and Distress? Exploring What Service Users Say*. York: Joseph Rowntree Foundation. https://www.jrf.org.uk/report/towards-social-model-madness-and-distress-exploring-what-service-users-say Accessed: 29 June 2020.

Beresford, P, Perring, R, Nettle, M and Wallcraft, J (2016) *From Mental Illness to a Social Model of Madness and Distress*. London: Shaping our lives. https://www.shapingourlives.org.uk/wp-content/uploads/2016/05/FROM-MENTAL-ILLNESS-PDF-2.pdf Accessed: 29 June 2020.

Branfield, F (1998) What Are You Doing Here? 'Non-disabled' People and the Disability Movement: A Response to Robert F. Drake. *Disability & Society* 13(1), 143–144. https://doi.org/10.1080/09687599826966

Brown, N and Leigh, J (2018) Ableism in Academic: Where are the Disabled and Ill Academics? *Disability & Society* 33(6), 985–989. https://doi.org/10.1080/09687599.2018.1455627

Crow, L (1996) Including All of our Lives: Renewing the Social Model of Disability. In C. Barnes and G. Mercer (eds) *Exploring the Divide*. Leeds: The Disability Press. Available at: https://disability-studies.leeds.ac.uk/wp-content/uploads/sites/40/library/Crow-exploring-the-divide-ch4.pdf Accessed: 29 June 2020.

Davar, B V (2015) Disabilities, Colonisation and Globalisation: How the Very Possibility of a Disability Identity was Compromised for the 'Insane' in India. In H. Spandler, J. Anderson and B Sapey (eds) *Madness, Distress and the Politics of Disablement*. Bristol: Policy Press.

Drake, R F (1997) What Am I Doing Here? 'Non-disabled' People and the Disability Movement. *Disability & Society* 12(4), 643–645. https://doi.org/10.1080/09687599727173

Graby, S (2015) Neurodiversity: Bridging the Gap Between the Disabled People's Movement and the Mental Health System Survivors' Movement. In H Spandler, J Anderson and B Sapey (eds) *Madness, Distress and the Politics of Disablement*. Bristol: Policy Press

Ferrie, J and Watson, N (2015) The Psycho-social Impact of Impairments: The Case of Motor Neurone Disease. In T Shakespeare (ed) *Disability Research Today International Perspectives*. London: Routledge.

Finkelstein, V. (2001) *The Social Model of Disability Repossessed*. https://disability-studies.leeds.ac.uk/wp-content/uploads/sites/40/library/finkelstein-soc-mod-repossessed.pdf Accessed: 29 June 2020.

Goodley, D (2017) *Disability Studies: An Interdisciplinary Introduction*. London: Sage.

Hunt, J (2019) *No Limits. The Disabled People's Movement: A Radical History*. TBR Imprint: Manchester. https://www.gmcdp.com/no-limits Accessed: 29 June 2020.

Ingram, R A (2016) Mad Studies: Making (Non)Sense Together. *Intersectionalities: The Journal of Social Work Analysis, Research, Polity and Practice* 5(3), 11–17. https://journals.library.mun.ca/ojs/index.php/IJ/article/view/1680 Accessed: 29 June 2020.

LeFrancois, B Menzies, R, Reaume, G (eds) (2013) *Mad Matters: A Critical Reader in Canadian Mad Studies*. Toronto: Canadian Scholars' Press.

McWade, B and Beresford, P (2015) *Mad Studies and Neurodiversity – Exploring Connections* https://madstudies2014.wordpress.com/archive/mad-studies-neurodiversity-symposium-archive/ Accessed: 29 June 2020.

McWade, B Milton, D and Beresford, P (2015) Mad Studies and Neurodiversity: A Dialogue. *Disability & Society* 30(2), 305–309. https://doi.org/10.1080/09687599.2014.1000512

Meyer, J and Land, R (2003) *Threshold Concepts and Troublesome Knowledge: Linkages to Ways of Thinking and Practising within the Disciplines*, Enhancing Teaching–Learning Environments in Undergraduate Courses Project Occasional Report 4 [online]. http://www.etl.tla.ed.ac.uk//docs/ETLreport4.pdf Accessed: 13 June 2011.

Morgan, H (2012) Threshold Concepts in Disability Studies: Troublesome Knowledge and Liminal Spaces in Social Work Education. *Social Work Education* 31(2), 215–226. https://doi.org/10.1080/02615479.2012.644964

Morgan, H (2018) *In the Wake of the Social Model: Engaging with Policy, Theory and Practice*. Unpublished PhD Thesis. Lancaster: University of Lancaster.

Oliver, M (1990) *The Politics of Disablement*. Basingstoke: Macmillan.

Oliver, M (1996) *Understanding Disability: From Theory to Practice*. London: Macmillan.

Oliver, M (2004) The Social Model in Action: If I Had a Hammer. In C. Barnes and G. Mercer (eds) *Implementing the Social Model of Disability: Theory and Research*. Leeds: The Disability Press. https://disability-studies.leeds.ac.uk/wp-content/uploads/sites/40/library/Barnes-implementing-the-social-model-chapter-2.pdf Accessed 29 June 2020.

Oliver, M (2013) The Social Model of Disability: Thirty Years On. *Disability & Society* 28(7), 1024–1026. https://doi.org/10.1080/09687599.2013.818773

Oliver, M and Barnes, C (1997) All We Are Saying is Give Disabled Researchers a Chance. *Disability & Society* 12(5), 811–814. https://www.tandfonline.com/doi/abs/10.1080/09687599727074

Oliver, M and Barnes, C (2012) *The New Politics of Disablement*. Basingstoke: Palgrave Macmillan.

Plumb, A (1994) *Disability or Distress? A Discussion Document*. Manchester: Greater Manchester Coalition of Disabled People.

Reeve, D (2015) Psycho-emotional Disablism in the Lives of People Experiencing Mental Distress. In H Spandler, J Anderson and B Sapey (eds) *Madness, Distress and the Politics of Disablement*. Bristol: Policy Press.

Roulstone, A and Morgan, H (2009) Neo-Liberal Individualism or Self-directed Support: Are we all Speaking the Same Language on Modernising Adult Social Care. *Social Policy and Society* 8(3), 333–345. https://doi.org/10.1017/S1474746409004886.

Ryan, F (2019) *Crippled: Austerity and the Demonization of Disabled People*. London: Verso Books.

Scambler, S (2012) Long-term Disabling Conditions and Disability Theory. In N Watson, A Roulstone and C Thomas (eds) *The Routledge Handbook of Disability Studies*. Abingdon: Routledge.

Scott-Hill, M (2003) Deafness/Disability – Problematizing Notions of Identity, Culture and Structure. In S Riddelll and N. Watson (eds) *Disability, Culture and Identity*. Harlow: Pearson Education.

Sheldon, A (2006) Disabling the Disabled People's Movement? The Influence of Disability Studies on the Struggle for Liberation. https://disability-studies.leeds.ac.uk/wp-content/uploads/sites/40/library/Sheldon-disabling-the-dps-movement.pdf Accessed: 29 June 2020.

Sherry, M (2016) A Sociology of Impairment. *Disability & Society* 31(6), 729–744. https://doi.org/10.1080/09687599.2016.1203290

Slater, J and Liddiard, K (2018) Why Disability Studies Scholars Must Challenge Transmisogyny and Transphobia. *Canadian Journal of Disability Studies* 7(2). https://doi.org/10.15353/cjds.v7i2.424.

Spandler, H and Poursanidou, K (2019) Who is Included in the Mad Studies Project? *Journal of Ethics in Mental Health* 10, 1–20. https://jemh.ca/issues/v9/documents/JEMH%20Inclusion%20iii.pdf Accessed: 29 June 2020.

Swain, J and French, S. (2000) Towards an Affirmation Model of Disability. *Disability & Society* 15(4), 569–582. https://doi.org/10.1080/09687590050058189

Thomas, C (1999) *Female Forms. Experiencing and Understanding Disability*. Buckingham: Open University Press.

Thomas, C (2007) *Sociologies of Disability and Illness. Contested Ideas in Disability Studies and Medical Sociology*. Basingstoke: Palgrave Macmillan.

Union of the Physically Impaired Against Segregation (UPIAS) (1976) *Fundamental Principles of Disability*. London: Union of the Physically Impaired Against Segregation. https://disability-studies.leeds.ac.uk/wp-content/uploads/sites/40/library/UPIAS-fundamental-principles.pdf Accessed: 29 June 2020.

Watson, N, Roulstone, A and Thomas, C. (eds) (2012) *Routledge Handbook of Disability Studies*. Abingdon: Routledge.

Watson, N and Vehmas, S (2020) Disability Studies: Into the Multidisciplinary Future. In N Watson and S Vehmas (eds) *Routledge Handbook of Disability Studies*. 2nd Edn. London: Routledge.

14

WEAPONIZING ABSENT KNOWLEDGES

Countering the violence of mental health law

Fleur Beaupert and Liz Brosnan

Introduction

Woman on the Edge of Time by Marge Piercy tells the story of Connie Ramos, a woman who is detained in a psychiatric hospital after she defends her niece against a violent assault (Piercy, 2016a). The assaulter, her niece's boyfriend, has her detained by claiming *she* attacked him and her niece, knowing that her history with mental health services will lead the doctors to believe him and not her. A passage describing how she is physically restrained shortly after the admission interview captures the essence of the multifaceted violence that is wielded by mental health law. This violence is physical or material, on the one hand, and epistemic or symbolic, on the other (Roper, 2018):

> Connie writhed on the bed, pinned down with just enough play to let her wriggle. They had pushed her into restraint, shot her up immediately. She had been screaming— okay! Did they think you had to be crazy to protest being locked up? Yes, they did. They said reluctance to be hospitalized was a sign of sickness, assuming you were sick, in one of these no-win circles (Piercy, 2016a: 12).

Mental health law is primarily devoted to establishing mechanisms for forcing mental health interventions on people, by detaining them in mental health facilities or placing them on out-patient orders – or 'community treatment orders' – mandating their compliance. These two categories of involuntary status pave the way for specific drugs and procedures to be administered to an individual against their will. Voluntary support and service use tends to receive scant attention in this body of law.

Statutory objectives suggest that mental health law is concerned with providing 'care' and 'treatment'. The experiences of mental health service users and psychiatric survivors, however, indicate that the interventions are often physically violent and harmful, in both the short and long term (Lee, 2013: 110–113; Ashe, 2017). Involuntary measures revolve around incarceration, whether in one's own body through the action of mind-altering and incapacitating psychotropic medication (Fabris, 2011: 115; Fabris and Aubrecht, 2014), or in the traditional sense of confinement in a physical institution.

DOI: 10.4324/9780429465444-17

Mental health services coerce people into acceptance of mental health or psychosocial norms and treatments in both explicit and implicit ways. Informal coercion occurs in the way mental health services use many forms of containment and an environment of surveillance to create a culture of compliance; Sjöström discusses how staff in inpatient wards use threats and locked doors to control voluntary patients (Sjöström, 2006). Invisible power can be said to be most effective when the oppressed believe oppressive regimes operate in their best interests, or that alternative possibilities do not exist (Gaventa, 2006; Brosnan, 2012). However, for many this power is not invisible but takes the overt form of threats to control access to finances, subsidized housing and even to their children, or which force compliance to avoid imprisonment, outpatient commitment or involuntary hospital admissions (Canvin et al, 2013). Mental health law is a central enabler of the coercive practices permeating mental health services because the threat of an involuntary order is an unspoken constant.

The coercive functions of mental health law are intertwined with acts of epistemic violence and symbolic violence which suppress users' and survivors' individual and collective ways of knowing and making meaning. Epistemic violence in this context involves psychiatric institutions and practices operating to invalidate psychiatrized people's 'knowledge, and ways of knowing and, consequently, efface their ways of being' (Liegghio, 2013: 122). The symbolic violence of psychiatry refers to the way in which the dominant biomedical paradigm monopolizes society's understandings of, and responses to, madness and distress and associated discrimination and social injustice, while marginalising other ways of making meaning about these phenomena (LeBlanc and Kinsella, 2016; Lee, 2013). Mental health law facilitates and compounds this process of symbolic violence, embedding it deeply within socio-political structures and individual lives (Beaupert, 2018a).

When Connie Ramos speaks of 'reluctance to be hospitalized' being read as a 'sign of sickness', *Woman on the Edge of Time* gives voice to the way in which the symbolic violence of mental health (law) may merge into 'ontological violence'. Ontology deals with the nature of being; ontological violence occurs when a dominant ideology imposes an interpretation that 'determines the very being and social existence of the interpreted subjects' (Žižek, 2008: 62).

Mental health law sanctions processes of ontological violence, whereby psychiatry tells a person that they are 'sick' and reads any resistance to this interpretation as more profound evidence of 'sickness' (Hamilton and Roper, 2006: 420; Beaupert, 2018b: 769–771). It demands capitulation to these interpretations, including through the forced administration of drugs and procedures that alter the person's psyche, body and social relations (Minkowitz, 2007: 421). In so doing, mental health law cultivates the ontological nullification of its subjects (Beaupert, 2018a: 19). This is a denial of humanness – designation to a nonentity category unworthy of being treated with dignity and having one's experiences respected and acted on (Roper, 2018: 92–93).

In the first part of this chapter we reflect on the politics and ideologies underpinning mental health law and its violent practices. We approach this topic with a sense of alarm, since the coercive aspects of mental health law are expanding in many respects, while simultaneously becoming less overt and more insidious in others. For example, community treatment orders which extend formal coercion beyond the walls of mental health facilities, are well-embedded and increasingly over-used in jurisdictions such as the UK, Australia and New Zealand, and gradually being introduced in new jurisdictions around the world. There has been a recent push too by prominent psychiatrists to introduce community treatment orders in Ireland (Brosnan, 2018).

The policy justification for introducing outpatient commitment is that this is a 'less restrictive alternative' to detention. In fact, these orders may 'roll over' for many years, compared to shorter periods of detention. They can constrain a person's ability to live where they choose, travel and negotiate the workplace successfully. They facilitate the prolonged forced administration of psychotropic drugs which 'restrain the body and create dependency … which results in an indefinite form of detention' (Fabris and Aubrecht, 2014: 186). In some jurisdictions, residency conditions in orders can result in people being placed in secure 'community' residential facilities which operate much like institutions.

The socio-political forces that impel the introduction of more coercive mental health laws are often a fortuitous coalition of media induced moral panic whipped up by sensationalist journalism after some tragedy associated with failed mental health supports. The psychiatric professional lobby weigh in promising reduced risk of further tragedy if only politicians place their trust in the profession and give them more legal power to forcefully treat people who pose potential, assumed risks to themselves or others (Fabris, 2011: 97–98). Yet there is no reliable science behind risk assessment; literature on risk modelling in mental health demonstrates a consistent inability of professionals to accurately predict risk in individual cases, as distinct from statistical modelling (Large et al, 2016).

We also offer our reflections with a sense of hope, born out of the knowledge that Mad people and communities resist and persist in the face of violent and discriminatory practices (Costa et al, 2012). In the second part of the chapter, we sketch some developments which may illuminate and assist the Mad Studies 'project of inquiry, knowledge production, and political action' (Menzies et al, 2013: 13), and of probing interactions with other systems of oppression affecting differently positioned Mad and marginalized subjects. Liz explores possibilities opened up by Boaventura de Sousa Santos' analyses of power relations, anti-colonialism and the 'sociology of absences'. Fleur turns attention to the international human rights landscape and the emancipatory potential (and limitations) of instruments including the Convention on the Rights of Persons with Disabilities.

Both of us have been subjected to mental health laws and services, and while our experiences differed we share a commitment to resist the oppressions of mental health norms and institutional practices, consistent with Mad movements and theories. These oppressions work with, within and upon racist, heteropatriarchal, colonial and capitalist logics through collusions, which are integral to the Mad Studies project of inquiry (Gorman et al, 2013; Gorman & LeFrançois, 2018), and in relation to which we have different privileged and marginalized social positions. We write from privileged positions including as academics who have worked as part of the coercive apparatus of mental health law. It is this final orientation as former agents of mental health law that informs our first section reflecting on how the law is complicit in the dehumanising violence of psychiatry.

Legal capture and complicity: Sanctioning violence

Liz: My involvement with mental health law spans the past three decades. My initial encounters were involuntary, until I realized that accepting the status of voluntary patient was preferable to detention and forced treatment. Many years later, having extracted myself from services and following active involvement in the user/survivor movement, I was privileged to act as a lay member on Irish mental health tribunals over seven years, and witness the procedures surrounding reviews of involuntary detention orders.

I sought to become a lay member because some of us in the user movement believed that legal review of the practice of detaining people based on a definition of 'mental disorder' would not stand up to legal scrutiny. Such scrutiny, we hoped, would change the landscape of mental health services, because legal focus on the lack of scientific validity underpinning the diagnostic labels used to justify involuntary detention and treatment would herald a new dawn of freedom. What we failed to consider was how the legal profession would become captured by psychiatric hegemony, and align, for the most part, with the mental health system. The legal profession, with a few exceptions, accepted unquestioningly the status quo, the medico-legal paradigm of the Mental Health Commission ('MHC') and the mental health establishment. What promised for a brief period of time in 2006 to be an opportunity for reform, was quickly absorbed into a mental health system fundamentally resistant to change.

What is obvious looking back is the lack of dissenting perspectives provided to the incoming panel members. Mainstream psychiatric knowledge pervaded the training provided by the MHC to incoming tribunal members. A module was delivered by a peer advocacy organization, the Irish Advocacy Network. This aimed to humanize the 'patient', to sensitize tribunal members to the human experience of distress. The feedback from tribunal panel participants taking this session was that it was helpful preparation for their roles. Yet, at best this may have provided some insight and empathy for people experiencing distress, but failed to unsettle the medico-legal apparatus assembled to adjudicate on involuntary detention and treatment of people against their will with psychotropic medications.

The Irish Mental Health Act 2001 did not incorporate many provisions to facilitate the meaningful participation of the person at a tribunal. There was provision for consulting with the person, and for their attendance at the hearing but not of offering them any choices as to who might support them. The MHC appointed a legal representative unknown to the individual, who they might meet with briefly before the tribunal convened. This is the only advocate mentioned in the legislation: no mention of peer advocates or other possibilities for supported decision-making.

Under Irish legislation mental health tribunals are tasked with determining if the detention is legal or not. The tribunal cannot offer opinions on what other options for treatment might be beneficial, or less restrictive. The tribunal solely determines if the person 'suffers from a mental disorder' and would benefit from treatment, which de facto is provided in an institutional setting. Clinical assessments that a person 'suffers from a mental disorder' are impossible to counteract, because the twin constructs of 'lack of insight' and 'lacking capacity to consent' are deployed once a 'patient' disagrees with their diagnosis, fails to accept they are mentally disordered, and/or displays non-compliance with their treating psychiatrist's treatment directives (Brosnan and Flynn 2017; Hamilton and Roper, 2006: 420–421). The weight of medical authority renders the patient an unreliable witness, thus ontologically nullified.

Fleur: My first encounters with mental health services, unlike Liz, were voluntary and culminated in a hospitalization which I did not experience as traumatizing. These experiences led me to develop an interest in mental health law while studying law and to embark on socio-legal research exploring Australian mental health tribunals. A few years after completing my law degree I worked for a year as a solicitor with New South Wales (NSW) Legal Aid's Mental Health Advocacy Service, a specialist legal service providing representation in mental health law matters. In most cases I represented clients at the first legal review following their detention in a facility to decide whether to approve further involuntary treatment. At that time, initial hearings were conducted by magistrates in NSW, and subsequent reviews by the Mental Health Review Tribunal. During the magistrates proceedings the person was often referred to as 'the patient' by the presiding magistrate. In fact, some people would introduce themselves with: 'I'm the patient'.

While the patient role in general healthcare is infused with the promise of informed consent, the character of this role is effectively inverted in mental health services. The implicit promise is of coercion extending to the use of physical force, rather than respect, as a first response to decisions that others perceive as risky or unwise. Mental health law plays a pivotal role in producing and sustaining this informal coercion, fostering a culture of compliance – regardless of whether the 'patient' has voluntary or involuntary status (Beaupert, 2018a: 17). It was some years after my mental health lawyering experience, and following an involuntary hospitalisation, that I came to understand my ongoing 'voluntary' interactions with mental health services as being fundamentally coercive. This was based on not being given adequate information about the effects of drugs my body would become dependent on, not being offered support (other than drugs) to navigate altered states of consciousness and realising that deferral to medical norms and interventions was preferable to an involuntary order.

It is perhaps unsurprising that legal professionals working in this field may become captured by the mental health hegemony. Commenting on civil commitment proceedings in the US thirty years ago, Decker suggested that key difficulties providing effective legal representation in these matters were due to the almost impenetrable barrier 'psychiatrists' organizationally-situated knowledge' presented to asserting alternative perspectives (1987: 169). This surfaced unmistakably on one occasion when my arguments against clinical views about the allegedly high risk of violence posed by one of my clients prompted the tribunal's legal member to ask, 'Are you questioning the expert opinion?' – as if this was an unthinkable course of action. Rigorously challenging the other party's evidence is *expected* of lawyers working in most other fields. Even rigorous legal advocacy in mental health law matters is only sometimes accompanied by a determination at odds with the recommendation of the consultant psychiatrist.

Legal professionals are often complicit, albeit sometimes reluctantly, in the symbolic violence of psychiatry and the operation of sanist practices through mental health law. Research has consistently shown that 'relaxed' legal adjudication styles, characterized by reliance on clinically oriented proxies for legal tests (Peay, 1989; Perkins, 2003) and uncritical deference to clinical opinion (Parry et al, 1992; Hiday, 1981; Carney et al, 2011: 209–217), become normalized in mental health law matters. Lawyers who take an adversarial approach may find themselves cut short because of the way in which 'therapeutic jurisprudence' is applied by some Australian mental health tribunals.

Therapeutic jurisprudence seeks to maximize the 'therapeutic' effects of the law while upholding principles of justice, applying insights from the social sciences and psychology (Winick, 2005: 6). The following quote in the leading NSW textbook on mental health law demonstrates one influential interpretation of this approach:

> while some hearings may require robust questioning and advocacy, strident advocacy is rarely appropriate, and lawyers should ensure that they maintain an appropriate demeanour and tone that does not undermine a positive therapeutic relationship between the patient and their treating team.
>
> *(Howard & Westmore, 2018: 55)*

Such interpretations jar with the concern of therapeutic jurisprudence to protect individual self-determination because of beneficial impacts on psychological wellbeing (Winick, 1992). Nonetheless, a focus on relaxing adversarial processes within therapeutic jurisprudence can reinforce 'existing distributions of power in the relationship between the treated and the treater', while ostensibly promoting autonomy (Arstein-Kerslake and Black, 2020).

Mental health law is arguably intrinsically 'anti-therapeutic'. It assumes that deprivation of liberty and violence are legitimate means of ensuring that people deemed dangerous and disordered due to 'mental illness' receive 'needed treatment'. Yet little may be offered in the way of real help and support and the force applied is a one-way street: the State cannot be ordered to provide the spectrum of social supports a person may seek.

Housing was an issue for one of my clients, another assessed as being particularly dangerous. During the hearing I put forward arguments that the legal criteria for his continued detention were not met. The arguments I presented on his behalf included his explanation for tipping a cup of coffee on his case worker. This incident was being used as evidence that he posed a risk of serious harm to others. He said that the case worker not only failed to help him with housing but also laughed at him when he asked about securing accommodation. I ultimately regretted drawing attention to this backstory. The magistrate responded: 'But was it reasonable to throw coffee on your case worker?'

This example is emblematic of injustices which may be inextricably linked to experiences that come to be labelled as mental illness (Kinouani, 2018), and which therefore underly the legal encounter. Attempts to articulate the struggles that a person may be encountering in their daily lives are generally disavowed if explicitly raised, including concerns about harmful effects of drugs or a desire for more holistic support services. Although some Australian tribunal members or panels may be sympathetic and make non-binding recommendations in response (which may never be followed through), the legal 'brief' is highly circumscribed as Liz has discussed.

Mental health law sanctions forced interventions revolving around drugging individual bodies against a backdrop of inadequate systems for the provision of 'care' (Shimrat, 2013) and a culture of silence around the severe harms caused by psychiatric interventions (Whitaker, 2002). In this way the law is complicit in the physical and symbolic violence that is unleashed through the mental health paradigm, while simultaneously constructing the official 'truth' that effective 'treatment' is being provided via involuntary orders.

Recovering and weaponizing absent knowledges

Liz: In seeking new ways to understand and resist the operation of symbolic violence in medico-legal discourse it is enlightening to find writings from other fields of emancipatory scholarship, offering new lenses to dissect and dismantle the crushing hegemony. Anti-colonialism is one such promising perspective for Mad scholars and students, because it looks at how a small elite in a particular time and place in Europe developed so much power that their worldview dominated the world. They did this as much, if not completely, through how they thought of themselves and regarded the rest of humanity. Santos is one writer whose work offers us a way of understanding the power relations that determine what, and whose knowledge matters. What follows is a very brief truncated account of his work on how Eurocentric thinking and science dominate the global structures of power and resource extractions.

Epistemologies are philosophies about how we know what we know, or think we know, and Santos (2018) uses the term 'Epistemologies of the North' to refer to the most taken for granted ones that influence us all in many ways most are not aware of. The 'North' is the term used because geographically all colonial systems arose in Europe, and spread outwards to conquer and settle the rest of the world, usually referred to as the 'South'. However, both 'North' and 'South' are much more than geographical designations. The North refers to an overarching structure of power from which all other more familiar oppressive structures, such as racism, sexism and classism, get their power to designate one group and worldview as superior over others. So the term 'North' designates structures of power located within the centre (the metropolis), as distinct from the local, rural and remote, colonized and Indigenous peoples and others at the bottom of oppressive hierarchies, including predominantly racialized people incarcerated in the modern psy/prison industrial complex (White, 2018). These latter constitute the majority of humanity who populate the 'South': a designated space that renders those occupying it as sub-human, non-knowers and objects to be ignored or exploited to enrich those enjoying the privileges of the North. Indeed, in the geographical South, there are elites in all societies who may have more in common with elites in the North, than with the marginalized, dispossessed in their own societies.

What is most useful for Mad activists to take from decolonial scholars such as Santos is the explanations of how the dominant ways of knowing are rooted in western enlightenment traditions which privilege whiteness, reason and rationality, order, strength, individualism, science, and the heteropatriarchal worldview. Epistemologies of the North underpin the oppressions of capitalism, colonialism and patriarchy and are promulgated by political systems, the academy and the rule of law – structures which regulate and reproduce systems of belief which shore up the dominant structures of power. Building on these understandings, Mad activists may seek to explore how the symbolic violence of psychiatry informs, operates through or otherwise interacts with a range of oppressions.

Santos (2018) theorizes a dividing line between those radically excluded by these epistemologies, which he calls the abyssal line. Many of the justice and equality struggles of oppressed peoples situated within the apparently positive side of the North/South abyssal line use the tools and thinking of the very structures that subject them to oppression to seek advantages in their struggles for recognition and fairer access to resources. These oppressed peoples are deemed inferior but still human by the controlling structures of those on the privileged side of the line. So, feminists, unionized workers and anti-racist activists are somewhat less human with less access to power, privilege and resources within this hierarchy, but believe in (and are technically afforded) their birthright to be full citizens in many countries. These struggles occur on the 'Northern' side of the line. And conversely some positioned geographically in the so called Global South, as distinct from the theorized South, partake of the privileges of the North, in that their status and power is upheld by their relationship to Eurocentric thinking and the Academy, and indeed white privilege.

However, those positioned on the Southern side of the abyssal line are differently positioned, regarded as non-human, with sub-human status, mere objects. Abyssal thinking renders 'nonexistent, irrelevant or unintelligible all that exists on the other side of the line' (Santos, 2018: 84). Such lives have no value to the elites and their knowledges are therefore absent or silent because they are not regarded as having any of the features that make knowledge valuable: reason and rationality, systematic, scientific, and masculinist. Oppressed people located on the Northern side of the abyssal line may be rendered sub-human in some respects and contexts. For example, Santos (2018) observes that an African American student studying at a prestigious university may hope to succeed despite institutional racism but will encounter a radical and lethally different level of assigned non-humanity if he is stopped by racist police officers on his way home.

Applying these ideas to mental health activism we can see that those of us labelled with mental ill-health, and active in knowledge creation about the first-hand experience of coercive responses to distress, can obtain some trickle-down benefits. In our struggles to reform intolerable systems of sanist oppression (LeBlanc and Kinsella, 2016), and the total dominance of brain malfunction explanations (i.e. Santos' 'Epistemologies of the North') above embodied, social and relational explanations (i.e. ways of knowing of those far from the centre of power), we can believe in (and achieve) some precarious success on the advantageous side of the divide. However, if we become 'unwell', display symptoms of distress or confusion and are deemed 'incompetent', 'irrational' or otherwise 'mad' – particularly when formal or informal coercion is applied in response – we may fall over the other side of the divide (Santos' abyssal line), with epistemic and legal agency removed. We therefore walk a tightrope each time we take up some of the many new roles opening up in the psy-industrial complex as the embodied mad.

There are connections between our struggles against the dehumanizing ideologies and structures of psychiatry and the struggles of other marginalized groups confronting differing oppressions. Indeed many of us face the impact of being oppressed in other ways as well as, prior to, or interlocking with psychiatry, of struggling in capitalist, colonial or heteropatriarchal worlds. In fact, for many of us our earlier experiences of oppression and trauma led us into the world of the psychiatric industrial complex (Kinouani, 2018; White, 2018). In *Woman on the Edge of Time*, for example, Connie Ramos' experiences and socio-political positions as a Chicana single mother on welfare are integral to her capture by this complex.

Santos speaks of the 'sociology of absences' – turning absent subjects into present subjects – as the foremost condition for identifying and validating new and different knowledges, which can reinvent social emancipation and liberation (2018: 2). The 'absent' is produced through very unequal relations of power, so that recovering the absent is an eminently political gesture. Giving space to these absent knowledges is part of the emerging Epistemologies of the South which challenge the dominance of the de-humanizing processes of the North's worldview. This process of recovering the absent is evident in the mental health field through the emergence of both survivor-controlled research and Mad Studies. By bringing the knowledges of those sub-ject to mental health services to the fore, by focusing on the deliberately absented knowledge of those subjected to mental health law, we can reinvent social emancipation and liberation from the symbolic violence of mental health law.

Fleur: Human rights are one set of tools that may be wielded to further the project of recovering the absent, including the knowledges of those subjected to mental health services and laws. Recent evolutions in the international human rights landscape hold potential for asserting rights claims, and developing approaches, which may shift the oppressive epistemo-logical structures of mental health law and help to bring about their disruption. The fact that human rights discourse can shore up dominant systems of power does not prevent the strategic use of human rights mechanisms by Mad individuals and constituencies to expose discrimin-atory institutional arrangements and work towards genuinely inclusive societies.

The overt positioning of psychiatrized people as rights holders within the international disability human rights law framework with the advent of the Convention on the Rights of Persons with Disabilities ('CRPD') is one development providing valuable new lines of resist-ance. The relationship between madness and disability is contested; not all users and survivors identify as disabled (Russo and Shulkes, 2015). However for others, including some commu-nities in the Asian region (Davar, 2015; Davar, 2018), the CRPD offers an inspiring paradigm, free from the constraints of laws (and activism) oriented around the coercive medical model. The social model of disability is a foundational tenet of the CRPD deriving from disability studies, whose relevance for madness and distress is an area of ongoing exploration (Beresford et al, 2010). With its emphasis on the ideological construction of disability and the social and environmental conditions that oppress disabled people (Erevelles, 2011: 151), this model is arguably equally – if differently – relevant to 'mental health'.

One revolutionary aspect of the CRPD is how it rejects the dichotomy between mental capacity and incapacity in the disability law context (Minkowitz, 2007: 408), which has trad-itionally been validated by international human rights law (Steele, 2016: 1014). This dichotomy aligns with Santos' abyssal line. Historically, disabled and Mad people were often placed auto-matically on the sub-human side of this divide through legal determinations or societal practices effectively casting these oppressed peoples as 'incompetent' (United Nations, 2014: 2), including institutionalization under lunacy laws. These practices took away a person's ability to make a range of decisions about their life and body based solely on their deemed status as disabled or, in the case of madness, attributions of 'disorder' and 'dangerousness'. Of course, mental health laws continue to have the same effect. However, today's laws incorporate legal standards which assume a mantle of objectivity – such as 'mental illness', 'harm to self or other' and 'in/capacity' – buttressed by clinical concepts and opinions of their applicability in a particular case (Dhanda, 2007: 431–432).

According to Article 12 of the CRPD, enshrining the right to equal recognition before the law, such practices involve the denial of 'legal capacity', which encompasses the ability to hold and exercise legal rights and duties (Minkowitz, 2007: 408–410; United Nations, 2014). Article 12 prohibits the discriminatory denial of legal capacity, where the legal personhood of people with disabilities is singled out for arbitrary removal in purpose or effect (United Nations, 2014: 6). The Committee on the Rights of Persons with Disabilities ('CRPD Committee'), the United Nations body responsible for monitoring the CRPD, has determined that forced mental health interventions contravene Article 12 and that only voluntary support measures are acceptable (2014: 11). In fact numerous CRPD provisions operate in tandem to prohibit forced interventions, including Article 15 (freedom from torture), Article 16 (freedom from exploitation, violence and abuse), Article 17 (protecting the integrity of the person) (United Nations, 2014: 11), Article 14 (liberty and security of the person) (United Nations, 2015) and Article 25 (right to health) (United Nations, 2017: 14–15).

The CRPD Committee's interpretation of Article 12 has meant that numerous governments have been considering for the first time whether forced mental health interventions are intrinsically discriminatory and incompatible with human rights standards. This interpretation has generally been resisted by parties to the Convention, through interpretive declarations stating their understanding that involuntary orders are permissible as a last resort subject to safeguards. Even so, the debates around the CRPD and connected developments signal a dislocation of dominant discourses surrounding mental health law which can be capitalized on to fuel the demand for change.

The CRPD's rearticulation of human rights standards has also contributed to renewed understandings of the measures needed to protect rights contained in other core international treaties. For example, the Special Rapporteur on torture has increasingly drawn attention to mistreatment in disability and health service settings, including situations in which forced psychiatric interventions amount to torture (United Nations, 2008; 2013). This extended to a recommendation for an 'absolute ban' on non-consensual psychiatric interventions in 2013 (United Nations, 2013: 23). A ground-breaking 2017 report of the Special Rapporteur on the right to health pointed to: failures of research to confirm concepts supporting the biomedical model; harms caused by power imbalances in psychiatry; and the imperative to research and develop 'psychosocial, recovery-oriented service and support and non-coercive alternatives to existing services' (United Nations, 2017: 5–8).

To date, much scholarship and thinking about the CRPD in the Global North has considered Article 12 and provisions prescribing how the State should *not* intervene. Yet the spectrum of CRPD rights envisions numerous actions that should be taken to support and empower people with disabilities, including Article 9 (accessibility) and Article 19 (living independently and being included in the community) (Davar, 2018), in addition to Article 12 itself which enshrines a 'support model' in the requirement that people be provided with 'the support they may require in exercising their legal capacity' (Minkowitz, 2010: 157–166). For Davar and Transforming Communities for Inclusion Asia, 'legal capacity' and 'voluntary and informed consent' are limited in their capacity to effect positive change, whereas the wider

CRPD framework revolving around Article 19 is one of 'mutual respect, interdependence and support', calling for investments in 'community based inclusion practices for their heuristic value' (Davar, 2018).

The global reach of the CRPD as an international instrument is critical considering that mental health agendas are increasingly imposed on countries around the world under the banner of the Global Mental Health Movement (Wildeman, 2013). This trend towards establishing a global hierarchy in which psychiatric classifications are unassailable risks the further erosion of diverse local knowledges about distress, madness and psychiatrization (Mills, 2018), and suppression of Indigenous practices of healing and experiences of colonization (Tam, 2013). However, the limitations of the CRPD are also heightened in countries where there is deep socio-economic inequality and governments may not recognize the status of people with psychosocial disabilities as rights holders – within or separate to (other) constituencies of disabled peoples. The manner in which the oppressions confronting people with disabilities may be inseparable from life-threatening injustices of poverty, inadequate social welfare, capitalism, occupation or war in parts of the world (Erevelles, 2011; Puar, 2017) should be of central concern for the project of Mad Studies.

The CRPD provides for people with psychosocial disabilities to exert influence on certain government processes, a position which may be used to frame and drive local, regional and international advocacy initiatives. According to the CRPD people with disabilities, including children with disabilities, through their representative organisations must be closely consulted and actively engaged in the development and implementation of laws and policies affecting them (Art 4(3)), and shall 'participate fully' in the process of monitoring the Convention's implementation (Art 33(3)). The CRPD Committee has emphasized that Art 4(3) places the 'effective and meaningful participation of persons with disabilities … at the heart of the Convention' (United Nations, 2018: 1). Importantly, these provisions are about how meaning is made and how knowledge is built, validated and activated. They mandate the creation of more authoritative roles for the fast-growing knowledges of psychiatrized people within domestic law and policy reform processes.

On the one hand, these CRPD requirements fall short of the goals of ensuring ownership and control (Sweeney, 2016), or even co-production (Roper et al, 2018), in research and policy making initiatives. On the other, this is a moment of unprecedented confluence between the agendas of Mad Studies, survivor research and the CRPD in their privileging of user and survivor perspectives, epistemologies and expertise – vis-à-vis professional medical and psy epistemologies – which offers opportunities for alliance building and collaborative action.

Conclusion

On the future society in which the heroine of *Woman on the Edge of Time* is able to find some refuge, Marge Piercy writes: '[W]hat we imagine we are working toward does a lot to define what we will consider doable action aimed at producing the future we want and preventing the future we fear' (Piercy, 2016b). We are drawn to Mad Studies because of the exciting possibilities it opens up for imagining and building futures in which we can control and nurture our own minds and bodies within community spaces offering real help and support, and assert our diverse social needs and political demands without fear that they will be redefined as illness and disorder. We have suggested that interrogating and exposing the symbolic violence of mental health law – and how this body of law renders its subjects unworthy of having their ways of being, knowing and making-meaning taken seriously through a process of ontological nullification – is a vital part of this enterprise.

Our comments on the anti-colonial work of Boaventura de Sousa Santos and international human rights trends focused on the Convention on the Rights of Persons with Disabilities have been offered in the spirit of inquiry, seeking to highlight synergies that exist between different fields from which Mad Studies may draw methods and approaches for research and activism. These developments indicate the deep extent to which individual and collective user and survivor knowledges have been absented and subverted, but also offer tools for change aligned with the Mad Studies' enterprise to recover, foster and produce knowledges that will – 'transform oppressive languages, practices, ideas, laws and systems, along with their human practitioners, in the realms of mental "health" and the psy sciences, as in the wider culture' (LeFrançois et al, 2013:13).

References

Arstein-Kerslake A and Black J (2020) Right to Legal Capacity in Therapeutic Jurisprudence: Insights from Critical Disability Theory and the Convention on the Rights of Persons with Disabilities. *International Journal of Law and Psychiatry* 68: 101535.

Ashe L (2017) *Knowing Violence: Psychiatric Hegemony and the Corruption of Care*. Presentation at the European Association of Social Anthropologists, Medical Anthropology Network Conference. Lisbon, Portugal.

Beaupert F (2018a) Freedom of Opinion and Expression: From the Perspective of Psychosocial Disability and Madness. *Laws* 7(1) (3). DOI: 10.3390/laws7010003. Accessed: 16 December 2018.

Beaupert F (2018b) Silencing Prote(x)t: Disrupting the Scripts of Mental Health Law. *University of New South Wales Law Journal* 41(3): 746–781.

Beresford P, Nettle M and Perrin R (2010) *Towards a Social Model of Madness and Distress? Exploring What Service Users Say*. York: Joseph Rowntree Foundation.

Brosnan L (2012) Power and Participation: An Examination of the Dynamics of Mental Health Service-User Involvement in Ireland. *Studies in Social Justice* 6(1): 45–66.

Brosnan L and Flynn E (2017) Freedom to Negotiate: A Proposal Extricating 'Capacity' from 'Consent'. *International Journal of Law in Context* 13(1): 58–76.

Brosnan L (2018) Who's Talking About Us Without Us? A Survivor Research Interjection into an Academic Psychiatry Debate on Compulsory Community Treatment Orders in Ireland. *Laws* 7(4) (33). DOI: 10.3390/laws7040033. Accessed: 10 December 2018.

Canvin K, Rugkåsa J, Sinclair, J and Burns T (2013) Leverage and Other Informal Pressures in Community Psychiatry in England. *International Journal of Law and Psychiatry* 36(2): 100–106.

Carney T, Tait D, Perry J, Vernon A and Beaupert F (2011) *Australian Mental Health Tribunals: Space for Fairness, Freedom, Protection & Treatment*. Sydney: Themis Press.

Costa L, Voronka J, Landry D, Reid J, McFarlane B, Reville D and Church K (2012) Recovering our Stories: A Small Act of Resistance. *Studies in Social Justice* 6(1): 85–101.

Davar B (2015) Disabilities, Colonisation and Globalisation: How the Very Possibility of a Disability Identity was Compromised for the 'Insane'. In H Spandler, J Anderson, J and B Sapey (eds) *Madness, Distress and the Politics of Disablement*. Bristol: Policy Press, 215–228.

Davar B (2018) From 'User Survivor' to 'Person with Psychosocial Disability': Why we are 'TCI Asia'. *Mad in Asia*. https://madinasia.org/2018/07/from-user-survivor-to-person-with-psychosocial-disability-why-we-are-tci-asia/. Accessed: 9 March 2019.

Decker F H (1987) Psychiatric Management of Legal Defense in Periodic Commitment Hearings. *Social Problems* 34(2): 156–171.

Dhanda A (2007) Legal Capacity in the Disability Rights Convention: Stranglehold of the Past or Lodestar for the Future. *Syracuse Journal of International Law and Commerce* 34(2): 429–462.

Erevelles N (2011) *Disability and Difference in Global Contexts: Enabling a Transformative Body Politic*. New York: Palgrave Macmillan.

Fabris E (2011) *Tranquil Prisons: Mad Peoples Experiences of Chemical Incarceration Under Community Treatment Orders*. Toronto: University of Toronto Press.

Fabris E and Aubrecht K (2014) Chemical Constraint: Experiences of Psychiatric Coercion, Restraint, and Detention as Carceratory Techniques. In L Ben-Moshe, C Chapman and A C Carey (eds) *Disability*

Incarcerated: Imprisonment and Disability in the United States and Canada. New York: Palgrave Macmillan, 185–200.

Gaventa J (2006) Finding the Spaces for Change: A Power Analysis'. *IDS bulletin* 37(6): 23–33. http://bulletin.ids.ac.uk/idsbo/article/view/898. Accessed: 10 December 2018.

Gorman R and LeFrançois B A (2018) Mad studies. In B H Z Cohen (ed), *Routledge International Handbook of Critical Mental Health.* London: Routledge, 107–114.

Gorman R, Sainia, A, Tam, L, Udegbe, O and Usar, O (2013) Mad People of Color – A Manifesto. *Asylum* 20(4): 27.

Hamilton B and Roper C (2006) Troubling "Insight": Power and Possibilities in Mental Health Care. *Journal of Psychiatric and Mental Health Nursing* 13(4): 416–422.

Hiday V A (1981) Court Discretion: Application of the Dangerousness Standard in Civil Commitment. *Law and Human Behavior* 5(4): 275–289.

Howard D and Westmore B (2018) *Crime and Mental Health Law in New South Wales.* Chatswood: Butterworths, 55.

Kinouani G (2018) *Injustice: The Root Cause of Psychological Distress?* Keynote presentation at the 8th Service User Academia Symposium. Melbourne, Australia, 15–17.

Large M, Kaneson M, Myles N, Gunaratne P and Ryan C (2016) Meta-Analysis of Longitudinal Cohort Studies of Suicide Risk Assessment among Psychiatric Patients: Heterogeneity in Results and Lack of Improvement over Time. *PLOS ONE* 1(6). DOI: 10.1371/journal.pone.0156322. Accessed: 13 December 2018.

LeBlanc S and Kinsella E A (2016) Toward Epistemic Justice: A Critically Reflexive Examination of 'Sanism' and Implications for Knowledge Generation. *Studies in Social Justice* 10(1): 59–79.

Lee J (2013) Mad as Hell: The Objectifying Experience of Symbolic Violence. In B A LeFrançois, R Menzies and G Reaume (eds) *Mad Matters: A Critical Reader in Canadian Mad Studies.* Toronto: Canadian Scholars Press, 105–121.

LeFrançois, R Menzies and G Reaume (eds) *Mad Matters: A Critical Reader in Canadian Mad Studies.* Toronto: Canadian Scholars Press.

Liegghio M (2013) A Denial of Being: Psychiatrization as Epistemic Violence. In B A LeFrançois, R Menzies and G Reaume (eds) *Mad Matters: A Critical Reader in Canadian Mad Studies.* Toronto: Canadian Scholars Press, 122–129.

Mental Health Act 2001. Dublin: Irish Statute Books.

Menzies R, LeFrançois B A and Reaume G (2013) Introducing Mad Studies. In B A LeFrançois, R Menzies and G Reaume (eds) *Mad Matters: A Critical Reader in Canadian Mad Studies.* Toronto: Canadian Scholars Press, 1–22.

Mills C (2018) The Mad are like Savages and the Savages are Mad: Psychopolitics and the Coloniality of the Psy. In B H Z Cohen (ed) *Routledge International Handbook of Critical Mental Health.* London: Routledge, 205–212.

Minkowitz T (2007) The United Nations *Convention on the Rights of Persons with Disabilities* and the Right to Be Free from Nonconsensual Psychiatric Interventions. *Syracuse Journal of International Law and Commerce* 34(2): 405–428.

Minkowitz T (2010) Abolishing Mental Health Laws to Comply with the Convention on the Rights of Persons with Disabilities. In B McSherry and P Weller P (eds) *Rethinking Rights-Based Mental Health Laws.* Oxford: Hart Publishing, 157–166.

Parry C D H, Turkheimer E and Hundley P L (1992) A Comparison of Commitment and Recommitment Hearings: Legal and Policy Implications. *International Journal of Law and Psychiatry* 15(1): 25–41.

Peay J (1989) *Tribunals on Trial: A Study of Decision-Making under the Mental Health Act 1983.* Oxford: Clarendon Press.

Perkins E (2003). *Decision-Making in Mental Health Review Tribunals.* London: Policy Studies Institute.

Piercy M (2016a) *Woman on the Edge of Time.* New York: Ballantine Books.

Piercy M (2016b) Woman on the Edge of Time, 40 Years on: 'Hope is the Engine for Imagining Utopia'. *The Guardian* 30 November. https://www.theguardian.com/books/2016/nov/29/woman-on-the-edge-of-time-40-years-on-hope-imagining-utopia-marge-piercy. Accessed: 9 March 2019.

Puar J (2017) *The Right to Maim.* Durham: Duke University Press.

Roper C (2018) Capacity Does Not Reside in Me. In C Spivakovsky, K Seear and A Carter (eds) *Critical Perspectives on Coercive Interventions: Law, Medicine and Society.* London: Routledge, 85–96.

Roper C, Grey F and Cadogan E (2018) *Co-production: Putting Principles into Practice in Mental Health Contexts.* https://recoverylibrary.unimelb.edu.au/__data/assets/pdf_file/0010/2659969/Coproduction_putting-principles-into-practice.pdf. Accessed: 9 March 2019.

Russo J and Shulkes D (2015) What We Talk about When we Talk about Disability: Making Sense of Debates in the European User/Survivor Movement. In H Spandler, J Anderson and B Sapey (eds) *Madness, Distress and the Politics of Disablement*. Bristol: Policy Press, 27–42.

Santos B (2018) *The End of the Cognitive Empire: The Coming of Age of Epistemologies of the South*. Durham: Duke University Press.

Shimrat I (2013) The Tragic Farce of "Community Mental Health Care". In B A LeFrançois, R Menzies and G Reaume (eds) *Mad Matters: A Critical Reader in Canadian Mad Studies*. Toronto: Canadian Scholars Press, 144–157.

Sjöström S (2006) Invocation of Coercion Context in Compliance Communication—Power Dynamics in Psychiatric Care. *International Journal of Law and Psychiatry* 29(1): 36–47.

Steele S (2016) Court Authorised Sterilisation and Human Rights: Inequality, Discrimination and Violence against Women and Girls with Disability. *University of New South Wales Law Journal* 39(3): 1011–1015.

Sweeney A (2016) Why Mad Studies Needs Survivor Research and Survivor Research Needs Mad Studies. *Intersectionalities: A Global Journal of Social Work Analysis, Research, Polity, and Practice* 5(3): 36–61.

Tam L (2013) 'Mad Nation?' Thinking Through Race, Class, and Mad Identity Politics. In B A LeFrançois, R Menzies and G Reaume (eds) *Mad Matters: A Critical Reader in Canadian Mad Studies*. Toronto: Canadian Scholars Press, 269–280.

United Nations (2008) *Interim Report of the Special Rapporteur on Torture and Other Cruel, Inhuman or Degrading Treatment or Punishment*. Sixty-third session. A/63/175. https://unispal.un.org/UNISPAL. NSF/0/707AC2611E22CE6B852574BB004F4C95. Accessed 5 December 2018.

United Nations (2013) *Report of the Special Rapporteur on Torture and Other Cruel, Inhuman or Degrading Treatment or Punishment*. Twenty-second session. A/HRC/22/53. https://www.ohchr.org/ Documents/HRBodies/HRCouncil/RegularSession/Session22/A.HRC.22.53_English.pdf. Accessed 5 December 2018.

United Nations (2014) *General Comment No. 1. Article 12: Equal Recognition before the Law*. CRPD/ C/11/4 (Committee on the Rights of Persons with Disabilities). https://tbinternet.ohchr.org/_ layouts/15/treatybodyexternal/Download.aspx?symbolno=CRPD/C/GC/1&Lang=en. Accessed 4 December 2018.

United Nations (2015) *Guidelines on article 14 of the Convention on the Rights of Persons with Disabilities – The Right to Liberty and Security of Persons with Sisabilities*. Fourteenth session (Committee on the Rights of Persons with Disabilities). https://tbinternet.ohchr.org/_layouts/15/treatybodyexternal/Download. aspx?symbolno=A/72/55&Lang=en. Accessed 4 December 2018.

United Nations (2017) *Report of the Special Rapporteur on the Right of Everyone to the Enjoyment of the Highest Attainable Standard of Physical and Mental Health*. Thirty-fifth session. A/HRC/35/21. https://ap.ohchr. org/documents/dpage_e.aspx?si=A/HRC/35/21. Accessed 5 December 2018.

United Nations (2018) *General Comment No 7 (2018) on the Participation of Persons with Disabilities, Including Children with Disabilities, Through their Representative Organizations, in the Implementation and Monitoring of the Convention*. CRPD/C/GC/7 (Committee on the Rights of Persons with Disabilities). https:// tbinternet.ohchr.org/_layouts/15/treatybodyexternal/Download.aspx?symbolno=CRPD/C/GC/ 7&Lang=en. Accessed 5 December 2018.

White W (2018) *Crazy Lives Matter Too: Imagining a World Where Everyone Is Valued*. Keynote presentation at the Alternatives 2018 Conference – On Our Own: Transforming the Future Together. Washington DC, United States.

Whitaker R (2002) *Mad in America: Bad Science, Bad Medicine, and the Enduring Mistreatment of the Mentally Ill*. New York: Basic Books.

Wildeman S (2013) Protecting Rights and Building Capacities: Challenges to Global Mental Health Policy in Light of the Convention on the Rights of Persons with Disabilities. *The Journal of Law, Medicine & Ethics* 41(1): 48–73.

Winick B J (2005) *Civil Commitment: A Therapeutic Jurisprudence Model*. Durham, North Carolina: Carolina Academic Press, 6.

Winick B J (1992) On Autonomy: Legal and Psychological Perspectives. *Villanova Law Review* 37(6): 1705–1777.

Žižek S (2008) *Violence: Six Sideways Reflections*. Profile Books.

PART 3

Mad Studies and knowledge equality

15

THE SUBJECTS OF OBLIVION

Subalterity, sanism, and racial erasure

Ameil Joseph

As Sherene Razack has described,

> When we depend on storytelling, either to reach each other across differences or to resist patriarchal and racist constructs, we must overcome at least one difficulty: the difference in position between the teller and the listener, between telling the tale and hearing it … wherever storytelling is used, that it should never be used uncritically, and that its potential as a tool for social change is remarkable, provided we pay attention to the interpretive structures that underpin how we hear and how we take up the stories of oppressed groups.
>
> *(Razack 1998:36–37)*

I often find myself thinking about my connections and affinities to Mad Studies, critical disability studies, studies of colonialism and critical race theory in research, teaching and in practice. I remember sitting at an event on white privilege where an all-white panel took turns sharing stories of how they learned about their unearned sane, abled, gendered, class privilege and histories complicit with racism. They did this through expressions of guilt, acknowledging the privilege attached to their obliviousness and how systems of education as well as structures around them contributed to how this was possible. As they spoke, I recall feeling a mix of sadness and rage. A feeling that is all too familiar. I thought about how my entire life has been forged within the relations that they seemed oblivious to in my world around me. My experiences of racism in schools, by police, in mental health and healthcare, as a child of immigrants to Canada from Guyana. I felt that teaching others that they were oblivious to these contemporary forms of discrimination and violence often set up a situation where trainings and workshop are the answer. This answer is inadequate.

Often, I attend to the confluence of problematic themes that flow together from common historical trajectories that are still maintained within professional distinctions, pedagogical practice, policy, law and totalizing regimes of taxonometric knowing (Joseph 2016).

I am drawn to the ways perspectives and experiences that are lived realities have been engaged for their fundamental disruptive power to dominance and subjectivity with the intent of transformation (LeFrançois et al. 2013; Faulkner 2017; Castrodale 2017; Ingram 2016; Aho

DOI: 10.4324/9780429465444-19

et al. 2017). I am also drawn to consideration of how historical discourses of innocence are forged and claimed through the appropriation of this counter-knowledge (Beresford and Russo 2016). This is carried out by the same structures of dominance and oppression that have historically erased the histories, lives, knowledge and experiences of people who are the very subjects and objects of these erasures and extractions (Russo & Beresford 2015; Voronka 2017).

I have learned a great deal from those who have calculated through experience how to speak back into the darkness of their own erasure, the ways in which these erasures are deeply connected to historical projects of incarceration, eugenics, eradication, and genocide (Ingram 2016; Leblanc & Kinsella 2016; Ben-Moshe et al. 2014; Reville & Church 2012; Sweeney 2016; Friedlander 2001). I have also learned a great deal from those who have shared the importance of attending to how these practices, social relations, discourses and technologies have become embedded within contemporary manifestations of professions, their regimes of knowledge, and pedagogical practices (Poole et al. 2012; Thomson 2010; Liegghio 2013; Joseph 2019; Kanani 2011; Patel 2014).

What I continue to struggle with are the ongoing forms of historical erasure/exclusion/silence that continue to carry out the work of global projects of elimination and how some of these practices are still quite connected to historical/contemporary projects of racial and eugenic projects of eradication (Pickens 2019; Mitchell & Snyder 2003; Meerai et al. 2016; Gramaglia 2009; Smith 2014). All of this is also deeply connected to me.

When confronted with ableism, sanism, eugenics, and white supremacy a common response is to acknowledge how oblivious some people, professions, disciplines and forms of knowledge are, and this then becomes a distancing from complicity. This is frequently presented as individualized privilege, bias and stigma, sometimes implicit or unconscious rather than systemic and structural infrastructure established to perpetuate ongoing forms of transnational denial and colonial violence (Belenen 2016; Howe 2010; Graham 2016; Torino 2018; Case & Rios 2017; Bamgbade et al. 2016; Schwartz 2019).

Often the language of invisibility is associated with white, sanist, ableist privilege. A continuation of the pedagogical practice of Peggy McIntosh encouraging an audience (presumed to be white) to unpack their privileges in order to see them and appreciate them (McIntosh 1988, 2015). Leslie Margolin among others has directly named how this pedagogical formation, while intended to challenge racism, produces complacency (2015). Specifically, as a method of anti-Blackness Margolin notes that,

> by focusing on personal identity (whites' personal identity) over institutional structures, by paying more attention to whites' experiences than to Blacks', by falsely claiming that the confession of white privileges leads to social action beneficial to Blacks, and by restoring and expanding whites' sense of moral rightness.
>
> *(2015:1)*

I would argue that this ethos is continued with Robin DiAngelo's commentary on white fragility highlighting how white reactions of "anger, fear, and guilt and behaviours such as argumentation, silence, and withdrawal" when confronted with racism are a product of the fact that people who are white are intolerant of "racial stress" in daily life and this is "born of superiority and entitlement" (2018:2).

I am concerned with how these ideas continue to supplant the perspectives of those who do not experience racism as invisible, who do not see reactions of anger to naming racism *as* fragility but active manifestations of projects of complicit erasure, denial and violence. These projects not only participate in the manufacturing of innocence broadly, they do so in very concrete ways. Specifically, these projects enable the continuation of historical projects of eugenic and racial erasure via their reliance on discourses of obliviousness as an individualized product, while maintaining control over the forms of knowledge, voice and experience permissible in these conversations (by overdetermining that which might be required to be known in order to confront the invisible). This process contributes to the ejection of subjects outside of the realm of what is most often rendered for palatability, and consumption for innocence-making – who are rendered as unknowable, unseen, rendered into oblivion.

Here, I intend to highlight how Mad Studies, critical disability studies, critical race theory and perspectives on colonialism via intergenerational knowing, can and do contribute to pedagogical practices that undermine a focus on obliviousness that renders the Other into oblivion by challenging the historiographies of invisibility/innocence as ongoing projects of white supremacy. This pedagogical practice also provides a way of exemplifying how Mad Studies, critical disability studies, critical race theory and postcolonial, decolonization studies can be applied in practice, in teaching for transformative ends.

Invisibilizing complicities and manufacturing innocence through obliviousness

In Mad Studies, histories and experiences of those who challenge psy disciplines often evade a presentation of violence by exposing ongoing forms of dehumanization and violence as symbolic, epistemic, relational, individual, systemic and structural. When I was a teenager and was taken to hospital and was immediately treated with Narcan (Naloxone – the anti-opioid overdose drug) as an assumption that I had overdosed, and later questioned about my parents' abilities, I was able to put my experience into a broader context. A context that appreciates the racial assumptions that are automated within professional mental health and health practice (Nestel 2012; Metzl 2010; Keating 2016).

When learning about critical race theory, I learned about how racism is instituted in daily life, in law, and space. When I was pulled over too many times to count while driving to my placement in grad school, I was able to look back on this while thinking about why. Was it because I was driving past Westmount Golf and Country Club, did I stand out driving through that white neighborhood? Was I going too fast every day? These ideas already had roots. Was I really that bad of a kid in elementary school? Reading Charles Mills (2014), bell hooks (2003), Patricia Hill Collins (2002), Kim Crenshaw (1990), Sherene Razack (1998) and Derrick Bell (2004) helped me appreciate historical continuities and structures that can be challenged and that are acknowledged as having life and death consequences. I challenged my driving charges after the fact and won. My parents called a race relations counsellor who confronted my principal and teacher in my elementary school, and I was moved into another class. In my example, I survived, I am still alive.

Through critical disability studies, I learned that my experiences with my mothers' progressive supranuclear palsy, and being denied basic human dignity were not isolated incidents related to particular individuals but deeply connected to systems of dehumanization, and institutionalization, problems of access and professionalism over experience (Castrodale 2017; Nabbali 2009; Beresford 2000).

Through studies of colonialism I learned about how Ranajit Guha and Gayatri Spivak (1988) transformed the Gramscian concept of the *subaltern* referring to those who have been historically jettisoned outside the lines of social mobility across the globe and often at the same time have been forced to internalize interests outside of (and often oppositional to) their own interest. When attempting to trace change and erasures by attending to the lived experiences of those rendered historically invisible, complexities continue to entangle the relations through which we are forced to be strategic about how we navigate existing oppressive, violent systems and structures, while not serving them. Simultaneously, we need to be ever critical of positions taken under the banner of resistance that perpetuate ongoing outcomes of oblivion. I thought about this concept of the subaltern specifically in relation to those who have been historically and contemporality speaking back into the voids rendered through colonial projects of obliviousness and innocence making.

Spivak also used the term "sanctioned ignorance" in her book *Death of a Discipline* (2003) and Eber Hampton talks about "perverse ignorance" in the book, *The Circle Unfolds* (1995). I thought about how I never learned about slavery and indentureship and colonialism, my histories or my stories and how these are still rendered into oblivion or crafted into palatable products for consumption divorced from ideas of complicity and ongoing violence to address white able, sane obliviousness. I think about Sarah Isabel Wallace's work on South Asian immigration exclusion based on ideas of fitness and that immigrants carry some sort of contaminating hereditary defectiveness and how this is also bound to histories that saw us as beast of burden, and carriers of lack, to be eradicated through eugenic policy, practice and law (2017). I also think about Achille Mbembe's idea of necropolitics, that appreciates that "to exercise sovereignty is to exercise control over mortality and to define life as the deployment and manifestation of power" (2008:152).

I am grateful for all these contributions and analyses. I sought them out and continue to do so as they help me to cope, struggle with, frame and interrogate the ways in which I am made to feel that my experiences are a series of coinciding products of individual bias or discrimination. Common to them are the critical practice of storytelling for transformation.

My ongoing struggle is to appreciate the confluences of analyses and ideas that help me to name my experience within nationalist and transnational context across time and space.

I think about how my experiences with my mom's progressive supranuclear palsy, racism in school, racism by police, racism in mental health and healthcare, someone screaming at my dad to go back to his country in a drive through, writing the n word on his license plate, these all already had roots related to the practices that render subjects into oblivion.

My great-grandmother was born on a boat named *Temple*, which sailed from Calcutta to Guyana in 1889. On my grandfather's birth certificate, she is identified by the boat she was born on and a registration number without a last name. Her history is actively suppressed by the technologies of eradication that actively authorized dehumanization for the specific purposes of colonial nation building and exploitation. She was brought over with a group of indentured labourers to toil in sugar cane fields. With indentureship, colonialism and empire came the erasure of languages, the supplanting of faith, belief, religion and knowledge, inferiorization, dehumanization and abject humiliation. Extreme poverty and subjugation also came with disease, violence experienced inside and outside the home, systemic alcohol use tied to sugar production, and structural exclusion. My mother grew up in a shack on stilts with cow dung flooring, whose survival depended on a story rendered into oblivion by the intentional obliviousness of the powers that crafted our circumstance. All of these tied to global projects of conquest, colonial, eugenics and national building and the establishment of human hierarchy. I have come to appreciate that this is not a story for consumption nor innocence making, but one that helps me challenge historiographies from the place of oblivion. A key contribution by subaltern studies specifically has been the contestation of erasures within historiographies of change. Rather than accepting the dominant discourses of change as transitions or progressions, we must actively work to name these as sites of struggle or "confrontation". This critical acknowledgement positions these conversations in relation to broader contexts and "histories of domination and exploitation" (Guha & Spivak 1988:3). As Spivak notes, "The most significant outcome of this revision or shift in perspective is that the agency of change is located in the insurgent or the 'subaltern'" (Guha & Spivak 1988:3). This form of attention resists appropriating maneuvers by hegemonic entities that claim progress, exploit identity and experience, and operate to reclaim positions of innocence or obliviousness to avoid transformation. It acknowledges that our circumstances of racism in daily life are bound to histories that crafted a people worthy of death and argued that this was all necessary for a more supreme people to exist.

I also think about this as someone who, worked for mental health, criminal justice and immigration organizations and agencies complicit with systems of violence that reproduce ideas of human hierarchy and professional innocence. I have come to appreciate that my own experiences are places of knowing. That Mad Studies, critical disability studies, critical race studies and studies of colonialism were a way to help me grapple with this aspect of my own struggles for liberation. I was intergenerationally born into violence rather than coming to know it afterwards via a profession or discipline and field of study. I am also complicit in ongoing practices of historical and contemporary obliviousness and innocence making that are deeply connected to colonial relations of racial and eugenic eradication.

In my research, teaching and practice I now wield this respect for intergeneration, transnational contexts of necropolitics alongside the fields that have also respected the voices, knowledges and experiences of those deemed mad, the subaltern, those actively worked against in a-historical, individual, simply local ways and into oblivion. This begins with critically reappraising historiographies of ableism, sanism, white supremacy as a confluence actively working to forge subjects of oblivion. This begins from intergenerationally lived experience and embodied knowing as epistemic disobedience. Not within an innocence-making project nor through the confrontation of obliviousness in consumable ways but rather to undermine these projects across professional and disciplinary hegemonies, while actively confronting complicity. I have learned to listen and look into the erasures of oblivion and see histories of survival and struggle, of nuanced complexities of intergenerational transnational emancipation. These are the stories I want to tell, stories resistant to appropriation, and consumption but with transformative potential.

References

Aho, T., Ben-Moshe, L., & Hilton, L. J. (2017). Mad futures: Affect/theory/violence. *American Quarterly* 69(2): 291–302.

Bamgbade, B. A., Ford, K. H., & Barner, J. C. (2016). Impact of a Mental Illness Stigma Awareness Intervention on Pharmacy Student Attitudes and Knowledge. *American journal of Pharmaceutical Education* 80(5): 80.

Belenen. (2016). Medium. *Mental Health Privilege Checklist (Neurotypical Privilege through the Lens of Mental Illness)*. https://medium.com/@belenen/mental-health-privilege-checklist-neurotypical-privilege-through-the-lens-of-mental-illness-6403b1bb43ad Accessed: 29.06.2020.

Bell, D. A. (2004). *Race, Racism, and American Law*. Aspen Pub.

Ben-Moshe, L., Chapman, C., & Carey, A. C. (Eds.) (2014). *Disability Incarcerated: Imprisonment and Disability in the United States and Canada*. Palgrave Macmillan.

Beresford, P. (2000). What Have Madness and Psychiatric System Survivors got to do with Disability and Disability Studies? *Disability & Society*, 15(1): 167–172.

Beresford, P., & Russo, J. (2016). Supporting the sustainability of Mad Studies and preventing its co-option. *Disability & Society* 31(2): 270–274.

Case, K. A., & Rios, D. (2017). Educational Interventions to Raise Awareness of White Privilege. *Journal on Excellence in College Teaching* 28(1): 137–156.

Castrodale, M. A. (2017). Critical Disability Studies and Mad Studies: Enabling New Pedagogies in Practice. *The Canadian Journal for the Study of Adult Education* 29(1): 49. https://cjsae.library.dal.ca/index.php/cjsae/article/view/5357.

Collins, P. H. (2002). *Black Feminist Thought: Knowledge, Consciousness, and the Politics of Empowerment.* Routledge.

Crenshaw, K. (1990). Mapping the Margins: Intersectionality, Identity Politics, and Violence Against Women of Color. *Stanford Law Review* 43: 1241.

DiAngelo, R. (2018). *White Fragility: Why it's so Hard for White People to Talk about Racism.* Beacon Press.

Faulkner, A. (2017). Survivor research and Mad Studies: The role and value of experiential knowledge in mental health research. *Disability & Society* 32(4): 500–520.

Friedlander, H. (2001). The exclusion and murder of the disabled. In R. Gellately & N. Stoltzfus (eds). *Social Outsiders in Nazi Germany*. Princeton University Press, 145–164.

Graham, M. (2016). The Invisible Backpack of Able-Bodied Privilege Checklist. https://melissagraham.ca/2009/10/12/the-invisible-backpack-of-able-bodied-privilege-checklist/ Accessed:29.06.2020.

Gramaglia, L. (2009). Colonial Psychiatry in British Guiana: Dr Robert Grieve. In K. White (ed). *Configuring Madness: Representation, Context and Meaning*. Inter-Disciplinary Press, 191–206.

Guha, R., & Spivak, G. C. (1988). Selected Subaltern Studies. *New York*.

Hampton, E. (1995). Towards a redefinition of Indian education. In M A Battiste & J Barman (eds). *First Nations Education in Canada: The Circle Unfolds*. University of British Columbia Press, 5–46.

hooks, b. (2003). *Teaching Community: A Pedagogy of Hope* 36. Psychology Press.

Howe, B. (2010). Able-bodied Privilege: Unpacking the Invisible Knapsack. http://billhowe.org/MCE/able-bodied-privilege-unpacking-the-invisible-knapsack/ Accessed: 29.06.2020.

Ingram, R. A. (2016). Doing Mad Studies: Making (non) Sense Together. *Intersectionalities: A Global Journal of Social Work Analysis, Research, Polity, and Practice* 5(3): 11–17.

Joseph, A. J. (2016). *Deportation and the Confluence of Violence within Forensic Mental Health and Immigration Systems*. Springer.

Joseph, A. J. (2019). Contemporary Forms of Legislative Imprisonment and Colonial Violence in Forensic Mental Health. In A. Daley, L. Costa & P. Beresford (eds). *Madness, Violence, and Power: A Critical Collection*. University of Toronto Press, 169–183.

Kanani, N. (2011). Race and Madness: Locating the Experiences of Racialized People with Psychiatric Histories in Canada and the United States. *Critical Disability Discourses/Discours critiques dans le champ du handicap*, 3.

Keating, F. (2016). Racialized Communities, Producing Madness and Dangerousness. *Intersectionalities: A Global Journal of Social Work Analysis, Research, Polity, and Practice* 5(3): 173–185.

Leblanc, S., & Kinsella, E. A. (2016). Toward epistemic justice: A critically reflexive examination of 'sanism' and implications for knowledge generation. *Studies in Social Justice*, 10(1): 59–78.

LeFrançois, B. A., Menzies, R., & Reaume, G. (Eds.). (2013). *Mad Matters: A Critical Reader in Canadian Mad Studies*. Canadian Scholars' Press.

Liegghio, M. (2013). A Denial of Being: Psychiatrization as Epistemic Violence. In B. A. LeFrançois, R. Menzies & G. Reaume (eds). *Mad Matters: A Critical Reader in Canadian Mad Studies*. Canadian Scholars' Press, 122–129.

Margolin, L. (2015). Unpacking the Invisible Knapsack: The Invention of White Privilege Pedagogy. *Cogent Social Sciences* 1(1): 1.

Mbembe, A. (2008). Necropolitics. In S. Morton & S. Bygrave (eds). *Foucault in an Age of Terror*. Palgrave Macmillan, London, 152–182.

McIntosh, P. (1988). White Privilege: Unpacking the Invisible Knapsack. https://files.eric.ed.gov/fulltext/ED355141.pdf?utm#page=43 Accessed: 29.06.2020.

McIntosh, P. (2015). Extending the Knapsack: Using the White Privilege Analysis to Examine Conferred Advantage and Disadvantage. *Women & Therapy* 38(3–4): 232–245.

Meerai, S., Abdillahi, I., & Poole, J. (2016). An Introduction to Anti-Black Sanism. *Intersectionalities: A Global Journal of Social Work Analysis, Research, Polity, and Practice* 5(3): 18–35.

Metzl, J. M. (2010). *The Protest Psychosis: How Schizophrenia Became a Black Disease*. Beacon Press.

Mills, C. W. (2014). *The Racial Contract*. Cornell University Press.

Mitchell, D., & Snyder, S. (2003). The Eugenic Atlantic: Race, Disability, and the Making of an International Eugenic Science, 1800–1945. *Disability & Society* 18(7): 843–864.

Nabbali, E. M. (2009). A "Mad" Critique of the Social Model of Disability. *International Journal of Diversity in Organisations, Communities & Nations* 9(4): 1–12.

Nestel, Sheryl (2012). *Colour Coded Health Care: The Impact of Race and Racism on Canadians' Health*. Wellesley Institute.

Patel, S. (2014). Racing Madness: The Terrorizing Madness of the Post-9/11 Terrorist Body. In L. Ben-Moshe, C. Chapman & A. Carey (eds) *Disability Incarcerated*. Palgrave Macmillan, 201–215.

Pickens, T. A. (2019). *Black Madness: Mad Blackness*. Duke University Press.

Poole, J., Jivraj, T., Arslanian, A., Bellows, K., Chiasson, S., Hakimy, H., ... & Reid, J. (2012). Sanism, 'Mental Health', and Social Work/education: A Review and Call to Action. *Intersectionalities: A Global Journal of Social Work Analysis, Research, Polity, and Practice* 1(1): 20–36.

Razack, S. (1998). *Looking White People in the Eye: Gender, Race, and Culture in Courtrooms and Classrooms*. University of Toronto Press.

Reville, D., & Church, K. (2012). Mad Activism Enters its Fifth Decade: Psychiatric Survivor Organizing in Toronto. In A. Choudry, J. Hanley & E. Schragge (eds) *Organize*, 189–201.

Russo, J., & Beresford, P. (2015). Between Exclusion and Colonisation: Seeking a Place for Mad People's Knowledge in Academia. *Disability & Society* 30(1): 153–157.

Schwartz, S. (2019). Education Week. *Next Step in Diversity Training: Teachers Learn to Face Their Unconscious Biases*. https://mobile.edweek.org/c.jsp?cid=25919951&rssid=25919141&item=http://api.edweek.org/v1/ew/index.html?uuid=19748B1A-7332-11E9-9D99-B4F258D98AAA Accessed:29.06.2020.

Smith, L. (2014). *Insanity, Race and Colonialism: Managing Mental Disorder in the Post-emancipation British Caribbean*. Springer, 1838–1914.

Spivak, G. C. (2003). *Death of a Discipline*. Columbia University Press.

Sweeney, A. (2016). Why Mad Studies Needs Survivor Research and Survivor Research Needs Mad Studies. *Intersectionalities: A Global Journal of Social Work Analysis, Research, Polity, and Practice* 5(3): 36–61.

Thomson, M. (2010). Disability, Psychiatry, and Eugenics. In A. Bashford & P Levine (eds) *The Oxford Handbook of the History of Eugenics*. Oxford University Press, 116–133.

Torino, G. C. (2018). Examining Biases and White Privilege: Classroom Teaching Strategies that Promote Cultural Competence. In A. Dottolo & E. Kaschak (eds) *Whiteness and White Privilege in Psychotherapy*. Routledge, 129–141.

Voronka, J. (2017). Turning Mad Knowledge into Affective Labor: The Case of the Peer Support Worker. *American Quarterly*, 69(2): 333–338.

Wallace, S. I. (2017). *Not Fit to Stay: Public Health Panics and South Asian Exclusion*. UBC Press.

16

INSTITUTIONAL CEREMONIES?

The (im)possibilities of transformative co-production in mental health

Sarah Carr

Introduction

This chapter is a critical examination of 'transformative co-production' in mental health services and systems, with a particular focus on British mental health policy and practice. The policy critique is located within the discipline of Mad Studies. I am writing both as a survivor and an academic, discussing the challenges for co-production operating both within and beyond the limits of psychiatric culture, institutions and clinical paradigms. I look at the origins of co-production, the purportedly radical approach to service, system and social reform, and the associated policy construction, which occurred outside the service user and survivor movement. Inherent power asymmetries and risk of co-option and neutralization within traditional mental health services are explored, with reference to the precedents of recovery and peer support. The effect of the historical legacy of the asylum on the possibility of achieving co-production between service users and survivors and mental health service staff and managers within psychiatric systems is critically examined using Rosenhan's study of psychiatric hospitals and Goffman's theory of the 'total institution'. Finally, I conclude with the argument that co-production will not work without thorough attention to the underlying epistemic injustices that continue in the mental health structures and systems it is supposed to transform, and that Mad Studies offers an important new development here.

The faulty policy

The meanings and origins of co-production as a general concept are somewhat complex and contested. It has been critiqued for its 'excessive elasticity' (Needham and Carr, 2009). This has often proven to be problematic for its practical application in health and social care research, policy and practice, leading to frequent and repeated attempts to define the approach. Nonetheless this 'elasticity' can open up a space for critical discussion of co-production and the possibility of its applications in mental health. Farr has noted that 'the theoretical roots of … concepts of co-production and co-design are distinct from other radical participatory literatures that have politically emancipatory aims such as feminist, post-colonial, indigenous knowledge and critical theory' (Farr, 2018:625). Mental health has been the most challenging field for co-production to gain traction and have an impact on the ability of politically positioned service

DOI: 10.4324/9780429465444-20

users and survivors to determine and lead on system transformation (Carr, 2016). However, there is some agreement, based in evidence and policy analysis for mental health, that co-production between service users/ survivors and practitioners as equals means 'the transformation of power and control' (Slay and Stephens, 2013:4) and it is therefore a 'potentially transformative way of thinking about power, resources, partnerships, risks and outcomes, not an off-the-shelf model of service provision or a single magic solution' (Needham and Carr, 2009:1). This implies that the co-production project is not just to improve mental health service provision and research, but to fundamentally transform systemic power relations. The challenges here are clear, given the 'power asymmetries' that persist in mental health systems and biomedical psychiatry, most recently highlighted by the UN Special Rapporteur on the right to health. He reported that three major obstacles stood in the way of mental health reform: power asymmetries, the biased use of evidence in mental health research and the dominance of the biomedical model. Of power asymmetries he noted that 'at the clinical level, power imbalances reinforce paternalism and even patriarchal approaches, which dominate the relationship between psychiatric professionals and users of mental health services' (UNHRC, 2017:6). Nonetheless he recommended that States 'ensure that users are involved in the design, implementation, delivery and evaluation of mental health services, systems and policies' (UNHRC, 2017:21). But is this possible given the relational, systemic and structural power asymmetries?

Elsewhere I have explored the origins of co-production in US and UK public administration and health service reform (Carr, 2018). It is important to understand this aspect because such a critical analysis reveals some of the fault lines inherent in co-production policy construction, not least because it largely excluded the knowledge and contributions of the service user and survivor movement (Beresford, 2019), and has its roots in a different place (Carr, 2014). It could even be argued that co-production was imposed by the British government on health and social care service users. Here, I will briefly outline two key points from my examination of the policy of co-production: public service delivery vs. social justice and the problems of control and citizenship.

Firstly, it appears that two conflicting models of co-production were absorbed into British health and social care policy in the late 2000s. One is concerned with citizens engaging with public services to improve delivery and outcomes, and the other has a more radical and broader focus on social justice and achieving a 'core economy' where social and emotional contributions are valued as much as financial ones. The model developed by the economist Elinor Ostrom in the 1970s determined the importance of relationships between public services and citizens because the latter has valuable knowledge that is important for the effective and efficient operation of those services. This requires certain relationships and behaviours from the human actors within the system (Ostrom, 1996; Garn, 1973). This type of co-production is led by public service administrators and professionals, with the citizen and service user role determined by them (Bovaird, 2007). The later approach was developed by US legal academic and citizen advocacy campaigner, Edgar Cahn whose experiences as a hospital patient following a heart attack made him critical of the operation of a health and care system in which he felt 'declared useless' and which created 'throw-away people' (Cahn, 2000). Rather than improving service efficiency and effectiveness, his focus was on relocating power and worth with the service user or patient as a citizen and fundamentally challenging the services and systems that declared them useless. He argued for the disruption of the conventional power relations between service users or patients and professionals, promoting 'reciprocity: stop creating dependencies and devaluing those whom you help whilst you profit from their troubles'; 'an asset perspective: no more throw-away people' and 'social capital: no more disinvesting in families, neighbourhoods and communities' (Cahn, 2008:31). There is a basic tension between the two approaches: while one calls for the system to be improved, the other calls for the system to be dismantled. However, based on both these models, a 'hybrid version of co-production coalesced as a core health and social care reform concept' in the UK (Carr, 2018:79), with Edgar Cahn's model as the policy brand but Ostrom's approach implemented in practice. By 2008 co-production had entered into the 'language of the ruling regime' (LeFrançois et al, 2013:25). As Beresford observed in his historical account of the co-production of knowledge and change in health and social care, this tension is reflected in, and perhaps related to, the inherent conflicts between 'consumerist and democratic' participation where the shared language of participation 'disguises fundamental difference between them, which have blurred and confused the issues' (Beresford, 2019:6).

The second point concerns control and citizenship. The case of the contested and partial citizenship of the mental health service users/survivors has been well made, by describing the 'illusion of citizenship' for those with a diagnosis of 'mental illness' (Sayce, 2000). This is a particular impediment to achieving political citizenship as 'people with mental health challenges do not have the same legal rights as other citizens: in particular the UK's mental health laws permit compulsory treatment of people even when you have "capacity"' (Sayce, 2015:4). Despite this, policy makers assumed that mental health service users/survivors could fulfil the role of active citizen or pseudo-management consultant (Scourfield, 2007; Carr, 2014). They are expected to act as 'patient leaders' and be willing to collaborate, ostensibly in equal partnership with professionals, to 'improve the patient experience', rather than challenge systemic and wider structural problems. This was despite the fact that service hierarchies, 'current system configurations … and processes can actively prevent them from exercising their citizenship' (Carr, 2014:31). Such a tendency towards the 'mobilisation of bias' (Farr, 2018) and the imposition of 'normative citizenship' (Voronka, 2017) was foreseen by Brudney in 1985 who warned that it may

> …lead to service delivery arrangements in which citizens undertake activities that fit administrators' preferences for citizen involvement and/or for the convenience of their present positions – rather than those that might augment service effectiveness or contribute to a restoration of communitarian values and citizenship.
>
> *(Brudney, 1985:252–253)*

A key obstacle to achieving the 'restoration of communitarian values and citizenship' for mental health service users/survivors is the continued absenting and marginalization of user-led organizations from both the original policy conceptualization and the active implementation of co-production. Both remain led by professionals with their own collective power bases and organizations (Carr, 2018). Pestoff has argued that co-production is not entirely possible without the collective, independent power bases and separate platforms provided by user-led and community organizations, saying that they 'can prove very important for facilitating the participation of persons with serious physical, mental or social problems and for retaining their participation over time' (Pestoff, 2013:394). However, the Ostrom-Cahn tension has been borne out in practice, as Farr observes

> service user movements may create more disruptive innovations that challenge institutions, whereas co-production and co-design processes tend to work within institutions. The emphasis on partnership with public service institutions may overlook the importance of observable conflict, agonism and contentious opposition.
>
> *(Farr, 2018:626)*

This reflects Cahn's assertion that 'hell-raising is a critical part of co-production' (Cahn, 2008:4).

The neutralizing formula

Of academia and Mad Studies, LeFrançois warned of 'what might happen when partnerships harm more than help, or when our goals lose their initially unabashed political grounding, or when we become corrupted by a hierarchical and competitive ... culture detached from the mad community and people's everyday lives' (Le François, 2016:vii). In mental health systems there are a number of precedents to the co-option and neutralization of transformative co-production where radical, transformative ideas in mental health originating with service users and survivors have been absorbed and defined by hierarchical mental health services, administrative systems and biomedical understandings (Carr, 2016). This of course includes the value placed on and the acceptance of, survivor knowledge (Beresford, 2019). A classic example of this is personal recovery in mental health, which like co-production, services and professionals have found 'difficult to define' (Le Boutillier et al, 2015). Despite this, the approach has been absorbed into the mainstream and in Britain at least, administratively splintered into three different types of 'recovery': clinical recovery with the defining power remaining with the clinician who determines recovery in terms of symptom reduction; personal recovery in line with original thinking on hope, identity, autonomy, social recovery and citizenship; and service-defined recovery with the practice determined according to the 'service goals and financial needs to the organisation' (Le Boutillier et al, 2015:1). The ultimate challenge of recovery, as defined by pioneer US survivor and disability rights activist, Deegan (1987) and others, was to mental health and psychiatric theories, systems and structures, which require 'a transformation of services, practices *and the paradigm* within which they are delivered' (Slade et al, 2014:12) (emphasis added). However, that paradigm is yet to shift. This situation has led Morrow to set out a critique of the co-option of recovery in Canada, in which she explores the implementation of recovery frameworks in 'neoliberal political regimes' and governmentality. Her analysis reveals a very similar situation to that of co-production where there are competing and incompatible models and where 'recovery as a concept and a paradigm is poised to either disrupt biomedical dominance in favour of social and structural understandings of mental distress or to continue to play into individualistic discourses ... which work against social change' (Morrow, 2013:323). Just as co-production which only serves to 'improve the patient experience' within services and is unable to progress broader social justice issues, Morrow argues that 'recovery suffers from its individualistic framing as a personal journey which has neglected a wider analysis of social and structural relations in mental health that signal systemic discrimination...' (Morrow, 2013:325). Drawing on her critical recovery research with service users and survivors, Morrow surfaces the continued importance placed on independent peer support in recovery by people who experience mental and emotional distress.

Mad Studies scholars have also analysed the journey of peer support from its roots in mutually supportive service user and survivor relationships, networks and initiatives as a response to experiences of powerlessness and the harms of the biomedical model, to its co-option and operationalization in traditional mental health systems and hierarchies (Russo and Sweeney, 2016). Research from the Netherlands on the experience of peer workers in mainstream mental health services suggests that their work can be impeded by professional routines and concepts of 'good care' and that they can struggle with a conflicted sense of identity, crisis oriented cultures without service user involvement and with administrative procedures that compromise peer support values (Vandewalle et al, 2015). Elsewhere research has shown that the rules and constraints of mainstream mental health services are at odds with the recovery philosophy as rooted in the service user and survivor movement (Gillard et al, 2014). This situation has led Brown and Stastny to ask if peer support is a 'transformative or collusive experiment' (Brown and Stastny, 2016:183). In their examination of the co-option of survivor knowledge, Penney and Prescott focus on peer support and the familiar dynamics when

> movements for social justice by marginalised and oppressed groups often face the challenge of co-optation by powerful institutions seeking to protect the status quo … [it] is a process by which a dominant group attempts to absorb or neutralize a weaker opposition that it believes poses a threat to its continued power.
>
> *(Penney and Prescott, 2016:35)*

Consistent with the research cited here, the authors discuss the challenges of maintaining peer support practices that are rooted in the service user and survivor movement in traditional psychiatric environments where practitioners do not understand the foundational value base of the approach and its original transformative ambitions are undermined. Further to this Voronka asserts that involvement and co-production determined by mental health professionals and systems, specifically peer support, amounts to madness, mad identities and marginalized knowledge being 'harnessed as a commodity for exchange in neoliberal care and service markets' (Voronka, 2017:334). According to Voronka, mad movements have been turned into 'models' to be co-opted by dominant mainstream mental health services and practices, where 'our inclusion does little to disrupt structural violence, and rather allows psy powers to proceed' in managing, controlling and administering madness (Voronka, 2017:336).

In an attempt to answer the question 'are mainstream mental health services ready to progress transformative co-production?' I assessed the mechanisms for the co-option and neutralization of service user and survivor originated ideas for fundamentally transforming understandings of madness and mental distress, along with the support for people experiencing these. I examined the fates of empowerment, personal and social recovery, service user and survivor participation and direct payments. On the basis of this analysis I concluded that despite or because the aim of transformative co-production is to dismantle institutions, it is at risk of being absorbed into traditional mental health service culture and of becoming 'part of institutionally or professionally defined procedure' (Carr, 2016:1). Even though the transformative co-production project is to 'transform power and control' thereby involving professionals in the process of disruption, 'institutional control in the form of traditional rules and roles can negatively affect the way practitioners can work equally and collaboratively with service users and survivors' (Carr, 2016:2). It appears, from the evidence examined here, that the continued operation of the 'total institution' and its control and administration of madness is one of the biggest challenges for achieving transformative co-production in mental health.

The legacy of harm

The New Zealand survivor activist Mary O'Hagan has described the 'legacy of harm' left by psychiatry and its institutions, and the consequent continuation of psychiatric harm in contemporary practice and community settings (O'Hagan, 2016). Does this historical legacy of harm make co-production largely impossible unless it is recognised and addressed in the process, particularly where mental health service users/survivors and professionals are expected to work together to transform concepts of and responses to madness and distress? Scull wrote in his book on the experimental atrocities carried out in 'mad-houses' by the American 'mad-doctor' Henry Cotton in the early twentieth century: 'cultures and … institutions cling to retrospective illusions, substitute them for a fuller record of the past, and fiercely resist reconstructions that would disturb and displace the myths we … live by' (Scull, 2007:274). In researching and writing the book his stated aim was to promote an understanding of the history of material and structural violence in psychiatry to avoid inflicting symbolic violence in the present day. Voronka and other Mad Studies scholars are very clear that structural and symbolic violence against mad people continues in mental health services (Voronka, 2016; LeFrançois et al, 2013). To understand the origins of this structural violence that makes equal partnerships between professionals and service users/survivors (or mad people and mad doctors) almost unrealizable for co-production, it is worth revisiting two foundational critiques of psychiatry and its institutions – those of the sociologist Goffman and the psychologist Rosenhan. Both authors have attracted criticism (Cummins, 2017), but their research and theories remain useful for analysing the problems the historical legacy of the institution poses for transformative co-production in mental health.

In 1877, L S Forbes Winslow wrote and published a slim volume for use by British county asylum and hospital staff called *Handbook for Attendants on the Insane* (Forbes Winslow, 1877). This manual set out a strict set of rules for treating and administering 'lunatics' in the institution, from restraint and seclusion to force feeding via the mouth, nose and rectum, to bathing and corpse dressing. Although Forbes Winslow instructs against the gratuitous 'ill-treatment of patients', the manual clearly sets out the rules for material violence in asylums and the associated tasks and roles for staff. Violence was part of the everyday working routine and patients were entirely powerless and dehumanized. Nearly a century later Rosenhan revealed the continuation of this legacy in his famous psychological experiment 'On Being Sane in Insane Places' (Rosenhan, 1973), research which would probably not be ethically permissible today. The study focused on the experiences of eight 'pseudopatients' who had tricked their way into various American psychiatric institutions and received 'sticky' and stigmatizing psychodiagnostic labels that determined how their behaviour was perceived by staff and resulted in dismissal and depersonalization. Among other things, Rosenhan concluded that staff operated in a hierarchical institution which caused the depersonalizing responses to patients and where nurses and attendants were subordinate to frequently absent or removed psychiatrists who retained the most power and influence. He asked readers to 'consider the structure of the typical psychiatric hospital. Staff and patients are strictly segregated…staff keep to themselves, almost as if the disorder that afflicts their charges is somehow catching' (Rosenhan, 1973:254). In his re-reading of Rosenhan, Cummins argues that the findings of the experiment are still relevant for understanding 'relational attitudes within institutional settings', dividing practices' and 'toxic organisational cultures' in the 'closed worlds' that still exist in mental health systems today (Cummins, 2017:9–10). Such 'toxic cultures' and 'closed worlds' remain sites for contemporary examples of depersonalisation and abuse in the psychiatric system, from difficulties for patients raising safety concerns (Berzins et al, 2018) and reporting incidences of sexual violence on wards (Foley and Cummins, 2018) to the targeted violence and abuse of people with mental distress by staff in closed environments and in the community (Carr et al, 2019).

The themes of segregation, administration and dehumanization continue in Goffman's seminal volume, 'Asylums' (Goffman, 1961). In it he describes the function and operation of the 'total institution' (of which the asylum is one) its discourses and structures of power and how staff and 'inmates' are expected to behave within it: 'all phases of the day's activities are tightly scheduled, with one activity leading at a prearranged time into the next, the whole sequence of activities being imposed from above by a system of explicit formal rulings and a body of officials' (Goffman, 1961:17). Important for understanding the extent to which equal collaboration or alliances can be achieved between staff and service users/survivor in the transformative co-production project is Goffman's assertion that 'total institutions vary … in the amount of role differentiation found within the staff and inmate groupings, and in the clarity of the line between the two strata' (Goffman, 1961:110). Like Rosenhan's research findings, Goffman's theory is that asylums had very clear lines of differentiation between staff and patients and operated on dominance and subjugation, with discipline and punishment power dynamics throughout the hierarchy. Communication was limited and strictly formalized where 'not only will acts be required, but also the outward show of inward feelings. Expressed attitudes ... will be explicitly penalised' (Goffman, 1961:108). If we are to accept Goffman's analysis and theory, it can provide an explanation for the situation in service user/survivor involvement and consequently co-production where discussion and deliberation is subject to 'a significant exercise of power ... in the context of an institutional setting ... where the ability to exercise power in a meeting is linked to the institutional power relations in operation' (Hodge, 2005:174). Furthermore, the service users/survivors whose expressions are testimonial, emotional or disruptive during mental health involvement initiatives can be penalized by being discredited and marginalized (Barnes, 2002; Carr, 2007).

The question of (in)justice

Among many other aspects of Mad Studies, other chapters in this book explore the important idea of 'epistemic injustice', a theory that is highly relevant for our assessment of the possibilities for transformative co-production to work in mental health. The most basic 'epistemic practice' is 'the practice of gaining knowledge by being told' (Fricker, 2003:154). Developed by the philosopher Fricker (2007), the theory of epistemic injustice is a way of explaining how and why some people's knowledge is given less credibility than others based on social and individual prejudice. Fricker argues that this often happens to people who are the most powerless in society. This powerlessness and the damaging social identities given to certain groups of people (such as those deemed mad or those who are racialized) makes speaking and asserting their knowledge problematic. Epistemic injustice therefore happens when someone is 'wronged specifically in her capacity as a knower' (Fricker, 2007:18). In other words, a person's status and social identity determines whether or not their knowledge is seen as reliable and credible, and the decision about what is legitimate and true is often made by the more powerful in society (Fricker, 2003). Fricker describes this as 'testimonial injustice' which arises when 'prejudice on the part of the hearer leads to the speaker receiving less credibility than he or she deserves' (Fricker, 2003:154) and is a form of oppression or even 'epistemic violence' (Dotson, 2011). According to Fricker if a 'hearer's prejudice wrongly deflates her judgement of credibility, then the flow of knowledge is blocked, and truths fail to flow from knower to inquirer' (Fricker, 2008:69). Fricker also describes 'hermenutical injustice' as part of epistemic injustice, which LeBlanc and Kinsella explain as being 'the art of interpretation, which affects people's ability to express themselves or to be understood' (LeBlanc and Kinsella, 2016:67). They assert that 'hermenutical injustices are revealed in the lack of opportunities for Mad persons to participate in the generation of interpretive resources for making sense of madness' (LeBlanc and Kinsella, 2016:67). Although this theory is relevant for exploring the shortcomings of co-production to generate new understandings of and responses to madness, for the purposes of our exploration of transformative co-production, the notion of 'testimonial injustice' is most relevant because in the co-production process we are looking at 'testimonial exchange' where the speakers' knowledge can be discredited in the process by hearers (inquirers) who retain particular social and individual prejudices about the speakers (knowers).

Newbigging and Ridley argue that 'the testimony of people experiencing mental distress is ... at high risk of being viewed as irrelevant or unreliable and, therefore ignored, downgraded or rejected' (Newbigging and Ridley, 2018:37). Not being believed and having 'voices of less eligibility' when people are victims of crime is an example of this (Carver et al, 2017). The same could be said of the co-option, neutralization and 'silencing' of service user/survivor generated approaches such as recovery and peer support, which are not deemed credible until controlled by professionals. If the service user/survivor is the discredited speaker in the co-production process (as the evidence here suggests), then the professional fulfils the role of the hearer. For formulating explanations for mental distress with the service user in clinical settings, Lakeman asserts that 'forms of epistemic injustice can be perpetuated in subtle ways, but with far-reaching consequences. Obviously health professionals need to be scrupulous in their determinations of decisional capacity and acknowledge its dynamic nature' (Lakeman, 2010:152). The same is even truer of transformative co-production between service users/survivors and professionals in mental health working in culturally institutional environments with historical legacies of material violence and continuing problems with structural and symbolic violence, and where people have been accorded social otherness and dehumanized because of their psychodiagnostic labels. Resisting systematic epistemic injustice in such an environment will be overwhelmingly challenging, particularly if madness tropes such as 'hysterical' are being used to dismiss women's testimony in general circumstances (Fricker, 2003). Fricker makes an important point about the position of the hearer in moving towards epistemic justice, when she says: 'But it is not simply a matter of failure to properly accommodate the speaker's social identity ... the hearers fail to adjust for the way in which their *own* social identity affects the testimonial exchange' (Fricker, 2003:169) (emphasis added). This is played out in LeBlanc and Kinsella's argument about epistemic justice and 'sanism' where service users/survivors have a received social identity of 'pathological' and professionals' received social identity is 'normal' (LeBlanc and Kinsella, 2016). In terms of epistemic injustice, one is accorded a 'credibility deficit' and the other, a 'credibility excess'. If we return to Rosenhan's assertion that staff in the psychiatric hospital fear of catching madness and so strictly segregate themselves from the patients and refuse to listen to them, we can see how this was engrained in everyday practice and the legacy will affect co-production. This illustrates how 'stereotypes informing testimonial exchange will tend to imitate relations of social power at large in the society' (Fricker, 2003:164), a society which has demanded the incarceration and segregation of the mad. So is there any way to overcome this epistemic injustice to achieve the type of testimonial exchange needed for transformative co-production for mental health?

Farr has argued that co-production requires 'constant critical reflective practice and dialogue ... to facilitate more equal relational processes' (Farr, 2018:623). Again we can look to Fricker for a theoretical solution to the epistemic injustice potentially inherent in the transformative co-production project. Her idea of 'reflexive critical openness to the word of others' appears to offer a helpful perspective on solving the seemingly intractable ethical and practical problems between professionals and service users/survivors in the testimonial exchange. This openness relies on what she calls 'testimonial sensitivity'. She writes that 'an appropriately trained testimonial sensibility enables the hearer to respond to the word of another with the sort of critical openness that is required for a thoroughly effortless sharing of knowledge' (Fricker, 2003:163). Testimonial sensibility is influenced by the hearers' socialization and through their individual experience. Fricker clarifies that 'testimonial sensibility, then, needs to be shaped by collective and individual experiences described in rich, socially specific terms relating to the trustworthiness of the speakers of different social types in different contexts' (Fricker, 2003:161). For transformative co-production, then, the professionals involved in co-production need to be aware of the context in which they are operating. They also need to be aware of their own position as hearer and remain sensitive to their own influences and socialization in institutional practice on their perception of the speaker and the degree of credibility accorded to their knowledge.

Fricker says this sensibility is also dependent on the cultural-historical setting of the testimo-nial exchange, such as that of the asylum where there was no meaningful critical awareness of the institutionalized prejudices that led to epistemic injustice and violence. In this case Fricker would argue the staff were not yet in a position to know better. Arguably professionals are now in a position to know better, despite the reproduction of the dynamics of the asylum in con-temporary mental health practice, and in co-production.

Conclusion

Perhaps the fundamental question for transformative co-production is, 'how can professionals and service users/survivors exist within an institutional system with such a track record and his-torical legacy as discussed here, and then be expected to function as allies and equals within the same system in order to dismantle it?'. The operation of rules and roles in institutional cultures and hierarches, past and present can also be damaging to professionals. Goffman describes the 'institutional ceremonies' such as social events held in the asylum and the 'role release', which may occur as staff–patient boundaries become momentarily blurred: 'Given the usual roles, given the pervasive effect of inmate-staff distance, any alteration in the direction of expressing solidarity automatically represents a role release' (Goffman, 1961:90). The notion of the role release is an important one, but co-production cannot work as an 'institutional ceremony'. Needham's research with housing officers and tenants showed that co-production needs to be facilitated away from institutional cultures or service settings. Service users/survivors and ally professionals need to 'move away from the point of delivery and create forums in which officials and citizens can articulate service experiences [and] recognise common ground' (Needham, 2008:229). Additionally, professionals may have their own experiences of mental distress that they cannot disclose in their institutionalized role. In his commentary on Rosenhan, Cummins notes that 'there is a danger of using only one aspect of a person's identity as a means of classifi-cation. All of us have many roles and identities' (Cummins, 2017:9). In this respect Mad Studies could offer a way of developing radical forms of co-production because it 'treats survivors' first hand knowledge with equality', but 'is a venture we can all work for together in alliance. So it includes the experiential knowledge/wisdom of workers and the knowledge of those offering support...' (Beresford, 2019:10). With an emphasis on plurality, the discipline operates beyond the limits of the biomedical model and the psychiatric paradigm. It can therefore challenge and resist the oppressive rules and roles that are the legacy of the institution as described here, and promote equal collaboration with mad-positive allies and scholars. As LeFrançois has argued, 'this form of knowledge production and activism also acknowledges not needing to resist and toil wholly on our own to dismantle what has become an all too economically powerful and deeply entrenched psychiatric system' (LeFrançois, 2016:v).

Transformative co-production in mental health can be usefully reframed as an ethical project, underpinned by epistemic justice and the idea of the testimonial exchange in the co-productive process. In order to undertake this exchange with service users/survivors, professionals who are the hearers need to exercise what Fricker calls 'testimonial sensibility' in order for the speaker's knowledge to be rendered credible in the exchange. Awareness of the historical legacy of the asylum as total institution and the associated power dynamics between staff and patients where strict rules and roles applied and violence was permitted as standard practice must inform the development of this testimonial sensibility. Attentiveness to the mechanisms of co-option and neutralization to resist disruption as forms of epistemic injustice is equally important. Finally, professionals should retain a sensitivity to their own testimonies and experiences in the exchange, particularly if those relate to their own experiences of mental distress. These factors still affect the positioning of the hearer and speaker and the credibility accorded to their relative testimonies and knowledge in co-productive processes within the phantom institutions of contemporary mental health services. They must therefore be overcome before service users/survivors and our allies can begin to collaborate on the dismantling of our contemporary institutions because ghost asylums still haunt our actions and our minds.

References

Barnes M (2002) Bringing difference into deliberation? Disabled people, survivors and local governance. *Policy & Politics* 30 (3), 319–331.

Beresford P (2019). Public participation in health and social care: Exploring the co-production of knowledge. *Frontiers in Sociology* 3 (41), 1–12.

Berzins K, Louch G., Brown M, O'Hara J & Baker J (2018). Service user and carer involvement in mental health care safety: Raising concerns and improving the safety of services. *BMC Health Services Research* 18 (644).

Bovaird T. (2007). Beyond engagement and participation: User and community coproduction of public services. *Public Administration Review September/October 2007*, 846–860.

Brown C & Stastny P (2016). Peer workers in the mental health system: A transformative or collusive experiment? In Russo J and Sweeney A (2016). *Searching for a Rose Garden: Challenging Psychiatry, Fostering Mad Studies*. Monmouth: PCCS Books, 183–191.

Brudney J L (1985). Coproduction: Issues in implementation. *Administration and Society* 17 (4), 243–256.

Cahn E (2000). *No More Throw-away People: The Co-production Imperative*. Washington: Essential Books.

Cahn E (2008). Foreword: A commentary from the United States. In L Stephens, J Ryan-Collins and D Boyle (eds.). *Co-production: A Manifesto for Growing the Core Economy*. London: New Economics Foundation.

Carr S (2007). Participation, power, conflict and change: Theorizing dynamics of service user participation in the social care system of England and Wales. *Critical Social Policy* 27 (2), 266–276.

Carr S (2014). Personalisation, participation and policy construction: A critique of influences and understandings in Beresford, P. (ed.) (2014). *Critical and radical debates in social work: Personalisation*. Bristol: Policy Press, 27–32.

Carr S (2016). *Are Mainstream Mental Health Services Ready to Progress Transformative Co-production?* Bath: NDTi.

Carr S (2018). Who owns co-production? In P Beresford & S Carr (eds.) *Social Policy First Hand*. Bristol: Policy Press, 74–83.

Carr S, Hafford-Letchfield T, Faulkner A, Megele C, Gould D, Khisa C, Cohen R & Holley J (2019). "Keeping control": A user-led exploratory study of mental health service user experiences of targeted violence and abuse in the context of adult safeguarding in England. *Health and Social Care in the Community* https://doi.org/10.1111/hsc.12806. Accessed: 05.07.2020.

Carver L, Morley S and Taylor P (2017). Voices of deficit: Mental health, criminal victimization and epistemic injustice. *Illness, Crisis and Loss* 25 (1), 43–62.

Cummins I (2017). Rereading Rosenhan. *Illness, Crisis & Loss* https://doi.org/10.1177/1054137317690377. Accessed: 05.07.2020.

Deegan P (1987). Recovery, rehabilitation and the conspiracy of hope. https://www.patdeegan.com/sites/default/files/files/conspiracy_of_hope.pdf. Accessed 30.05.2019.

Dotson K (2011). Tracking epistemic violence, tracking practices of silencing *Hypatia* 26 (2), 236–257.

Farr M (2018). Power dynamics and collaborative mechanisms in coproduction and co-design processes. *Critical Social Policy* 38 (4), 623–644.

Foley M & Cummins I (2018). Reporting sexual violence on mental health wards. *Journal of Adult Protection* 20 (2), 93–100.

Forbes Winslow L S (1877). *Handbook for Attendants on the Insane*. Leopold Classic Library.

Fricker M (2003). Epistemic injustice and a role for virtue in the politics of knowing. *Metaphilosophy 34* (1/2), 154–173.

Fricker M (2007). *Epistemic Injustice: Power and the Ethics of Knowing*. Oxford: Oxford University Press.

Fricker M (2008). Forum on Miranda Fricker's "Epistemic Injustice: Power and the Ethics of Knowing": Précis. *Theoria: An International Journal for Theory, History and Foundations of Science 23* (1), 69-71.

Garn H A (1973). Public services on the assembly line. *Evaluation 1* (36), 41–42.

Gillard S, Edwards C, Gibson S, Holley J & Owen K (2014). *New Ways of Working in Mental Health Services: A Qualitative, Comparative Case Study Assessing and Informing the Emergence of New Peer Worker Roles in Mental Health Services in England: Health Services and Delivery Research No. 2.19.* Southampton (UK): NIHR Journals Library.

Goffman I (1961). *Asylums.* London: Penguin.

Hodge S (2005). Participation, discourse and power: A case study in service user involvement. *Critical Social Policy 25* (2), 164–179.

Lakeman R (2010). Epistemic injustice and the mental health service user. *International Journal of Mental Health Nursing 19*, 151–153.

Le Boutillier C, Chevalier A., Lawrence V, Leamy M, Bird V J, Macpherson R, Williams J & Slade M (2015). Staff understanding of recovery-orientated mental health practice: a systematic review and narrative synthesis. *Implementation Science 10* (87).

LeBlanc S & Kinsella E A (2016). Toward epistemic justice: A critically reflexive examination of 'sanism' and implications for knowledge generation. *Studies in Social Justice 10* (1), 59–78.

LeFrançois B (2016). Foreword. In J Russo and A Sweeney (2016). *Searching for a Rose Garden: Challenging Psychiatry, Fostering Mad Studies.* Monmouth: PCCS Books, v–viii.

LeFrançois B, Menzies R & Reaume G (2013). *Mad Matters: A Critical Reader in Canadian Mad Studies.* Toronto: CSPI.

Morrow M (2013). Recovery: Progressive paradigm or neoliberal smokescreen? In B LeFrançois, R Menzies and G Reaume (2013). *Mad Matters: A Critical Reader in Canadian Mad Studies.* Toronto: CSPI, 323–333.

Needham C (2008). Realising the potential of co-production: Negotiating improvements in public services. *Social Policy and Society 7* (2), 221–231.

Needham, C. & Carr, S. (2009) *Co-production: an emerging evidence base for adult social care transformation.* London: SCIE.

Newbigging K and Ridley J (2018). Epistemic struggles: The role of advocacy in promoting epistemic justice and rights in mental health. *Social Science & Medicine 219*, 36–44.

O'Hagan M (2016). Responses to a legacy of harm. In J Russo and A Sweeney (2016). *Searching for a Rose Garden: Challenging Psychiatry, Fostering Mad Studies.* Monmouth: PCCS Books, 9–13.

Ostrom E (1996). Crossing the great divide: Coproduction, synergy, and development. *World Development 24* (6), 1073–1087.

Penney D and Prescott L (2016). The co-optation of survivor knowledge: The danger of substituted values and voice. In J Russo and A Sweeney (2016). *Searching for a Rose Garden: Challenging Psychiatry, Fostering Mad Studies.* Monmouth: PCCS Books, 35–45.

Pestoff, V (2013). Collective action and the sustainability of co-production. *Public Management Review 16* (3), 383–401.

Rosenhan D L (1973). On being sane in insane places. *Science 179* (4070), 250–258.

Russo J and Sweeney A (2016). *Searching for a Rose Garden: Challenging psychiatry, fostering Mad Studies.* Monmouth: PCCS Books.

Sayce L (2000). *From Psychiatric Patient to Citizen: Overcoming Discrimination and Social Exclusion.* Basingstoke: Macmillan.

Sayce L (2015). *From Psychiatric Patient to Citizen Revisited.* Basingstoke: Palgrave Macmillan.

Slade M, Amerling M, Farkas M, Hamilton B, O'Hagan M, Panther G, Perkins R, Shepherd G, Tse S and Whitley R (2014). Uses and abuses of recovery: Implementing recovery-oriented practices in mental health systems. *World Psychiatry 13*, 12–20.

Scourfield P (2007). Social care and the modern citizen: Client, consumer, service user, manager and entrepreneur. *British Journal of Social Work 37* (1), 107–122.

Scull A (2007). *Madhouse: A Tragic Tale of Megalomania and Modern Medicine.* New Haven: Yale University Press.

Slay J and Stephens L (2013). *Co-production in Mental Health: A Literature Review.* London: New Economics Foundation/Mind.

UNHRC (2017). *Report of the Special Rapporteur on the Right of Everyone to the Enjoyment of the Highest Attainable Standard of Physical and Mental Health.* New York: UNHRC.

Vandewalle J, Debyser B, Beekman D, Vandecasteele T, Van Hecke A and Verhaeghe S (2015). Peer workers' perceptions and experiences of barriers to implementation of peer worker roles in mental health services: A literature review. *International Journal of Nursing Studies 60*, 234–250.

Voronka, J (2016). The politics of 'people with lived experience': Experiential authority and the risks of strategic essentialism. *Philosophy, Psychiatry and Psychology* 23 (3–4), 189-201.

Voronka, J (2017). Turning mad knowledge into affective labor: The case of the peer support worker. *American Quarterly 69* (2), 333–338.

17

"ARE YOU EXPERIENCED?"

The use of experiential knowledge in mental health and its contribution to Mad Studies

Danny Taggart

Introduction

Mad persons have historically been excluded from knowledge production in the field of mental health. Having our faculties of 'reason' fundamentally challenged necessarily placed people outside the arena where knowledge about mental health problems was produced. However recent years have seen a move towards valuing 'experiential knowledge' based on the work of people who have used psychiatric services. At a research, policy and practice level there is now a need to include experiential knowledge forms. This has led to some important advances in mental health but has come at a cost to many who have been asked to use and share their experience of often private and painful events.

My own perspectives on the topic of mental health are multi-faceted being a clinical psychologist, an academic and a survivor of institutional sexual abuse in childhood. Coming from a trauma survivor perspective, I am interested in thinking about how this sharing of 'experiential knowledge' impacts on us and what happens when our experience becomes a form of commodity that can be traded, debated and discarded. Firstly, I sketch out a brief history of experiential knowledge in mental health, before drawing on the work of the intellectual historian Martin Jay to explore how philosophical interpretations of the meaning and value of 'experience' have changed over time. Given that there are a number of ways that we can frame 'experience', I will conclude by discussing what the implications might be of different interpretations for 'experiential knowledge' producers in Mad Studies. Throughout the chapter I will refer to Mad Persons in various ways including their positioning as psychiatric patients. However this does not suggest endorsement of pejorative descriptors, it is instead an attempt to reflect the way we might be positioned in different contexts.

The use of experiential knowledge in mental health

A key feature of the emerging discipline of Mad Studies is the use of knowledge forms other than empirically grounded analyses to inform our understandings of what it is like to live with madness. This distinctive approach to knowledge formation has been described as differentiating between "so-called 'expert' and 'experiential' knowledge" (Beresford, 2016:25). Experiential knowledge can be loosely described as knowledge that is generated from people

DOI: 10.4324/9780429465444-21

with direct experience of the social issue under investigation, in this case living with madness and using mental health services, or indeed refusing to use those services.

The development of 'experiential knowledge' has come from the struggle of mental health service users over many decades to be recognized as having legitimate knowledge about the mental health and the psychiatric system. More recently this struggle for both epistemic recognition and a demand for experiential knowledge to inform mental health research, policy and practice has been described under the umbrella term Mad Studies. This struggle, that draws on civil rights movements both in terms of activist strategies and intellectual underpinning, has been in the face of a psychiatric orthodoxy that has viewed mental patients as lacking rationality. The fundamental 'irrationality' of the 'psychiatric patient' has been seen as reason in itself to discard any knowledge claims from them about their mental health and their treatment by the psychiatric system.

The system of Dr Tarr and Professor Fether

The unseemly phrase 'the lunatics have taken over the asylum' captures traditional views on mad people actually being listened to as purveyors of knowledge. The phrase itself is of uncertain etymology but is thought to originate in an 1845 Edgar Allen Poe short story called "The System of Dr Tarr and Professor Fether", where a new form of treatment is introduced known as the "system of soothing" in which patients are treated gently, their beliefs taken seriously and they are granted liberty as opposed to the norm of the time of punishment, accusations of lunacy and incarceration. A visitor who comes to the hospital is shocked and disappointed to find that the "system of soothing" has been abandoned on favour of a traditional, disciplinarian approach. Over the course of an increasingly bizarre dinner with a majority women staff, it becomes clear that the system of soothing has enabled the majority female patient body to take on the role of staff and to lock up the male staff as the newly anointed lunatics. One memorable phrase which makes clear the complexity of dividing lines between madness and sanity and the perverse logic of the psychiatric system is

> If he (the lunatic) has a project in view, he conceals his design with a marvellous wisdom; and the dexterity with which he counterfeits sanity, presents, to the metaphysician, one of the most singular problems in the study of mind. When a madman appears thoroughly sane, indeed, it is high time to put him in a straitjacket".
>
> *(Poe, 1845)*

The title of the story reveals to us what grizzly fate awaited the incarcerated staff at the hands of the recently liberated and vengeful patients – tarring and feathering. The story of origin for this phrase therefore reveals an ironic and macabre morality play that teases with how difficult it is to tell apart the sane from the mad in appearance and action, as well as a neatly satirising the gendered assumptions about mental health and professionalism that underpinned American society at that time. However what we are left with is a phrase of seedy reductionism that renders mad knowledge dangerous.

The anxiety for the protagonist in the Poe story about not being able to initially recognise the difference between mad and sane people, speaks to a broader set of fears in society about not being able to 'spot' difference. A black man 'passing' as white for much of his life was the basis for Philip Roth's novel on America's relationship with racism *The Human Stain* (2000). Jewish people 'passing' as Aryans was a preoccupation for the Nazis who were concerned about racial integration occurring covertly and enabling people to avoid persecution (Wallach, 2017).

What links these disparate threads is that preoccupations with difference is what fuels prejudice against minority groups, however when these differences become so invisible to be rendered meaningless, they call into question the agenda of 'essentialism' that discrimination is predicated on. In the case of mad people being indecipherable from their 'sane' counterparts, the lack of visible difference surely calls into question the validity of making these categorical distinctions at all. A Mad Studies perspective may serve to reify these differences from the other side but as we shall discuss later in the chapter group distinctions around mental health create as many problems as they resolve irrespective of who is doing the distinguishing. A better question to ask may be what and whose interests do these demarcations serve?

To conclude this section, what we see now in mental health services is in stark comparison to this phrase, at least at the level of rhetoric. Policy abounds with regards to the value that 'experience' brings to the field of mental health. So while those identifying as having experiential knowledge are not allowed to take over what little is left of the asylum in a post-institutional era, we are permitted to tinker with certain aspects of its administration.

The normalisation of some forms of experiential knowledge in mental health

In recent years, experiential or survivor knowledge in mental health has been used to inform and conduct research (Sweeney, 2009); contribute to health and social care education and training (Townend et al., 2008); provide a theoretical framework for peer support (Baillergeau and Duyvendak, 2016), and has framed critique of mainstream approaches in mental health services (Taggart, 2017). My own professional body the British Psychological Society has an Expert by Experience strategy 2018–2019 which describes them as; "service users, carers and members of the general public with direct or indirect experience of working with clinical psychologists, in a non-professional capacity". So in this case there is an emphasis not on the experiences that might bring us into contact with a psychologist in the first place but rather the experience of spending time with a psychologist in itself. The UK NHS Care Quality Commission describes Experts by Experience similarly as "people who have personal experience of using or caring for someone who uses health, mental health and/or social care services that we regulate" (CQC, 2020). Interestingly the Royal College of Psychiatry in the UK seem to have a more traditional, patient and carer involvement approach which does not grant any form of expertise to experience explicitly. This may reveal a more consumerist approach to involving service users, which positions their views as important by virtue of their service use. Whether this reveals an ideological objection to the idea of mad peoples having expertise or their experience being important is a worthwhile question. Internationally, Canada has a wealth of literature on the use of experiential knowledge forms in mental health services. Again there is, in the main, an emphasis on instrumental knowledge forms that can inform the development of policy and practice through a research agenda that prioritises practical change (for example Restall et al., 2011).

What emerges here is that the use of experiential knowledge in mainstream contexts appears to be more focused on using 'experience' as a way to enact instrumental change. The experience in this context is therefore part of a transaction between people with lived experience and the existing hierarchical structures, making any change piecemeal and inevitably co-opted into an essentially undisturbed orthodoxy. The Recovery movement is the most obvious example of this and has been critiqued extensively, almost to the extent that the critiques themselves have become oddly mainstreamed (see Harper and Speed, 2013 for an early iteration). My reading of Mad Studies thus far though seems to offer at least the possibility of different potentialities. The value of experiential knowledge forms seems to reach beyond the merely instrumental and to have space, in theory at least, for the telling and hearing of experience to have value in and of itself. The introduction to a key Mad Studies text *Searching for a Rose Garden* illustrates this distinction with the expression of an unusually poignant demand; "The main value of the rose garden might be our right to search for it ourselves, collectively and regardless of anyone's promises. That right cannot be denied to people labelled mad anymore" (Sweeney and Russo, 2016:9). This positions experiential knowledge as having the potential to be a collective good, which can lead to a reclaiming of rights independently of traditional power structures. It is in this sense that I want to consider experiential knowledge and more particularly what 'experience' might mean in this context. As I hope will become clear, what we mean when we talk about our 'experience' is not straightforward and leads to the sort of conceptual disagreements that can cause interpersonal misunderstandings, personal pain and dynamic splits between people interested and involved in Mad Studies work. As the poet Maggie Nelson puts it;

> when I think about it now I hear only the background buzz of our trying to explain something to each other, to ourselves, about our lived experiences thus far on this peeled, endangered planet. As is so often the case, the intensity of our need to be understood distorted our positions, backed us farther into the cage.
>
> *(2016:102)*

The trouble with experience

The idea that experiential knowledge in Mad Studies is a problematic category is not new, as Jijian Voronka (2016: 197) says in her paper on the complexities of being a "person with lived experience"; "Universalizing ourselves as 'experts by experience' belies the variances that our bodies carry, how we experience madness, and how mental health fields of power respond to us". As way of example, some people with experiential knowledge appreciate the validation, resource access and certainty of a diagnostic label, while others experience this categorisation as a form of violence. Now the reasons for these differences are complex and may be in part down to the relational and ethical context in which the diagnosis occurs. Nonetheless we can see situations whereby people's experiential knowledge can be invalidated by contradictory experiential knowledge of another person. Given the emotional labour it takes to describe aspects of our 'experience' this invalidation is likely to be personally costly for many. I think that part of our struggle here is finding it challenging to let go of the evidence of our own experience enough to hear another's that contradicts ours, as if their contrasting evidence threatens our truth. This dynamic seems to me to be empirical in nature – who's got the best evidence and who wins the argument. We will move on to consider the risks of translating experiential knowledge into empirical language later in the chapter after first considering one meaning of 'experience' in a Mad Studies context.

Jijian Voronka's 2016 Mad Studies paper offers a detailed and historically situated account of how the Expert by Experience identity came to be in mental health, what it offers in way of opportunities but also importantly what risks it carries in reducing down the rich diversity of experience in mental health to an homogenous whole. She cites at length a seminal paper in the area of experiential knowledge from a feminist historian perspective; Joan Wallach Scott's 1991 paper "The Evidence of Experience". In the paper, Scott emphasises the importance of 'visibility' in relation to the experiences of underground groups. She goes on to critique an ahistorical treatment of 'experience' as by necessity being framed within dominant discursive formations. A central passage is;

> It is not individuals who have experience, but subjects who are constituted through experience. Experience in this definition becomes not the origin of our explanation, not the authoritative evidence that grounds what is seen or known, but rather that which we seek to explain, that about which knowledge is produced. To think about experience in this way is to historicize it as well as to historicize the identities it produces.
>
> *(1991:780)*

As Diana Rose (2016) points out, this sensible need to historically situate experience and in doing so critically calibrate our receptiveness to it as a knowledge form needs to be undertaken sensitively, particularly in a Mad Studies context where the very reason for the existence of the field is to counteract the dismissal of experiential knowledge as inherently unreliable. However Scott's is only one, relatively recent take on 'experience' as a concept. She is not the first to be tempted to do away with it as being too vague and broad, nor is she the first to want to critically examine its claim to represent a form of knowledge that can be trusted. And yet it seems to me that the underpinning philosophy driving Scott's paper – that of post-structuralism is one dominant way in which Mad Studies seeks to understand what 'experience' means. While Scott's work adds much to the field in questioning the essential truth claims that 'experiential knowledge' carries as a form of evidence in mental health, it would be limiting to solely focus on this particular understanding of what experience is and what it could be for Mad Studies. Moreover, Scott's post-structuralist mistrust of experience being meaningful outside of discourse and historical context may have important implications for those of us using our experiential knowledge to inform Mad Studies but take different approaches to understanding ours and others experience. In this sense post-structuralist denigration of 'experience' as a natural category carries risks. By entirely merging experience and the language designed to describe it, there is a risk of denying people access to a more spiritually enriched and aesthetically poised experience that paradoxically might be exactly what separates out the value of experiential knowledge from the 1s and 0s of empirical science. In critiquing the category of experience we should be mindful of turning the solution to the categorical reductionism of psychiatric disorder into a linguistic reductionism.

The history of 'experience' as an idea

For the next section of the chapter, I have drawn on the work of the Intellectual Historian Martin Jay, in particular his 2005 book on the modern history of 'experience' – *Songs of Experience: Modern American and European Variations on a Universal Theme*. In this book Jay charts the differing ways that 'experience' has been conceptualised from political, scientific, artistic, religious and philosophical perspectives. In this 'history of an idea' Jay discusses various attempts to reform or even to do away with the concept of experience altogether, the example of Joan Wallace Scott being one we have touched on. More than anything what becomes clear when we delve into the area of 'experience' as an idea is that there is no one formation of experience that can properly capture it's different uses across time and place. So we are not exploring 'experience' here in order to understand what it is, so much as thinking about it's different meanings in order to examine their usefulness and limitations in the development of experiential knowledge forms in the field of Mad Studies.

"Experience itself is a scientific scandal ... the ordinary everyday human world ... is consigned by science to its slop bucket" (Laing, 1982:115). What RD Laing was voicing here, in his own inimitable style, is a longstanding and complex suspicion of experience as being an inferior form of knowledge than that gained through empirical investigation. Laing was interested in experience from an existentialist and phenomenological perspective and Mad Studies in some senses carries on the spirit if not the methodology of his approach, by continuing as he did to look for meaning in madness. In the *Politics of Experience and the Bird of Paradise* he went even further by saying that, "Experience is the only evidence" (1967:16), placing his philosophy of mental illness well and truly at odds with psychiatric scientific orthodoxy. This split between the experiential and empirical is broader than psychiatry, as the literary critic Terry Eagleton (2005) writes

"We live in the era of scientific rationalism, which is interested in weighing and measuring an object rather than registering its sinuous curve or peculiar tint. Science is the enemy of the sensuous. It is anchored in perception, but it also puts it into question. It looks as though the sun is coming up, but actually the earth is going down. A rift opens up between how things are and how we experience them. Since this is a rift inherent in reality itself, our experience of the world is bound to be a matter of *misrecognition* as well as knowledge.

(emphasis added)

I have highlighted the word misrecognition as we will return to it again later when we consider experience in the light of our current moment of identity politics, but for now I want to consider the gap he identifies between what we experience as mad persons and what science tells us is happening. One example of this in wider health research is that some researchers have welcomed the inclusion of experiential knowledge as a resource but only because it is 'wrong knowledge'. So in this case you ask non-experts for information about a health condition in order to find out how lay people wrongly understand them. This has been used to inform public health information around myths surrounding HIV and AIDS (Prior, 2003). While this is clearly different from the value attached to experiential knowledge in a Mad Studies context, it may provide some insight into how experience can be viewed from an empirical standpoint.

This inherent suspicion of knowledge derived from experience has a long history, dating back to Francis Bacon, described by Hegel as the father of empiricism and who sought to develop reliable ways of measuring phenomena that has been called the 'quest for certainty' (Jay, 2005). Bacon said "Experience is blind and silly, so that while men roam and wander around without any definitive course, merely taking counsel of things as happen to come before them, they range widely, yet move little forward" (Jay, 2005:78). In reading Bacon's critique of experience, I cannot help but notice the reference to 'aimless wandering' and two of the most knowledge enhancing walks in all of literature, those of Steven Deadalus and Leopold Bloom in James Joyce's Ulysses. The material for which came from, of course, Joyce's memories in exile of walking apparently aimlessly around Dublin. Now it seems to me that it is foolish to compare the wealth of knowledge about the human condition that can be learnt from a great work of art such as Ulysses and that which comes from systematic empirical scientific research. They are quite simply, different forms of knowledge. To return to mental health, Diana Rose makes the point that Mad Studies does not have to be restricted to one epistemological position, furthermore she says; "We do not have to worry about epistemology at all in one sense – it is part of the end of it that has been coming for some time" (2017:7). In this sense the use of experiential knowledge to inform the development of Mad Studies can side step the epistemological battles that have raged intermittently between experience and empiricism since Bacon's time. Joyce's work and that of other artists can point to one way in which Mad Studies can find a different direction in which to wander.

The value of experiential knowledge: Getting to the corners of madness science cannot reach

The author and literary critic David Lodge (2002) talks about the potential complementary use of art and science by using examples from neuroscience and the idea of qualia. Qualia refers to specific, individual subjective experience and Lodge points out that it highlights the limitations of science. While we can map which areas of the brain light up when a person eats an apple, we cannot describe scientifically what the experience is like of eating an apple. Lodge proposes literature as a way to fill this empirical gap and uses the example of poetry as the purest, distilled form of qualia. I would suggest that experiential knowledge offers another way to do what empirical science alone cannot – to capture the qualia of living with madness in all its multiplicity. In my own modest work I have tried to communicate one experience of living with trauma that tried to express something of what it is to be 'in it' (Taggart, 2016, 2017). This required a departure from purely psychological models of explanation and led to me citing varying figures from the musician John Coltrane to the plays of Samuel Beckett, to the Irish novelist Eimear McBride to try to get across what trauma is 'like'. It's flavour, texture, appearance and sound. This work was undertaken at least in part as a response to the woefully inadequate cognitive models of trauma offered by my profession of clinical psychology. While technically competent and in many cases clinically useful, psychological models of trauma in no way captured the wild injustices of abuse and the terrifying psychic consequences and social alienation that many survivors have to live with.

However, having undertaken this work it seems important not to think of it as directly comparable to empirical research and so downgrade it as a lesser form of knowledge as will inevitably happen if exposed to the same quality standards. It is simply different and necessary to reach the corners of madness that science cannot, and in the case of trauma often does not want to. Once we do this and do not make claims based on experiential knowledge that are similar to those from empirical research, then a lot of the historical tension between these two areas can disappear. One problem with locating experiential knowledge in the field of the humanities however is that most of us struggle to render our experience accessible to others in such a vivid and artful way. Much experience is humdrum and prosaic, and this is nowhere more true than in the case of living with debilitating mental distress under conditions of economic austerity as many are in the UK today. It seems important not to try to elevate it to artistry but to try to allow it to reflect the more ordinary beauty of everyday survival. However I do not think this is a problem for purveyors of experiential knowledge to resolve alone, disappointing though it may be not to write as well as great prose stylists, it ought not to exclude our experiential knowledge and does make it any less legitimate. Instead, responsibility must be shared with those who are listening to the experiential knowledge being spoken.

The ethics of listening to experiential knowledge: Towards a testimonial sensibility

In her work on epistemic justice Miranda Fricker (2003) extends the scope to include the responsibilities of those receiving experiential knowledge. She calls for ethics to rescue epistemology from a moral relativism that cannot distinguish between good knowledge and bad. This is surely an important idea in the field of mental health generally and Mad Studies specifically. One area where more attention needs to be paid to ethics and less to empiricism is aetiology, where varying evidence confounds the need for simplistic nature/nurture reductionisms but yet there is an insistence among some psychiatric researchers that the issue will be resolved in the genome. Although as Diana Rose points out it would be incorrect and strategically unwise to view all of psychiatry in a monolithic fashion (2017). An emphasis on genetic vulnerability masks structural and interpersonal abuses that lead people into distress and can also rob them of their agency. Greater humility about the limitations of genetic evidence could allow space for the sort of ethical listening that Fricker is referring to. In evaluating the quality of experiential knowledge, she warns against a reductionist binary choice between uncritical acceptance and intellectualist argumentation. Instead she calls for a 'critical openness' that is defined by a sensibility afforded by ethics.

This approach can promote certain ethical virtues including what Fricker describes as: "A testimonial sensibility, then, needs to be shaped by collective and individual experiences of testimonial encounters described in rich, socially specific terms relating to the trustworthiness of speakers of different social types in different sorts of contexts" (2003:161). She claims that the development of this sensibility can lead to an 'epistemic revolution' whereby previously held beliefs about the trustworthiness of certain groups can be transformed. It is not difficult for us to conclude that an epistemic revolution rooted in an ethical sensibility is needed in mental health and that those of us who are supposedly professional listeners have some way to go to achieve it. This critical openness does not require us to conclude that all experiential knowledge is true but instead that judged untrue or partially true, it is still important. I notice in my role as service user and carer involvement lead in my university, being tempted at times to pass over experiential knowledge that does not fit with the university's agenda. The tension between corporate branding in the neoliberal university and the unpleasant realities of patient and carer experiences can lead to the subjugation of their experiential knowledge. The challenge is to create spaces where professionals can develop a testimonial sensibility and avoid the strangely macho displays of authority that treats all conversations concerning mental health as if they are part of a debating society in a minor public school. Or to return to Sweeney and Russo's (2016) point earlier, maybe it is to create spaces where Mad Studies scholars can be protected from the ideological clamour altogether by developing their own paths.

Trauma based experiential knowledge

A feature of developing a testimonial sensibility in this area is that at times there is too much pain to bear in people's experience and so listeners turn away feeling overwhelmed and helpless. I think this is particularly true of trauma, where revulsion and disgust are common responses from listeners but often denied. We can in part understand psychiatry and the public's fixation with genetic research are in part a way to deny the realities of the abuses that often bring people into the mental health system. In creating a space where testimonial sensibilities can be nurtured and allowed to grow, Mad Studies needs to offer a conceptual framework in which traumatised experiential knowledge can tolerated. I would suggest this is a complex task and one that mainstream mental health services have largely failed to do, based on the low levels of asking about abuse histories by professionals (Xiao et al., 2016). Developments in this area need to be organic, but making a clear link between 'madness' and structural and interpersonal abuses can offer those of us who see our mental health in the context of trauma opportunities to forge experiential knowledge forms. Once trauma based experiential knowledge is honed in a Mad

Studies context it can then be exported to influence how the mainstream mental health field understands aetiology, while offering scholars some protection from the hostilities of trying to work alone in this area. For what can be a better antidote to trauma than the exercising of collective power and agency? For a recent example of Mad Studies scholars taking experiential knowledge forms into a mainstream context in order to influence debates around aetiology see Sweeney and Taggart (2018). There is also a converse problem which is the translation of all experience into a trauma narrative leading to what Fassin and Rechtman (2007) call the 'traumatisation of experience".

Now we have considered the ethical responsibilities of the listeners to experiential knowledge, we can return again finally to the purveyors of experiential knowledge. Although in the field of Mad Studies many will be both speakers and listeners at different points, making the need for a critical openness all the more urgent when faced by testimony that sits uneasily with ours. In this last section I want to consider what the risks are for those of us who use our experiential knowledge in the field of mental health, before concluding on how we might best navigate them individually and collectively.

The theft of experience

Experience in an age of commodification risks jeopardising an idealised version of our experiential knowledge through cheapening it to sell in, what gets described terrifyingly, as the marketplace of ideas. As the German philosopher Theodor Adorno said in the 1990s, "The marrow of experience has been sucked out: there is none, not even that apparently set at remove from commerce, that has not been gnawed away" (cited in Jay, 2005:346). In mental health we can see this in the work of Lucy Costa and colleagues (2012) who have written about challenging the appropriation of psychiatric survivors' experiential knowledge in the form of narratives. They talk about the risks of 'disability tourism' and 'patient porn' whereby the experiences of people can be co-opted and used to progress the interests of mental health services. In the context of this paper we can think of this as the *theft of experience*: the use of experiential knowledge as a commodity, which can be traded in a marketplace, and discarded when no longer needed. While I agree with Costa and colleagues in this analysis, I think it needs to go further. I think that in an age of identity politics we can commodify our own experience in a way that can paradoxically lead to us becoming alienated from it in the way Adorno alluded to. To turn back to Terry Eagleton (2005) again,

> Instead of wandering along Hadrian's Wall, we have the Hadrian's Wall Experience; instead of the Giant's Causeway, the Giant's Causeway Experience . ... Since what all of these packaged tourist spots have in common is the fact that they are experienced, they become, like commodities, interchangeable. Experience, a term which can mean an event of exceptional value, ends up as a dead leveller.

It is the use of experiential knowledge as a form of knowing that has exceptional value that needs to be developed by Mad Studies and the history of experience as an idea suggests that it often means more when not overly determined.

I think that a hard-line identity politics pushes us towards what Martin Jay refers to as 'overly claimed experience'. In other words experience that is too closely managed and presented, that is used to say too clearly who we are and who we are not. Experience that binds and limits us. The risks of misrecognition that we bookmarked earlier are heightened when we frame our experience and our identity in the same way. In my own case where at times I describe myself as a survivor/academic/clinician with not enough thought as to how those three aspects of identity interact and why in presenting those parts I leave out others – father, husband, record collector, Irish person etc. For while a traditional clinical psychology scientific method would see no reason for any of those identities to be named, an identity politics might leave me with the sense that without them I have no right to claim a space in the discussion. The costs for us having our experiential knowledge critiqued is much higher than when we place so much value in it as part of who we are. I think this is where a lot of the pain in this experiential knowledge work can come from. When our experiential knowledge is not treated with sufficient respect then we feel it is an attack on our identity and draw battle lines accordingly. This can easily slip into a pattern of seeing our experiential knowledge as a source of group identity that clearly demarcates who we are in comparison to others and can lead to the sorts of splits that have bedevilled survivor movements for years. It also has the effect of limiting our exposure to different experiences, we can become stuck in the role of service user, survivor or expert by experience when that identity is no longer serving us.

To return to Martin Jay one more time,

> the very notion of experience as a commodity for sale is precisely the opposite of what many … have argued an experience should be … *something which can never be fully possessed by its owner*. Instead because experiences involve encounters with otherness and open onto a future that is not fully contained in the past or the present, they defy the very attempt to reduce them to moments of fulfilled intensity in the marketplace of sensations.
>
> *(Jay 2005:405, emphasis added)*

Now one thing I think Jay is getting at here is that we can never really own our experiences and so experiential knowledge must be in constant movement, dynamic flux or else it ceases to be truly experiential at all. In short, this way of looking at experiential knowledge can enable Mad Studies to avoid the same objectification of experience that results in psychiatric diagnosis. In liberating our experience from our identity there is the possibility new, less dogmatic ways of thinking about mental health.

Conclusion

All of this leads me to the current position that can be briefly summarised as follows: in looking to a future not yet experienced, I try to ensure my experience of past traumas can be faithfully rendered in the present to inform an experiential knowledge, but not so much that they keep me stuck there. In thinking about the development of Mad Studies more broadly, metaphors of discovery, wandering and searching, whether for a rose garden or something else, seem an appropriate way to describe where we are at this juncture. Through drilling down into the complexity of experience as an idea spanning hundreds of years and many philosophical traditions, we can be forgiven for struggling to resolve the contradictions, inconsistencies and limitations of the use of experiential knowledge to inform the emergent field of Mad Studies. We can also see that we may at times use our experiential knowledge in different ways – at times empirically, at other times aesthetically or even to inform our sense of identity. This is not to promote a hard relativism whereby experience can mean whatever we want it to and therefore to end up meaning nothing. Rather it is to leave it open for Mad Studies to enable experiential knowledge to reflect the richness of the history of experience as an idea. A history that illustrates that the seemingly intractable question of what experience is, continues to endure because it is so central to the experience of being human. That alone, given the history of mad people being dehumanised, is reason enough for us to join such a great intellectual tradition in working at what experience means for Mad Studies and how it can enable the ongoing struggle to create new knowledge forms in mental health.

References

Baillergeau E and Duyvendak J (2016) Experiential knowledge as a resource for coping with uncertainty: Evidence and examples from the Netherlands. *Health, Risk & Society*, 18 (7–8), 407–426.

Beresford P (2016) The role of survivor knowledge in creating alternatives to psychiatry. In J Russo and A Sweeney (eds.) *Searching for a Rose Garden: Challenging Psychiatry, Fostering Mad Studies*. Monmouth: PCCS Books, 25–34.

Care Quality Commission (CQC) (2020, 8 December) Experts by experience program, https://www.cqc.org.uk/about-us/jobs/experts-experience.

Costa L, Voronka J, Landry D, Reid J, Mcfarlane B, Reville D and Church K (2012) Recovering our stories: A small act of resistance. *Studies in Social Justice*, 6 (1), 85–101.

Eagleton T (2005) Lend me a fiver. *London Review of Books*, 27 (12), 23–24, https://www.lrb.co.uk/the-paper/v27/n12/terry-eagleton/lend-me-a-fiver.

Fassin D and Rechtman R (2007) *The Empire of trauma: An enquiry into the condition of victimhood*. New Jersey: Princeton University Press.

Fricker M (2003) Epistemic injustice and a role for virtue in the politics of knowing. *Metaphilosophy*, 34 (1/2), 154–173.

Harper D and Speed E (2013) Uncovering recovery: The resistible rise of recovery and resilience. *Studies in Social Justice*, 6 (1), 9–26.

Jay M (2005) *Songs of Experience: Modern American and European variations on a universal theme*. Berkeley, CA: University of California Press.

Laing R (1967) *The Politics of Experience and the Bird of Paradise*. Routledge and Kegan Paul.

Lodge D (2002) *Consciousness and the novel: Connected essays*. London: Penguin Random House.

Nelson M (2016) *The Argonauts*. London: Melville House.

Poe E A (1845) The system of Dr Tarr and Professor Fether. *Graham's Magazine*, No 5.

Prior L (2003) Belief, knowledge and expertise: The emergence of the lay expert in medical sociology. *Sociology of Health & Illness*, 25, 41–57.

Restall G, Cooper J E and Kaufert J M (2011) Pathways to translating experiential knowledge into mental health policy. *Psychiatric Rehabilitation Journal*, 35 (1), 29–36.

Rose D (2016) Experience, madness theory and politics. *Philosophy, Psychiatry & Psychology*, 23, 3/4, 207–210.

Rose D (2017) Service user/survivor-led research in mental health: Epistemological possibilities. *Disability & Society*.

Roth P (2000) *The Human Stain*. Penguin Random House.

Scott J W (1991) The evidence of experience. *Critical Inquiry*, 17, 4, 773–797.

Sweeney A (2009) So what is survivor research? In A Sweeney, P Beresford, A Faulkner, M Nettle, D Rose (eds). *This is Survivor Research*. Monmouth: PCCS Books, 22–37.

Sweeney A and Russo J (eds) (2016) *Searching for a Rose Garden: Challenging Psychiatry, Fostering Mad Studies*. Monmouth: PCCS Books.

Sweeney A and Taggart D (2018) (Mis)understanding trauma-informed approaches in mental health. *Journal of Mental Health*, 27 (5), 383–387.

Taggart D (2016) Notes from the underground: Some reflections on clinical psychology's role in responding to historical and institutional child sexual abuse. *Clinical Psychology Forum*, 286, 6–9.

Taggart D (2017) Anatomised. *Asylum Magazine for Democratic Psychiatry*, 24 (1), 29–31.

Townend M, Tew J, Grant A and Repper J (2008) Involvement of service users in education and training: A review of the literature and exploration of the implications for the education and training of psychological therapists. *Journal of Mental Health*, 17 (1), 65–78.

Voronka, J (2016) The politics of 'people with lived experience': Experiential authority and the risks of strategic essentialism. *Philosophy, Psychiatry & Psychology*, 23 (3–4), 189–201.

Wallach, K. (2017) *Passing illusions – Jewish visibility in Weimar Germany*. Ann Arbor, MI: The University of Michigan Press.

Xiao C, Gavrilidis E, Lee S and Kulkarni J (2016) Do mental health clinicians elicit a history of previous trauma in female psychiatric inpatients? *Journal of Mental Health*, 25, 359–365.

18

DE-PATHOLOGISING MOTHERHOOD

Angela Sweeney and Billie Lever Taylor

Introduction: A mother's mind

This chapter is rooted in our own experiences of motherhood, mental health services and research. One of us (Angie) is a survivor researcher, the other (Billie) is a clinical psychologist and researcher, and we are both mothers. During pregnancy and whilst breastfeeding, Angie was under a mental health midwife team and monitored by a perinatal (pregnancy to one year post-birth) psychiatrist. Billie (coincidentally) worked in the same service as a psychologist and attended a therapeutic group with her daughter elsewhere. We have both worked on a qualitative study of women's experiences of perinatal mental health services, Billie as the main researcher, which we are calling the Perinatal Study. This study was based in the UK, and whilst the issues we describe reach beyond this context, much of the text relates to UK systems, policies and practices. Inevitably, we also write from our limited, partial positions as heterosexual, cis, working white mothers, with white or mixed race partners and children, living in a metropolitan city in the Northern hemisphere. Whilst we are aware of the important differences in the experiences of mothers who are straight, lesbian, transgender, single, co-parenting, poly-parenting and so on, our focus here is on the underlying structures that influence our varied experiences, and the ways in which gender norms can affect mothers beyond our social positionings. However, we also hope to inspire further research on motherhood from other positions and perspectives within Mad Studies.

Motherhood has, for both of us, been characterised by intense and conflicting emotions: of love and loss; exhaustion and elation; guilt and gratitude; fear and fracture; mayhem and monotony; connection and isolation; and, often, of failure. It is a relentless experience of giving and doing what it can feel beyond our resources to give and do, day after day – no matter how exhausted, how desperately in need of respite. It has also entailed huge transitions in our roles, identities and relationships. These experiences have occurred despite our current, relative socioeconomic privilege.

Faced with dominant cultural beliefs that, as women, we should naturally be nurturing and able to cope with the mothering role, we have often doubted ourselves: why am I struggling? Am I the only one? Am I harming my child? Am I mad? Why do I feel so angry? How can I keep going? We believe there is no one right way to parent and that we only need to be *good enough*, yet still feel we are falling short. We know that it is possible to *not be a good enough* mother too and to inflict enormous damage. We find motherhood hard to figure out, and to write about.

DOI: 10.4324/9780429465444-22

It is in this context, along with our clinical and research experiences, that we question psychiatric conceptualisations of maternal struggles as postnatal depression, postpartum psychosis, or a return/triggering of a pre-existing mental disorder. We have seen how this limits understandings of motherhood and narrows the way society responds. How it can make mothers fearful about discussing their difficulties, and coerce them into adhering to dominant gender norms. And how it promotes medical and individual treatments, whilst diverting attention from the need for broader community, social, political and structural responses.

Throughout this chapter, we include quotes from women who participated in the Perinatal Study. This study included interviews with 52 mothers (between 2015 and 2017), with 6–9-month-old babies, seen in NHS services in England for perinatal mental distress (UCL, 2019). The quotes we have chosen to include are from mothers who shared experiences that resonated with us, sometimes validating and at other times shaping, enriching or changing our evolving perspectives. Some women in the study felt that psychiatric diagnoses explained and validated their experiences, and enabled them to access treatment. Whilst the reasons for this should be considered too, our main focus here is on the voices who felt differently; who questioned the way services responded to their distress; or whose words, we felt, shed light on psychiatry's limitations.

Natural motherhood

In the UK and beyond, although legislation and mainstream narratives are shifting away from the notion that heterosexual couples are the only acceptable foundation of a family unit, historically and now, across a wide range of cultures, raising children primarily remains women's responsibility, with emphasis placed on the mother–infant bond and women's presumed natural ability to nurture. Although some societies have seen recent shifts towards increased paternal involvement, in both Northern and Southern hemispheres, social customs and arrangements tend to perpetuate women's role as the main caregivers.

This notion of motherhood as natural, innate and inevitable is fuelled by cultural images of the fulfilled mother with contented baby. Although there may be occasional (droll) popular cultural references to some of motherhood's challenges, like the need for extraordinary levels of multitasking, women are nonetheless depicted as having a natural capacity for this, with fathers at times painted as hapless, bumbling and in need of direction from women. Given this cultural context, women may justifiably expect motherhood to bring joy and contentment.

But this is often far from reality. Although some women may glide easily through motherhood – and experiences may be different in cultures with which we are less familiar – we suspect that the dominant experience can be one of simultaneous emotional extremes and unrelenting monotony alongside a fluctuating sense of fulfilment and struggle. Experiencing complex shifting emotions in cultures that characterise motherhood as natural, joyful and fulfilling whilst often ignoring its many challenges, can reinforce the idea that there is something personally wrong with us. Trying to get by, to be enough, rather than feeling gratitude and delight in these precious moments, can cause huge self-doubt. This is both created and fuelled by the culturally prescribed myth of the perfect mother – the expectation that we will be all, always; gentle, tender and nurturing. That strong negative, angry or ambivalent emotions are abnormal, unfeminine and a sign of illness.

Media analysis has shown that news stories about women experiencing perinatal distress often categorise them as either 'mad' or 'bad' (Dubriwny, 2010). Some women, who Dubriwny observes tend to be white, middle class and heterosexual, are depicted as 'diverted good mothers'. They are shown as having gone through an alarming and abnormal, but ultimately temporary disruption to their natural ability to mother, from which they later recovered. In these cases, there is usually a happy ending, showing them now delighting in motherhood in the expected way. Other mothers – particularly those who are lesbian, single and black and minority ethnic are either absent from news coverage or depicted as 'bad' rather than 'mad'.

(Who is) crossing the line

Recent years have seen increased media attention given to perinatal mental health. This is part of wider efforts to reduce stigma and increase help-seeking through public education about mental illness – 'an illness like any other'. We are told that 'baby blues' and tiredness are a normal part of early parenting, but that there is a line we can cross into postnatal depression or, more rarely, postpartum psychosis, and once crossed, it is essential that we seek help. For instance, in an article about the baby blues, The National Childbirth Trust (NCT[1]) states that post-birth:

> Symptoms might upset you at the time, but they are relatively mild and will usually pass within 10 to 14 days. If they hang around, become more severe or include manic symptoms, they could be signs of more serious postnatal illness. You should speak to your GP or health visitor about getting some help and support.
>
> *(NCT, 2018)*

The implication – sometimes stated overtly, sometimes implied – is that if we do not seek help, our children may be harmed through the impact of untreated mental illness. Clinicians have the responsibility of i) ensuring that those who are at risk, or who have crossed the line, are identified or educated so that they can appropriately seek help and ii) developing and delivering effective treatments and ensuring mum is monitored. The existence of diagnoses like postnatal depression goes unquestioned – they are seen as concrete, diagnosable, objective illness states afflicting individual mothers. Treatment, in turn, aims to modify a woman's body and mind – in a sense, to fit 'diverted mothers' back into society and the mothering role.

The National Institute for Health and Care Excellence (NICE) has produced clinical guidelines that UK clinicians are expected to follow for women who have crossed the line (2018). The guidelines clearly address difficulties in women rather than, for example, focusing on the wider familial or social context. Recommended treatments include facilitated self-help, cognitive behavioural therapy and medication, increasing to inpatient stays on mother and baby units. Monitoring of the baby becomes necessary for pregnant and breastfeeding mothers because of the potential for treatments, particularly medications, to harm infants.

Electroconvulsive therapy (in which under general anaesthetic, an electric current is passed to the pregnant woman's brain through electrodes, triggering a seizure) is recommended where a clinician judges that the physical health of the woman or baby is at risk, for instance through suicide. There is a bitter irony to this: a recent systematic review of international case studies found that ECT in pregnancy is associated with adverse outcomes for mother and baby, including foetal heart rate reduction, premature labour and neonatal death: "Lethal outcomes for the fetus and/or baby were stated to have diverse causes, in one case a long lasting severe

---

1 NCT is a respected, UK-based organisation that supports (predominantly middle class) parents through pregnancy, birth and early parenthood.

grand mal seizure (status epilepticus) induced by ECT" (Leiknes et al., 2015). In a rebuttal of the Leiknes review, the academic psychiatrist Donna Stewart counters that:

> [a] 2009 review of 57 case reports involving 339 pregnant women, included *only* 11 neonatal complications, which included *2 deaths* that were likely related to ECT.
>
> *(Anderson and Reti, 2009; Stewart, 2015 emphasis added)*

For Stewart and others, the risk to the mother and baby is so great that the risks from ECT, including death of the unborn child, do not warrant it being considered an unethical or dangerous treatment. Inevitably, judgement regarding what constitutes an acceptable risk falls on the clinician. The horror of this does not need stating. For those women who have lost unborn children to ECT, what might have been the personal, interpersonal and sociocultural contexts they were navigating? What might have been their personal stories?

Mind and body

> When a woman's distress is interpreted as symptomatic of a mental disorder, attention is likely to focus on her body to the neglect of her social circumstances.
>
> *(Stoppard 2000:101)*

In her doctoral research on postnatal depression, Paula Nicolson interviewed 24 British women during pregnancy and post-birth and found that almost all reported feeling depressed, anxious or tearful, but that:

> each gave detailed explanations of what led to their behaviours. They contextualised them within the varied events over the days and weeks following childbirth, making their own reactions logical and meaningful...
>
> *(1998:55)*

In the Perinatal Study, we found that mothers often faced overwhelming challenges including: poverty; homelessness; chronic sleep deprivation and exhaustion; relationship breakdown; isolation; turbulent and sometimes violent relationships; mothering after a traumatic childhood; lack of support; and traumatic birth experiences. It was common for mothers' distress to reflect changes going on *between* and *around* people as well as *within* them. Sarah, a young, single, white, working–class mother expressed some of these challenges.

> *I was in a good place before I got pregnant. And then when I found out I was pregnant, it knocked me sideways. And then, with everything that happened with his dad [leaving me], it was just a massive blow. So, within the space of a few months, I had lost his dad, fell pregnant, gave up my job, and I was just in a big hole …*
>
> *… You want to be on your game for your child, you want to be on the ball, perfect mum, and sometimes you just feel so low about yourself and the situation that you're in. When it's raining outside, you don't want to take your baby when you've got nowhere to go. You're not heading anywhere … You're on your own, you hardly see anyone … You try looking in a baby group or you try stepping in there and some of the women are just … They've never been in that situation … So, you go in there and you're either getting looked at or just dodgy looks …*
>
> *… There's nowhere that you can have respite, there's nowhere that you can just go, I just need an hour sleep, I'm just so tired.*

Sarah's isolation was intensified because she felt that her available ways of connecting with other mothers, such as through playgroups, were dominated by middle-class women living in traditional relationships and with more support. Whilst Sarah was desperate to be the perfect mother amidst poverty and isolation, her family doctor diagnosed her with postnatal depression and prescribed medication.

> *They tried giving me different medications at the doctors, and they just didn't help. If anything, they just made me feel sick ... A couple of the doctors' appointments were terrible. I'd sit there and I'll explain to them what's been going on, and they said, 'So what do you want us to do?' ... And it was just a case of, take some drugs. Take these, see how you feel, then come back to us and let us know ... You give up after a while.*

Whilst clinicians may agree that young, poor mums like Sarah need interventions beyond psychiatry, they may also consider those diagnosed with postpartum psychosis to be different, mad, unquestionably in need of psychiatric treatment. In postpartum psychosis, biology and physiological changes after birth are seen as causal, with symptoms including sleep problems and delusions. Remarkably, researchers at Cambridge University have likened maternal postpartum psychosis to female pigs biting their newborns to death, and are studying the chromosomes of affected pigs in a bid to identify candidate genes for postpartum psychosis (Quilter et al., 2008). In this model, pigs are equated with humans, postpartum psychosis with pig infanticide, and the role of environment (the pigs lived in harsh conditions) considered irrelevant to understanding behaviours.

Linda, a white British mother in the Perinatal Study (who was neither a pig nor considering biting her baby to death) with no previous contact with psychiatry, was hospitalised for post-partum psychosis shortly after giving birth when she became convinced that her partner and others were trying to harm her and her baby. Linda's account describes how hospital practices made her feel unsafe, helpless and unable to sleep in the run-up to diagnosis.

> *They decided that I was just so tired that I had to have an epidural. And I hadn't wanted to have an epidural. So they administered that and then that didn't, it only numbed part of my body ... I ended up with sort of two or three different cannula for different things ... I really felt like, immobilised by that ... I couldn't, when she was born I couldn't hold her to try and feed her ...*
>
> *The first couple of nights ... I was having trouble sleeping. Not necessarily because of my baby, but because of the people around me ... Eventually they got us a room so [my partner] could stay with me and, I mean, that was good, but ... all night there was the alarm ... beep beep ... And also the heating was broken ... And we couldn't open the window because the window was broken. So it was like this horrible mix of noise again and the kind of heat ...*
>
> *I was getting paranoid about [my partner's] ability to look after our baby while I was asleep because they'd asked me to put earplugs in. But I was finding that, when I put earplugs in, I became really paranoid ... I felt really sort of unsafe by putting them in ...*

Yet, despite Linda's vivid account of her environment, there was little attempt to understand her sleep problems and fears as anything other than 'symptoms' of a disorder. The role of hospital practices, familial support, or the normative social rules surrounding infant care were disregarded, and Linda was admitted to a psychiatric ward and then a mother and baby unit (MBU) and medicated.

Of all the services that women in the Perinatal Study had accessed, MBUs were amongst the most well liked. MBUs are a specialist model of inpatient care for women diagnosed with severe perinatal psychiatric difficulties that admit the mother and baby together. They enable a residential stay that takes women away from the stresses of parenting a newborn at home, often with little support, and can relieve women's concerns about providing for their babies, financially, practically and emotionally. Staff in MBUs help care for newborns, meaning that, for instance, women are able to shower or sleep, things they may have struggled to do at home. Mums often said they developed supportive relationships with other women who were struggling; this too was unique.

Even so, MBU admissions fragment families (although in a world of gender-based violence, this may sometimes be welcome), reinforcing the idea that the mother–infant bond should be prioritised above all others. Thomas Main, a pioneer of joint mother-baby admissions, wrote,

> Just as it seemed important to keep a man patient in touch with his job and to treat him for the difficulties he might meet there, so it seemed important that a mother should be kept in touch with her job, and the children who were part of it.
>
> *(Main, 1958:845)*

Whilst keeping mums and babies together is to be welcomed, MBUs risk simply returning 'diverted' mothers to their natural caring state. Wider social contexts are largely ignored, as described by Yvonne, a young, single, black British mother:

> *And then when she was around like five months I came back out [of the MBU] and things went well for quite a while. It was like the happiest I'd ever been. I had bonded with her and everything was really good. But I just felt, I don't know. I just felt kind of like this is not real life and it didn't really, I think I was on such a high and so comfortable and so bonded, but then when I went back out into the like real life when you have to cook and clean for yourself, wash clothes for yourself and look after your baby 24/7 yourself, it's like it was just a big shock. So I kind of broke down again.*

Yvonne had been diagnosed with postnatal depression in the context of a traumatic birth, relationship breakdown, homelessness and socioeconomic deprivation. She clearly valued the support and respite provided by the MBU. But the failure to address her wider context meant she soon struggled again. Her ongoing difficulties coping with her baby also resulted in child protection concerns, meaning she now risked moving from 'diverted mother' to 'bad mother', further increasing her distress and eroding her ability to cope.

Where is the justice

> *I grew up in a crack house. My mum was a crack user and my stepdad was a crackhead. My house was filthy. My house was … so filthy I couldn't invite people in … friends … A lot of dysfunction was going on in my house.…*
>
> *…I wasn't ready to be a mother. I was sexually assaulted at age thirteen, fourteen. I was told that I couldn't have children because he had damaged me so much down there. When I found out I was pregnant I was, I was shocked. My mum said she'll stand by me no matter what; if I want to keep it or termination. My mum did not stand by me. My mum taught me nothing. My mum never taught me about periods. She never taught me about nothing. All my mum*

taught me is how to use a crack pipe … Social services should've worked with me better. They say that they like to keep families together. I truly believe that I've just been set up…where is the justice in this world?

(Sheryl, a single, black British mother diagnosed with personality disorder whose baby had been taken into care)

Like Sheryl, several mothers in the Perinatal Study were diagnosed with borderline personality disorder, a diagnosis more commonly given to women. These women often described growing up, and now parenting, in acutely traumatic and socially deprived contexts, including relationship breakdown, violence and sexual abuse in child and adulthood, sex work and criminal justice involvement. It was in these contexts that some were feeling ambivalent towards their babies and struggling to parent.

The diagnosis of personality disorder – seen to include persistent or frequent angry feelings, unstable and intense interpersonal relationships, and an unstable sense of self – labelled these mothers' feelings of anger, distress and instability as abnormal; outside of the bounds of what it is reasonable for a woman to feel; a far cry from the mild restraint of the perfect mother. Many of these women felt that they were judged as unfit. These were not diverted mothers; they were bad mothers. There were few attempts to understand how their rage might be legitimate, or how expecting a woman to have a stable sense of self during the transition to motherhood might be unreasonable, especially under these circumstances (for a wider discussion see Rowan Olive 2019).

Several of these mothers felt that their diagnosis and/or a refusal to understand or accept that they could be good mothers, contributed to coercive and discriminatory behaviour against them, particularly by social workers. Serious child protection concerns had been raised in relation to the vast majority, and several had had children removed from their care. Whilst we are aware that, as parents, we can irrevocably harm our children, these mothers felt blamed for their difficulties, judged as inadequate and monstered. Little attention was paid to structural inequalities, trauma contexts, and their lack of access to adequate support. Many felt that they were set up to fail.

More broadly, women are at high risk of deprivation during motherhood (Rabindrakumar, 2018). UK austerity has meant that single parent families and those with three or more children are the most likely to use food banks, often driven by in-work poverty and welfare sanctions (Loopstra et al., 2018a, 2018b). Simone Du Toit (2017) analysed interviews from 11 low income mothers in South Africa diagnosed with postnatal depression and found that many were attempting to mother whilst unable to meet their children's basic needs for food, clothes and school fees. She writes:

> Kruger and Lourens (2016) points out that neoliberal discourse of self-sufficiency in solving one's own problems translates into women's feelings of guilt and shame when they fail to meet their children's needs. Ultimately, the tension between low-income women's constructions of ideal motherhood and their inability to meet these ideals due to poverty-related constraints mean that providing for children is not only a daily struggle but also a marker of personal failure.
>
> *(83)*

Women's twentieth century move into the workplace has not been accompanied by great changes in home set ups, with working mothers in heterosexual relationships typically undertaking the bulk of domestic and emotional labour. Unsurprisingly, mothers, especially with two or more children, are amongst the most stressed in the workplace, with a reduction in working hours within flexible patterns singularly found to reduce stress (Chandola et al., 2019). However, irrespective of personal preference, this is economically unviable for many.

Maternal struggles to provide and survive are juxtaposed with frequent calls by commentators and politicians for parents (mothers) to turn screens off, provide healthier food, read bedtime stories, with middle class parenting approaches – rather than their associated resources – seen as the gold standard. In a further injustice, women's psychiatric diagnoses are seen as a greater cause of damage to their children than their socioeconomic circumstances. Consider the findings of this study, blogged under the title 'Mothers' Depression more Harmful than Poverty for Children's Mental Health':

> there were very early signals that a child might develop symptoms of mental illness. For example, 3-year-olds with poor speech development or irregular bedtimes were more likely than other children to go on to develop symptoms of mental ill health at ages 5 and 11.
>
> *(UCL blog, 2017)*

The same study also found that fathers' mental health had little influence on children (Fitzimons et al., 2017), perpetuating the need for the diverted mother to become the perfect mother. But pathways to mental distress are not set in stone by variable bedtimes. Instead, these children, growing up in difficult circumstances, are being set on a path to having the realities of their lives permanently pathologised.

A different way

Returning to the mother who has lost her unborn child to ECT, what might her account of her distress have been, her personal story? Some of the issues that occur in the perinatal period – some of which we've touched on, some not – that can cause intense stress and distress, include: interpersonal and social transitions and conflicts; changes in social status, identity and employment; traumatic births; chronic sleep deprivation; exhaustion; isolation; lack of community; maternal poverty; mothering through grief; parenting following maternal childhood trauma; gender-based violence; raising children in unequal societies, including the contexts and impacts of racism and homophobia; and sociocultural expectations of women and motherhood including a fear of being honest about the challenges. These factors will come together in different ways for different women, and each will have a complex and shifting account of what is causing her distress (Nicholson, 1998) – her own personal narrative. Put simply, parenting is hard.

Women are socialised to keep going, to put one foot in front of the other, to give to others and ensure their needs are met before our own, to be perfect wives, mothers and colleagues. As we've described, when we deviate from these expected female behaviours – because we are unable to give more, because we are angry, exhausted and operating beyond our resources, because parenting feels like a near impossible undertaking – mental health services tell us we are ill and step in to return diverted mothers to good mothers through diagnosis, medication, hospitalisation and ECT. The bad mothers – those with diagnoses, emotional expressions and behaviours that we cannot accept – are policed and scrutinised.

As we noted in our introduction, some women in the Perinatal Study welcomed psychiatric diagnoses, arguably in part because this granted access to a blameless, diverted mother narrative, with services responsible for returning women to their natural caring state. Yet Dubriwny (2010) describes how this narrative turns attention away from the need to challenge the problematic discourse of the 'essential/good mother'. And how access to this narrative is not equitable, with white, middle-/upper-class women who experience perinatal distress likely to be seen as diverted, while 'out-group' women – typically those of colour, single, deprived, or otherwise mothering outside of dominant cultural norms – are rejected as 'bad mothers' and policed by social services and the criminal justice system. Dubriwny writes: "This replication of the mad/bad mother dichotomy in which a woman is either "afflicted by her hormones or by evil" has negative implications for all women" (2010:297).

In losing interpersonal and sociocultural understandings of the difficulties of motherhood, a focus on familial and sociocultural responses is also lost. Survivor-led and coproduced research could enable an understanding of women's perinatal experiences in their broader context. The aim should not be to impose a single model of understanding on women's experiences, or to produce outputs that re-educate people into a single way of thinking, but to engage with women's perspectives on their circumstances, the causes of their distress, the intersections with their support needs and the implications for whose needs are being met, whose are unmet, and how support gaps might be addressed. This should be underpinned by a fundamental belief in the potential for women's experiential knowledge to transform how distress is conceptualised and responded to, and include, and be led by, women who mother outside of mainstream norms. Whilst we do not want to predict the support that women need, our belief is that it should be trauma-informed, community-based and address structural inequalities (Becker-Bleasley, 2017). This includes implementing or strengthening policies that, for instance, lessen economic pressures on women and families; enable shared parental leave; ensure fair and timely access to welfare; and address discrimination and protect rights.

Whilst we do not naively assume that children would not be taken into care if mothers had adequate support, we do believe that without meaningful support and in an absence of social justice, this becomes inevitable for some. Isobel et al. (2018) found that intergenerational trauma can best be prevented by addressing parental trauma and supporting parent–infant attachments within an approach that includes individuals, families, communities and society. In the Perinatal Study, women at risk of having their children taken into care often valued the support of Parent–Infant Teams. Key is that this avoids simply becoming another way to return mad/bad mothers to their natural mothering role. A further example is provided by Smith and colleagues (2017) in the Norfolk Parent-Infant Mental Health Attachment Project which provides intensive, trauma-informed and systemic support to young families considered 'at risk' – and who would ordinarily be monitored by social services. The project significantly increased the number of children able to remain safely with their families.

Unsurprisingly, where they were able to, women in the Perinatal Study valued connecting with other mums who were struggling. Perinatal peer support has been found to create a sense of connection and validation, and a place to be heard (McLeish and Redshaw, 2017). However, much research into peer support focuses on structured approaches, typically peer support workers employed in the mental health system. We also advocate access to mutual, intentional and trauma-informed peer support outside of psychiatric systems (e.g. Blanch et al., 2012; Filson and Mead, 2016). This is particularly important for perinatal women who can experience distress and overwhelm as the norm in a cultural context of perfect mothers, and who need a place to be honest about their difficult feelings. Certainly, this would have helped us.

Afterword

A final word to our children: we want you to know how much love and joy you brought into our lives as your mums, without at the same time romanticising the task of motherhood.

If you, our daughters, choose the path of motherhood, know that you will make infinite mistakes against the backdrop of society's expectation that women are perfect nurturers, and that this will cause great angst. Know too that your distress, despair, doubt and emotional extremes are ok, and that any struggles you encounter in providing for your child matter. What you will need – what we all need – is compassionate, meaningful support. We hope that by the time you arrive at motherhood (if that is what you choose), that support is something that all women will have.

This chapter summarises independent research funded by the National Institute for Health Research (NIHR) under its Programme Grants for Applied Research (PGfAR) Programme (Grant Reference Number RP-PG-1210-12002). The views expressed are those of the authors and not necessarily those of the NIHR or the Department of Health and Social Care.

References

Anderson E and Reti I (2009). ECT in Pregnancy: a review of the literature from 1941 to 2007. *Psychosomatic Medicine*, 71(2), 235–242.

Becker-Blease, KA (2017). As the world becomes trauma–informed, work to do. *Journal of Trauma & Dissociation*, 18(2), 131–138, DOI: 10.1080/15299732.2017.1253401.

Blanch A, Filson B, Peneny D and Cave C (2012). *Engaging women in trauma-informed peer support: A guidebook*. National Center for Trauma-Informed Care, Rockville, MD.

Chandola T, Booker C, Kumari M and Benzeval M (2019). Are flexible work arrangements associated with lower levels of chronic stress related biomarkers? A study of 6,025 employees in the UK Household Longitudinal Study. *Sociology*. https://doi.org/10.1177/0038038519826014

Dubriwny T (2010). Television news coverage of postpartum disorders and the politics of medicalization. *Feminist Media Studies*, 10(3), 285–303.

Du Toit S (2017). The experience of postpartum distress in the transition to motherhood: A study of one group of low-income mothers in South Africa. Masters Dissertation: Stellenbosch University.

Filson B and Mead S (2016). Becoming part of each other's narratives: Intentional peer support. In J Russo and A Sweeney (eds.). *Searching for a Rose Garden: Challenging Psychiatry, Fostering Mad Studies*. Monmouth: PCCS Books, 109–117.

Fitzimons E, Goodman A, Kelly E and Smith J (2017). Poverty dynamics and parental mental health: Determinants of childhood mental health in the UK. *Social Science and Medicine*, 175, 43–51.

Isobel S, Goodyear M, Furness T and Foster K (2018). Preventing intergenerational trauma transmission: A critical interpretive synthesis. *Journal of Clinical Nursing*. https://doi.org/10.1111/jocn.14735. Accessed: 09 August 2020.

Kruger L and Lourens M (2016). Motherhood and the "madness of hunger": "…want Almal Vra vir My vir 'n Stukkie Brood" ("…because everyone asks me for a little piece of bread"). *Culture, Medicine and Psychiatry*, 40, 124–143.

Leiknes A, Cooke M, Jarosch-von Schweder L, Harboe I and Høie B (2015). Electroconvulsive therapy during pregnancy: A systematic review of case studies. *Archives of Women's Mental Health*, 18(1), 1–39. https://doi.org/10.1007/s00737-013-0389-0. Accessed: 09 August 2020.

Loopstra R, Lambie-Mumford H and Patrick R (2018a). *Family Hunger in Times of Austerity: Families using Food Banks across Britain*. Sheffield University: Sheffield.

Loopstra R, Fledderjohann J, Reeves A and Stuckler D (2018b). Impact of welfare benefit sanctioning on food insecurity: A dynamic cross-area study of food bank usage in the UK. *Journal of Social Policy*, 47(3), 437–457.

McLeish J and Redshaw M (2017). Mothers' accounts of the impact on emotional wellbeing of organised peer support in pregnancy and early parenthood: A qualitative study. *BMC Pregnancy and Childbirth*, 17, 28. https://doi.org/10.1186/s12884-017-1220-0. Accessed: 09 August 2020.

Main T (1958). Mothers with children in a psychiatric hospital. *Lancet*, 2, 845–847.

National Childbirth Trust (NCT) (2018). *The baby blues: What to expect*. https://www.nct.org.uk/life-parent/how-you-might-be-feeling/baby-blues-what-expect. Accessed: 09 August 2020.

National Institute for Health and Clinical Excellence (2018). *Antenatal and Postnatal Mental Health: clinical management and service guidance*. London: The British Psychological Society and The Royal College of Psychiatrists.

Nicolson P (1998). *Post-Natal Depression: psychology, science and the transition to motherhood*. London, New York: Routledge.

Quilter C, Gilbert C and Oliver G (2008). Gene Expression Profiling in Porcine Maternal Infanticide: a model for puerperal psychosis. *American Journal of Medical Genetics*, Part B 147B, 1126–1137.

Rabindrakumar S (2018). One in Four: a profile of single parents in the UK. Gingerbread: London. https://www.gingerbread.org.uk/policy-campaigns/publications-index/one-four-profile-single-parents-uk/. Accessed: 09 August 2020.

Rowan Olive R (2019). Feminist critiques of "BPD". http://rachelrowanolive.co.uk/wp-content/uploads/2019/01/feminist-critiques-of-bpd-1.pdf. Accessed: 09 August 2020.

Smith V, Pratt R, Thomas C and Taggart D (2017). Norfolk Parent-Infant Mental Health Attachment Project (PIMHAP) Working towards integration in attachment, mental health and social care in P Leach (Ed). *Transforming Infant Wellbeing: Research, Policy and Practice for the First 1001 Critical Days*. Oxon, New York: Routledge, 261–271.

Stewart D (2015). Electroconvulsive therapy during pregnancy revisited. *Archives of Women's Mental Health*, 18, 655–656.

Stoppard JM (2000). *Understanding depression: Feminist social constructionist approaches*. London: Routledge.

UCL Blog (2017). Mothers' depression more harmful than poverty for children's mental health, study finds. https://www.ucl.ac.uk/ioe/news/2017/mar/mothers-depression-more-harmful-poverty-childrens-mental-health-study-finds. Accessed: 09 August 2020.

UCL (2019). Stakeholders' views and experiences of perinatal mental health care: A qualitative study (STACEY). https://www.ucl.ac.uk/psychiatry/research/stacey/. Accessed: 09 August 2020.

19

THE PROFESSIONAL REGULATION OF MADNESS IN NURSING AND SOCIAL WORK

Jennifer Poole, Chris Chapman, Sonia Meerai, Joanne Azevedo, Abir Gebara, Nargis Hussaini, and Rebecca Ballen

Introduction

According to the Canadian Association of Social Workers' (CASW) Guidelines for ethical practice (2005), social workers *shall not discriminate* against any person

> on the basis of age, abilities, ethnic background, gender, language, marital status, national ancestry, political affiliation, race, religion, sexual orientation or socio-economic status.
>
> *(2005: 24)*

Social workers are also expected/encouraged to participate in social action by striving to

> identify, document and advocate for the prevention and elimination of domination or exploitation of, and discrimination against, any person…
>
> *(CASW, 2005: 24)*

Despite these very clear guidelines, our research has found that social workers may actively discriminate against each other both intentionally and unintentionally when it comes to issues of 'mental health', madness and distress. In the name of protecting 'public safety', some workers have been disciplined, and some barred from their profession when judged as 'unfit' to practice. Some have been publicly humiliated, named in professional communications and branded as 'incompetent'. All participants in our study have seen their own sense of health and wellbeing worsen or collapse. Indeed, we have argued (Chapman et al, 2016: 43):

> The regulation of who is and isn't 'fit' to practice as a helping professional connects up to a wider problematic or field of political, ethical, and scholarly concern. That problematic is this: although framed as apolitical scientific phemonena, in everyday real life psychiatric diagnoses morally and politically disqualify people from being imaginable

DOI: 10.4324/9780429465444-23

as "competent" human beings. Countless systems are implicated in this extralocal problematic, including many systems that are peopled by helping professionals.

It follows that in the province of Ontario, regulatory colleges for social workers, social service workers and nurses have a formal Fitness to Practice process, 'peopled' by those who seek to 'help'. Part III of the 1998 Social Work and Social Service Act (SWSSA) states:

> Fitness to Practice Committee will hold a hearing to determine any allegation of incapacity on the part of a member of the College. The Fitness to Practice Committee may, after a hearing, find a member of the College to be incapacitated if, in its opinion, the member is suffering from a physical or mental condition or disorder such that the member is unfit to continue to carry out his or her professional responsibilities.

Similarly, the CNO states:

> The Fitness to Practice Committee determines whether a nurse is incapacitated and suffering from a physical or mental condition or disorder that is affecting, *or could affect*, her or his practice.
>
> *(emphasis added)*

Both colleges, then, specifically name "mental condition or disorder" as a possible cause of unfitness. As such, the colleges' position themselves as guardians of public safety and position individual (psychiatrized) professionals as potentially "incapacitated" and dangerous (Chapman et al, 2016: 44).

About the study

Into this context of 'fitness' and 'regulation' was born our research study. Phase I[1] detailed the case studies of two nurses with suspected 'mental health issues' and how they were reported to and disciplined by their respective professional regulatory college in Ontario. The study charted the college reporting process and the subsequent serious health and social effects on the individuals (Chapman et al, 2016).

Using an approach informed by Institutional Ethnography, Phase II sought a wider pool of respondents to better understand the experience of nurses and social workers both prior to being reported to a 'fitness to practice committee' and after. We report on these findings in this chapter.

Literature and orientation

According to the Accommodation for Ontarians with Disabilities Act (AODA, 2005), a 'mental health issue' may be episodic or invisible, but it is a disability legally entitled to accommodation. According to Oldfield (2015), workers who are higher up in their organization's hierarchy will be more successful at gaining such accommodations (see also Dyck and Jongbloed, 2000). In contrast, workers in precarious, shift and contract jobs (as is often the case in allied health) are often less successful (Schultz et al, 2011). Literature on health and work for such allied health professionals highlights the high probability of work burnout, distress, compassion fatigue, as well as negative physiological and mental health outcomes (see Ketelaar et al, 2014; Ray et al, 2013; Skovholt and Trotter-Mathison, 2011; Veage et al, 2014). The literature also highlights the importance of self-care for such professionals (Oldfield, 2015). Yet we have found that if a nurse who is practicing self-care and seeking support discloses their mental distress at work, they may be reported to/by management, found 'unfit' to practice, 'disciplined' and suspended by their regulatory college. The subsequent adverse health and social effects of this include: an increase in distress, often resulting in costly emergency room visits and hospital stays and, if found 'unfit' to work by the college, a loss of wages/employment/housing resulting in economic distress and further precarity (Chapman et al, 2016).

At the same time, regulatory colleges may prioritize the 'duty to protect' the public over the duty to accommodate the mental disability of an allied health worker. This duty to protect is rooted in the notion that the issue or disability not only undermines the allied health worker's ability to perform but it also makes the worker a 'risk' to the public. Regulators need to make sure the public 'trusts' their professionals, that those professionals are 'well' enough to work and are 'managing' their own distress and/or feelings in 'productive' ways. In short, helping professionals are not allowed to feel, to 'hurt' or show distress. Especially at work, they are not actually supposed to be human. This dynamic interacts and interlocks with other forms of oppression in countless ways such as the notion that women, gay men, and transfeminine folks are "too emotional" for example. Additionally, Badwall (2015) notes how this dynamic also plays out for racialized social workers who experience racism on the job.

Importantly, and according to the Ontario Human Rights Commission, the practice of discounting accommodation and disciplining 'feelings' may be in violation of human rights and disability law. Allied health professionals are thus caught betwixt and between; coping with inevitable job/life mental distress yet living with the threat of report and suspension by their regulatory college if they disclose to seek support or accommodation.

We count ourselves into this group, for we all identify as 'health' or helping professionals living with various forms and experiences of (pathologizable) distress. Some of it has been diagnosed and documented, making some of us, like the workers in our study, into patients and users of the 'mental health' system. Some of it is related to the work we do, the trauma we have experienced and the oppressions that have shaped our lives. Some of the labels we have refused, when we could or had a choice, which is more possible the more privileged you are in interlocking arenas of oppression. This multiplicity of understandings and responses to 'mental health' is embraced in the field that is Mad Studies (LeFrançois et al, 2013), but we do not all identify as mad. As some of us have written elsewhere (Meerai et al, 2016), to identify as mad may also be possible only with access to white privilege. And yet, for the purposes of this chapter, our work is clearly informed by a mad stance, one that believes and honours the experience of those who have been othered, labelled or ostracized because of their past/present behavior or 'mental illness', diagnosis, distress, or the suspicion of its presence.

The research process

From this stance, we set about recruiting nurses and social workers/social service workers. We used non-probability sampling techniques and specifically snowball and convenience sampling through social media, flyers and word of mouth. Participants all had a reporting/accommodation/discipline experience in the workplace or with their professional colleges. Participants were diverse in terms of age (25–60), mostly Canadian citizens who identified as women, with Bachelor's and Master's degrees in social work (50% of our group) or nursing (50%). Eight participants identified as racialized and one identified as Indigenous. Over 50% of participants were registered with their respective college, but for some participants, registration with the college had been or was suspended.

The interviews were guided by the qualitative methodology known as Institutional Ethnography (IE). Utilized during Phase 1 and developed by Dorothy Smith (2005), Institutional Ethnography seeks to explore a 'problematic' such as being reported to a college, establishing the series of events that led to the problematic and making visible the 'regimes of ruling' that govern the process. Although we do not strictly follow IE in this chapter, it guided our mapping out of the 14 participants' experiences before, during and after being reported.

Findings part 1: Before the report is made

In this first section of our findings, we chart the common experiences that happen before a report to the college for a 'mental health issue'. Following Burstow (2015), the path to being reported is not linear or predictable, and yet the 14 participants related resonant experiences.

'Better not be broken': The pressure to manage one's own mental health

We start with what we call an expectation of self-regulation and management. Otherwise known in the literature as managerialism (and neoliberalism), this expectation demands:

> …alteration of the self, rather than the institution. Change is largely redirected from the collective to the individual actor.
>
> *(Clegg, 2008 as cited in Barnoff et al, 2017: 8)*

"In the neoliberal institution, the preferred subjectivity is for employees to become entre-preneurial, competitive, and self-governing individuals, characterized as self-sufficient, self-directing, and enterprising" (Clarke, 2010; Clegg, 2008; Morrish, 2014, as cited in Barnoff et al, 2017: 8).

This managerial focus on self-regulation and self-direction was described by most participants. For social/service workers who want to continue their membership with the college, for example,

> we have to do a self-evaluation every year where we write down our goals, and though we don't have to send it in, it can be audited at any time.

A similar process exists for nurses, with requirements to carry out learning plans and a warning about 'random' audits if members are not managing their own learning, evaluations and/or any issues that may arise. We come back to this random assessment later in the findings section.

Participants explained the expectation is "that you'd be able to handle it all and if you can't handle it then maybe you shouldn't be in this field". Another noted, "Sure, you can be a social worker, but you better not be a lemon, right? Better not be broken". They added that the message they had received time and again in the field was, "you know, you really should be keeping your personal stuff at home. We don't really want to see that at work".

These experiences often contradict the publicly expressed and often anti-oppressive values of the profession or employer, reminding us of the work of Wilson and Beresford (2000). As one participant summarized, staff just have to be doing the most work possible in the least amount of time. So, it's basically a factory. So, they don't have time for our, whatever issues we might have going on. Like they don't care. 'Cause all they hear is that we're not gonna be able to work at the speed that they want us to work at.

'Not here to protect us'

Given the neoliberal focus outlined above, it was not surprising to find that all the participants experienced a lack of accommodation and support either from their employer or from their college. A participant noted,

I was dealing with some anxiety from stuff in the past and then also from the stuff that I was dealing with at work. Instead of asking me if I needed accommodations, they told me that they didn't think I could do my job.

A social worker explained to us that

My doctor wrote them [the employer] more notes saying, 'You need to accommodate this person' … He was writing letters saying this employee is ready to return to work, if you could accommodate this … And they just refused. They would not even answer.

And a nurse who specifically asked their employer to be accommodated "was told that it-it could not accommodate me for less clients or less patients …". A social worker explained that without any accommodation or support, they wondered what the actual benefits of registering with a college might be:

they make that clear to us that it's in our best interest to be registered with a college. Legally, in many places, you can't work unless you are a registered social worker, but there are no benefits to us… the College is there to protect the public, not to protect us.

Fear of report to employer or college

With an emphasis on 'self-regulation' and a lack of accommodation/supports, it also came as no surprise to us that *all the participants* spoke about the fear of being reported (for the first time) or of being reported *again*. This fear of report was palpable in the interviews, shaping workers' ways of being at work and home, of relating, trusting as well as all aspects of their health and wellness. It also impacted where they were applying to work:

Even when I have applied to places at X, I was told don't disclose that you're a person with lived experience … they usually don't come out as having lived experience until they've been hired. That's what I was always told. Don't tell them before you're hired.

we're humans so … our mental health fluctuates … so whether we're going through something work related or personal related I would fear that if I was reported … that would be just, I don't actually have words to describe how awful that would be personally.

Similarly, a participant noted, "I don't think that I know of a single nurse that would ever claim to the college that they had a problem because they'd be too afraid of the repercussions of it".

'They taught me how to lie'

This fear can then lead to a set of common practices we call *strategic dishonesty*.[2] As described by one participant,

> I know that there have been times where I've not been fully honest enough, and saying I have a doctor's appointment where actually I need to go to a different type of appointment.

Another participant felt this practice was

> a lot more common than a lot of people talk about … people feel like they can't … really speak freely about needing accommodations. Without being stigmatized, without the idea of them not doing their jobs properly or being like lesser in regards to the work that they do.

Tragically, for one participant who did choose to be honest about their issues and disclose, "…if I had known it would play out like this, I would've never disclosed". This person had disclosed because they needed support, but "I didn't think, it would come with more serious repercussions". They added:

> The college has taught me how to lie; it's a horrible, horrible thing to say, it has taught me how to lie to people and how to be dishonest. Because me being honest, being upfront got me in trouble, more trouble so that's what taught me how to keep things close to my chest and how not to trust people.

After a similar experience, a nursing participant explained, "And I still don't trust people … That's what got me into trouble…". Detailing what the long-term effects of this disclosure and subsequent response entailed, this participant explained:

> Cause what ended up happening when something like this happens, you build shame. And then you start to be secretive about everything. And then you start living alone. And the more you live alone you start to make that the norm. And you don't open up. And the more you don't open up the more you bottle up inside. And the more you bottle up inside the worse it gets.

With such ramifications for being honest, it becomes very possible that a worker might practice the opposite. Summing up all the experiences that can lead to a report, one participant said, "It just feels like they just push until you know, rise to it or you go on medical leave or you quit or you get fired".

Findings part 2: Discipline without report to the college

To recap, we have explained that participants are pressured to self-manage, are working without support or accommodation and in great fear. Now we turn to the kinds of disciplinary experiences they shared with us that take place prior to or instead of a direct report to a regulatory college. It is crucial to note that all but one of the participants we met with had been disciplined or formally punished for experiencing 'mental health issues' in the present or in the past.

One form of discipline is the 'random' audit/assessment. As introduced earlier, nurses registered with the college do a learning plan every year. They can be randomly called for an assessment. According to one participant, this was part of a disciplinary response to their 'mental health issues'. The participant explained, "…they emailed me and said ya know your name's come up, we want to see your learning plan so I had to submit that". It did not feel particularly random.

A second common form of discipline is a 'warning' from an employer. A social worker explained that, "there's basically different levels of disciplining somebody … at my agency it's a verbal warning and then it's a written warning. And then it can go to a second written warning which then turns into the work plan sometimes. And if you don't end up doing well on the work plan then you're basically asked to leave, like you're fired". Again, please note that none of these participants had ever had a client, patient, or member of the public express concern about their work or behaviour. These disciplinary measures were in response only to concerns that supervisors or co-workers had upon hearing about a diagnosis, witnessing distress, or in response to a request for accommodation.[3]

Another participant explained what was in the warning letters from their employer. "There was stuff in the letters about maybe she shouldn't be working in this field. This field is very difficult, it's very challenging, and not everybody can do this kind of work". This same participant then had to go through a process called 'performance management' with weekly meetings with their manager and constant scrutiny of all their work:

> Every day she was on me … I've never heard of anybody else having to go through this. She would go through every single bit of my work, every pen stroke. Every single [week] I would have supervision with her. It would go from one in the afternoon until five PM. And I would have crying fits … And she wouldn't let me leave the room. She would say, 'Oh, no… you're just being too emotional, you need to just stay here. Just pull yourself together so we can get through this work'. It was so condescending and so humiliating…

The report and its aftermath

It is at this point, when workers are being assessed, warned or heavily 'managed' that they may also be reported to the college, and there are multiple ways for this to happen. Here we focus on two routes in particular; self-disclosure and manager report. It is crucial to note again that NONE of the participants in our study were ever reported to their employer or college by a patient or service user.

Further, by self-disclosure we do not mean that any of our participants decided to call their respective college and suggest they were unfit to practice. Self-disclosure can be a casual conversation between peers at work about an experience of distress long ago. Self-disclosure can be a conscious request for support or accommodation or, as explained below, it can also be prompted by an advisor or mental health professional.

> …it was recommended by my doctor, him and I had many conversations, and we decided to report, and I did. I told them what was going on and from there everything,

even though I was in recovery for a year and a half. They [the employer] still reported me to the college, and my colleagues then came to me and questioned my fitness to practice.

Similarly, a social worker described,

I thought if I was honest about the stuff that was going on in my life, they would probably be more understanding given the fact that we're a mental health agency. So that was thrown in my face real quick.

Additionally, a nursing participant agreed that telling her manager

wasn't well received ... I poured my heart out and I can still – she didn't support me. So, I went to my union rep and I suppose it all came out and resurfaced and it got to upper management it got to the chief nursing manager and they had to report me to the college of nurses ... I never had a patient complain in 33 years. And then it came to this.

Conversely, the report can be made directly by a manager, without any prior 'evidence' or documentation. In one case, a previously 'kind' nursing manager inquired as to a nurse's health after a bad fall at work and subsequently decided to make a report to the college.

The manager said, "Are you being followed?" And I made the mistake of saying, "Yes". And she said, "Well what are you doing?" And I said, "I'm taking medication". Even though it wasn't her right to know, she asked me, "What medication are you on?" And I said ... Right away that sent alarm bells, and red flags.

For nurses, any suspected fitness to practice issue related to mental health goes to:

the medical committee: the medical committee then decides what areas they have looked at and if this is a valid thing or it's not a valid thing. And suppose that it is a valid thing and there's evidence and it questions your practice it then goes on to another committee ... and then they respond whether they want to appear in front of the college ... most people will take whatever the college recommends and go from there, most people do not want to appear before the college.

Once brought before the college, the person is explicitly evaluated for fitness to practice, which partly involves the gathering of evidence from 'experts'. Shockingly, however, participants commonly described how their college would refuse any 'evidence' suggesting that they were fit to practice. One participant explained, "I got letters from a minster that I got counseling from, a psychologist, a clinical psychiatrist, a social worker that I was getting support after care, even the folks that I got treatment from, nothing, nothing was acceptable". For another, "They refused my doctor's diagnosis ... He is a psychiatrist that teaches at X. He is a practicing doctor with a license, right? But they refused to accept that". One participant detailed the grueling experience of being evaluated by her college's psychiatrist:

[The college's psychiatrist] interviewed me a total of four times. And interviews were anywhere from two to six hours long. I guess he just didn't find anything. And by the time I was kind of disoriented. You're doing 15-hour shifts, and then you're being asked all these psychological questions. So, I reached in for my bag, and he goes,

'What are you doing?' I'm like, 'Oh, I'm just getting Tylenol. My back's kind of sore.'
So, he writes in the interview, 'The client reaches into her bag for pain relievers'.
They watch your every move. They write everything about you from the minute you
walk into the door. The way you're walking. Your posture. How you're sitting. What
you're wearing.

For the participants in our study who were then found to be 'unfit' to practice, their names may
be publicly shared in various formats. For social workers/social service workers, we learned that
"We do have a College newsletter that writes you up and shares with other registered social
workers and social service workers who have lost their registration as a result of some indiscre-
tion". For some nurses in our study, their names were published on a web site: "…they have
a website called 'find a nurse'; what they would do is, they would publish your name on this
website, the entire world could see, your name would get published and they would also have
restrictions to practice…". For one nurse that had such restrictions on their practice for more
than five years:

I was unable to get a job because I had restrictions on my license … and that whole
time my life has been affected, and I was unable to work, unable to purchase a home,
unable to be in a relationship, fell into severe depression … tried to commit suicide,
like there was so many things that a committee makes one decision and doesn't realize
the effects it has on that person…

Indeed, all of the participants who had been reported to their college and found unfit because
of their 'mental health issues' experienced severe and lasting suffering. Listening to these stories
of denigration and violence, even in a research interview, was extremely difficult. Experiencing
it first-hand, of course, is much more devastating. Participants described it as "the most horrific
experience I've ever had to go through in my life", and "I probably have had some significant
traumatic events in my life, this, going through the college is probably the most, right up at the
top…". And the suffering is long-lasting:

I feel as though I'm still suffering. I feel as though I haven't really had a chance and I'm
going to feel as though I'm going to carry this until my death, and I want a chance to
properly heal because I don't want to take this until I die. It's right there sitting inside
me and I'm still suffering.

Discussion

Our study has thus far taught us many things. We have learned that the helping professions may
not be so very helpful when it comes to issues related to distress and disability. We have learned
that there is an active and well-designed system of discrimination directed at workers expected
to manage themselves in 'productive' ways. We have also learned that, in the name of public
safety, there may be no room to feel, no room to ask for support or accommodation and no
room for refusal or evidence that opposes the idea that those of us with 'mental health issues'
are unfit, incompetent or, worse, threats to society.

It would appear the helping professions are sites of what Procknow calls 'sane supremacy', as
this inevitably interlocks with white supremacy, cisheteropatriarchy, and capitalist denigrations
of precarious and working class people. We agree that "political, academic, social, and mainstream media realms" as well as employers and regulatory bodies "collude to shore up 'saneness'

as normative, and those falling outside the prescribed 'sane' boundaries are non-normative" (2017: 913)

In addition to sane supremacy, it would also appear that another 'regime of ruling' (Burstow, 2015) is at work. The discourse of 'protection of public safety' is a useful tool in settler states, providing cover for rights violations and legal discrimination against those imagined to pose a threat, whether real or perceived. No actual harm or threat to the public initiated any of the degradations and violence that our participants were subjected to. Rather, *perceived* threat is often used to justify the unfair treatment of people living in poverty, racialized people, and those with mental health diagnoses. This happens only based on stereotypes. In the absence of actual harm or threat, this is "mental health profiling", a legally recognized human rights violation (Ontario Human Rights Commission, nd).

> Mental health profiling is any action taken for reasons of safety, security or public protection that relies on stereotypes about a person's mental health or addiction instead of on reasonable grounds, to single out a person for greater scrutiny or different treatment.
>
> *(OHRC, nd)*

Such profiling can happen in conjunction with racial profiling or criminal profiling. It can also happen when behavior is judged as 'different' than a carefully constructed rational norm even though it does not present any concern for service users or the public. Without a doubt, our participants were subjected to mental health profiling. In a climate of neoliberal managerialism, they were surveilled and randomly assessed, with any hint of difficulty or distress taken as a reason to 'single out a person for greater scrutiny or different treatment'. That scrutiny has its own process and its own desired ends and is based on negative assumptions about mad folk and those with disabilities or experiences of distress. It assumes that we are a threat to 'public safety', relying on long debunked sanist stereotypes (Perlin, 1992) that persons with experiences of diagnosis or distress are more likely to perpetrate violence. Scholars of Mad and Disability studies have long provided evidence to the contrary, however: people with psychiatric diagnoses are considerably more likely to be the victims of violence but are not statistically any more likely to commit violence (Erevelles and Minear, 2010; Joseph, 2016; Spivakovsky, 2017; Steele, 2016).

This brings us to epistemic injustice. Citing Fricker (2007), LeBlanc and Kinsella (2016) explain epistemic injustice occurs in the helping professions when a person is insulted or wronged in their capacity as knower. Such a person or group of people will be 'unfairly depicted as intellectually inferior or lacking in credibility' (Medina, 2012) by those deemed more powerful. According to Fricker (2007, 2010), this can present itself as testimonial injustice or when a speaker's capacity to know and share their knowledge is in question because the hearer holds prejudicial feelings towards the speaker's identity. Epistemic injustice may also present as hermeneutical injustice when the same applies to groups of people trying to articulate their social experiences (Fricker, 2007; Medina, 2012). In our participants' accounts, when they were disciplined or reported to their regulatory colleges for sharing their distress or diagnosis, they were subjected to epistemic injustice; they were depicted as lacking in credibility, competence and 'fitness to practice' by hearers who had *already decided* that they – or people 'like them' – were dangerous and a threat to public safety. It does not matter what participants did or said, or what evidence they provided to the contrary, they had already been assumed guilty by a system founded on neoliberalism, managerialism, surveillance and interlocking forms of oppression including sane supremacy. They had already been found epistemically untrust-worthy, epistemically disposable and extraneous.

Conclusion

> Thank you so much for your work ... It [is] more a sense of relief that yes, there will
> be something out there for people like that. And just my heart was just shining, like
> alive to know that we haven't been forgotten.

For all these reasons, we seek epistemic justice for those we interviewed, for those reading this who share in these experiences and for all those who fear what may befall them as a result of being 'registered' helping professionals who dare to want support. Those who shared their time, experience and suffering speak the truth. They are to be heard and to be listened to very carefully, for they tell cautionary tales about the violence that the so-called helping professions are capable of. Lives are shattered by the disciplinary tactics of employers and regulators. When participants' experience with our professional bodies is so "horrific" that their recommenda-tion is to lie about their madness, it is clear that something is very wrong in nursing and social work. And if these professions are so harsh on their workers – how must they be on those who are patients? The resonance between these stories and those of others subjected to the gaze and regulations of the helping professions points to the fact that something is very wrong much more broadly. How is it that our social structures that appear to be set up to support, help, and accommodate are so frequently violent, intrusive, and oppressive? What must we take from these stories of helping professionals who have never had service users or patients formally complain about their work but who are nevertheless treated as a threat to the public? What can this teach us about how humans are regularly differentiated and siphoned into categories of worthy and unworthy, fit and unfit, valuable and disposable?

In terms of the future of this research, our next step will be to detail what participants suggested needs to happen now, how system-wide advocacy needs to bring regulatory law in line with disability law and how participants have imagined a radically distinct system based on caring for one another instead of naming and shaming. One participant summarized this as "let's get rid of the reporting and have supporting". We could not agree more.

Notes

1 We want to formally recognize the late Dr. Bonnie Burstow for bringing three of us together. By invitation from Dr. Burstow, Rebecca, Chris and Jennifer participated in a project focused on using Institutional Ethnography to better understand the machinations of psychiatry. Thus, began phase 1 of our work together, resulting in our joint publication in 2016.

2 This phenomenon is common among service users' navigations of unjust helping systems (see for example Dean Spade's (2013) work on trans surgeries or Jennifer Clarke's research (2012) on Afro-Caribbean moms 'cooperating' with child protection services.

3 In sharp contrast, research shows that service users/clients prefer to work with somebody who has lived experience of life difficulties and distress (see for example Jijian Voronka's work).

References

Accessibility for Ontarians with Disabilities Act, 2005, S.O. 2005, c. 11. (AODA) (2005) Toronto: Government of Ontario. https://www.ontario.ca/laws/statute/05a11.

Badwall H K (2015) Colonial encounters: Racialized social workers negotiating professional scripts of whiteness. *Intersectionalities: A Global Journal of Social Work Analysis, Research, Polity, and Practice* 3: 1–23.

Barnoff L, Moffatt K, Todd S, and Panitch M (2017) Academic leadership in the context of neo-liberalism: The practice of social work directors. *Canadian Social Work Review/Revue canadienne de service social* 34(1): 5–21.

Burstow, B (2015) *Psychiatry and the business of madness: An ethical and epistemological accounting*. Chicago: Springer.

Canadian Association of Social Workers (CASW) (2005) *Guidelines for ethical practice*. Ottawa: Canadian Association of Social Workers.

Chapman C, Azevedo J, Ballen R, and Poole J (2016) A kind of collective freezing-out: How helping professionals' regulatory bodies create "incompetence" and increase distress. In B Burstow (ed) *Psychiatry interrogated*. New York: Palgrave Macmillan, 41–61.

Clarke J (2012) Beyond child protection: Afro-Caribbean service users of child welfare. *Journal of Progressive Human Services* 23(3): 223–257.

Dyck I and Jongbloed L (2000) Women with multiple sclerosis and employment issues: A focus on social and institutional environments. *Canadian Journal of Occupational Therapy* 67(5): 337–346.

Erevelles N and Minear A (2010) Unspeakable offenses: Untangling race and disability in discourses of intersectionality. *Journal of Literary & Cultural Disability Studies* 4(2): 127–145.

Fricker M (2007) *Epistemic injustice: Power and the ethics of knowing*. Oxford: Oxford University Press.

Fricker M (2010) Replies to Alcoff, Goldberg, and Hookway on epistemic injustice. *Episteme* 7(2): 164–178.

Joseph A J (2016) *Deportation and the confluence of violence within forensic mental health and immigration systems*. New York: Springer.

Ketelaar S M, Nieuwenhuijsen K, Gärtner F R, Bolier L, Smeets O and Sluiter J K (2014) Mental Vitality @ Work: The effectiveness of a mental module for workers' health surveillance for nurses and allied health professionals, comparing two approaches in a cluster-randomised controlled trial. *International Archives of Occupational and Environmental Health* 87(5): 527–538.

Leblanc S and Kinsella E (2016) Toward epistemic justice: A critically reflexive examination of sanism and implications for knowledge generation. *Studies in Social Justice* 10(1): 59–78.

LeFrançois B A, Menzies R and Reaume G (eds) (2013) *Mad matters: A critical reader in Canadian mad studies*. Toronto: Canadian Scholars' Press.

Medina J (2012) Hermeneutical injustice and polyphonic contextualism: Social silences and shared hermeneutical responsibilities. *Social Epistemology* 26(2): 201–220.

Meerai S, Abdillahi I and Poole J (2016) An introduction to anti-Black Sanism. *Intersectionalities: A Global Journal of Social Work Analysis, Research, Polity, and Practice* 5(3): 18–35.

Oldfield M A (2015) *Staying in the Workforce with Fibromyalgia*. Unpublished PhD thesis. University of Toronto.

Ontario Human Rights Commission (nd). *Mental health profiling (fact sheet)*. http://www.ohrc.on.ca/en/mental-health-profiling-fact-sheet Accessed: 16.05.2020.

Perlin M L (1992) On sanism. *SMU Law Review* 46: 373.

Procknow G (2017) Trump, proto-presidency, and the rise of sane supremacy. *Disability & Society* 32(6): 913–917.

Ray S L, Wong C, White D and Heaslip K (2013) Compassion satisfaction, compassion fatigue, work life conditions, and burnout among frontline mental health care professionals. *Traumatology* 19(4): 255–267.

Schultz I Z, Milner R A, Hanson D B and Winter A (2011) Employer attitudes towards accommodations in mental health disability. In I Z Schultz and E S Rogers (eds) *Work accommodation and retention in mental health*. New York: Springer, 325–340.

Skovholt T M and Trotter-Mathison M (2011) *The resilient practitioner; burnout prevention and self-care strategies for counsellors, therapists, teachers, and health professionals*. New York: Routledge.

Smith D E (2005) *Institutional ethnography: A sociology for people*. Walnut Creek: Rowman Altamira.

Spade D (2013) Mutilating gender. In S Stryker and S Whittle (eds) *The transgender studies reader 2*. New York: Routledge, 331–348.

Spivakovsky C (2017) Governing freedom through risk: Locating the group home in the archipelago of confinement and control. *Punishment & Society* 19(3): 366–383.

Steele L (2016) Court authorised sterilisation and human rights: Inequality, discrimination and violence against women and girls with disability. *UNSW Law Journal* 39: 1002.

Veage S, Ciarrochi J, Deane F P, Andresen R, Oades L G and Crowe T P (2014) Value congruence, importance and success and in the workplace: Links with well-being and burnout amongst mental health practitioners. *Journal of Contextual Behavioral Science* 3(4): 258–264.

Wilson A and Beresford P (2000) 'Anti-oppressive practice': Emancipation or appropriation? *The British Journal of Social Work* 30(5): 553–573.

20

THE (GLOBAL) RISE OF ANTI-STIGMA CAMPAIGNS

Jana-Maria Fey and China Mills

Introduction

Within the global mental health assemblage (a diverse network of actors, organisations, technologies, policies and ideas that aim to scale up access to mental health services globally) stigma is a key point of focus. In this assemblage, mental distress is understood as illness and as universal, meaning that stigmatisation of "mental illness" is also thought to be universal, to be "worsening", and to be "the greatest obstacle to the improvement of the lives of people with mental illness and their families" (Kadri and Sartorius, 2005: 0597). As a response to this, there has been a rise and intensification of anti-stigma and mental illness awareness campaigns both nationally and internationally. Anti-stigma campaigns have increasingly become a feature of everyday public health initiatives around the world. By and large these campaigns aim to improve attitudes towards mental illness and end mental health discrimination by educating the public that mental distress is best understood and acted upon through biomedical and psychological explanations and interventions.

The focus of this chapter is the leading anti-stigma campaign in the UK – *Time to Change* (TTC), which launched in 2007, aiming to "change the way we all think and act about mental health problems" (TTC, n.d.). *Time to Change* is now part of a Global Anti-Stigma Alliance (GASA) which aims to "eliminate mental health stigma and discrimination around the world" (TTC, 2019).

In this chapter we draw upon scholarship from Mad Studies, survivor research and user-controlled research (and the necessary intersections between these diverse areas of scholarship) (Faulkner, 2017a; Sweeney, 2016), and including the scholarship of Mad people of colour, to provide an anti-sanist and intersectional analysis of the ways in which conceptualisations of stigma, and resultant anti-stigma campaigns, are constituted by and reproduce sanism. Sanism is understood here as a "system of discrimination and oppression" deeply embedded in western thinking and that underpins epistemic injustice and marginalises Mad ways of knowing (Leblanc and Kinsella, 2016: 61; Poole and Jivraj, 2015). Sanism is closely entwined with psychocentrism – the location of difference and transformation inside bodies and minds, instead of within socioeconomic and political structures (Rimke and Brock, 2012). In contrast, Mad studies "produces knowledge where the meaning-making of mad people is centred", against the societal debasement of mad people's knowledge (within and outside of academia)

DOI: 10.4324/9780429465444-24

(Leblanc and Kinsella, 2016). Yet sanism is not experienced in the same way by all Mad folks as it intersects with other forms of oppression, including racism and white supremacy (Gorman, et al, 2013; Meerai et al, 2016). McWade (2019) uses a Mad Studies analysis of anti-stigma campaigns that construct mental distress as illness to show how these representations are themselves productive of stigmatising psy-discourse – where stigma is understood as a form of power. This chapter makes the point that as anti-stigma gets done globally, it is important both to draw upon Mad knowledge to understand the potentially sanist practices of anti-stigma campaigns but also grapple with and challenge the whiteness of some Mad Studies scholarship. The chapter proceeds as follows: First, we provide a reflection on our positionality within the discipline of Mad Studies. Second, we sketch briefly the recent history of anti-stigma campaigns before introducing England's *Time to Change* campaign and the associated global anti-stigma alliance (GASA). We will contextualise the significance of these campaigns through observations of the way TTC is performed at key events (attended by one of the authors of this chapter), before exploring the assumptions about the workings of stigma made by TTC.

Who we are

Positionality is also part of anti-sanist praxis. As authors we want to avoid the temptation of succumbing to confessing our subject positions and then breathing a sigh of relief and carrying on as 'normal'. Yet it does matter who we are, and from where we write this chapter. It matters that we are two white, European women who have different relationships with distress and madness, but who do not identify as 'mad' or as 'survivors' (although our lives have been touched by both psychiatry and psychopharmaceuticals). It matters that our relationship is shaped by unequal power relations of student and academic 'supervisor'. It also matters that we write from locations within both the colonial University and UK University marketplace where book chapters such as this are seen to 'count' for nothing in the numerical ranking of research outputs. The western University is a site through which colonialism as a global project, and specifically colonial knowledge and hierarchies, is "produced, consecrated, institutionalised, and naturalised" (Bhambra et al, 2018: 5). This is significant because it highlights the potential limitations of critiques generated form colonial spaces, including some Mad Studies scholarship (discussed later).

Potted history of anti-stigma campaigns in the UK

This section introduces the development of anti-stigma campaigns in the United Kingdom through a discussion of the three principal mental illness awareness campaigns since the 1990s: *Defeat Depression* (1992–96), *Changing Minds* (1998–2003) and *Time to Change* (2007–2019/present). An exploration of the historical context and power dynamics in which these initiatives operate aids in illustrating how current campaigns have emerged to correspond with neoliberal and globalising logics of stigma and mental health.

The Royal College of Psychiatrists' (RCP) 4-year *Defeat Depression* (1992–96) campaign was a response to research that identified considerable reluctance and embarrassment (interpreted as due to stigma) in people to seek professional help when they feel depressed (Priest et al, 1995). The principal messages devised to address this perceived stigma were to show that depression is a common disorder amongst the population, and that professional help is easily accessible in the form of anti-depressants and psychiatric counselling (IJHCQA, 1995). Within the timeframe of this campaign, attitudes towards people with depression only shifted marginally in response, while the prescription of antidepressants increased by over 50% (Paykel et al, 1998). *Defeat Depression* was followed two years later by another RCP campaign on a larger scale: *Changing Minds* (1998–2003) was an attempt to educate the public (including GPs and the media) about the nature of mental illness as there was a perceived lack of understanding of the common occurrence of mental disorders, supposedly leading to stigma against those diagnosed. While people experiencing issues with substance-use were viewed as the most stigmatised, those suffering from depression or schizophrenia were generally depicted by the media as "violent, erratic and dangerous" (Luty et al, 2007: 327). Through 'factsheets', advertising campaigns and education packages sent out to newspapers, *Changing Minds* attempted to improve attitudes to mental disorders. The logic that followed this campaign was that – if mental illnesses are put on the same level as physical illnesses, not viewed as an individual's fault, and addressed through medication and correct treatment, then attitudes towards those experiencing mental distress would improve. While follow-up studies (e.g. Abraham et al, 2010; Sampogna et al, 2017) found little evidence that *Changing Minds* brought about significant positive changes in public attitudes, the campaign laid the groundwork for England's current *Time to Change* (TTC) campaign.

Time to Change (TTC) and the Global Anti-Stigma Alliance (GASA)

Time to Change was launched in 2007 and is jointly managed by the UK-based charities *Mind* and *Rethink Mental Illness*, both of which receive funding from the UK government. According to their website, mental health charity *Mind* (2018) received £1.9m funding from the government in 2018 alone to run *Time to Change*. This, and the fact that the government's current mental health strategy (Department of Health and Social Care, 2016) stresses the importance of combating stigma, suggests a long-term policy interest in constructing and responding to the rising diagnoses of mental illness in the UK as a public health issue. Moreover, the UK government continues to pledge increased funding in support of *Time to Change*.

In 2012, the Director of *Time to Change* – Sue Baker – became one of the co-founders of the Global Anti-Stigma Alliance (GASA). Currently combining the efforts of 17 countries, GASA was created with the aim to

> share learning, methodologies, best practice, materials, and the latest evidence in order to achieve better outcomes for people facing stigma and discrimination related to mental health issues.
>
> *(Time to Change, 2017: 2)*

Its secretariat and coordination lies with England's *Time to Change* campaign, and even though, at first glance, the Alliance appears to be a loose network of mental health anti-stigma campaigns around the globe, it has established itself as an arm-length body of *Time to Change* England through a strong presence on social media. In 2018 GASA released a short video "Time to Change Global – It's time to talk about mental health" which features mental health stories from around the world, including celebrity stories by Nadiya Hussain, a popular British TV chef and presenter, and Glenn Close, an American award-winning actress. Negative consequences of stigma are identified as creating barriers to employment and adequate psychiatric treatment, while stigma is described as "knowing no boundaries", affecting "all ages, all income groups and all cultures" and as deeply ingrained in all societies and that these must be transformed to put mental health on the same level as physical health. In the film, transformation is imagined through encouraging people to talk about their experience and diagnosis, which is presented as therapeutic.

Similarly to TTC, GASA puts a strong emphasis on the use of stories of lived experiences (so called 'leaders of change') and evidence-based programmes to eliminate mental health stigma and discrimination (TTC, 2019: 3). Despite GASA's insistence that approaches to tackle mental health discrimination "vary from country to country and are tailored according to need and culture as, as such, are not identical" (TTC, 2019: 2) the messages about mental illness that are communicated via GASA's social media presence mirror those which are used in the national context of England. For example, the idea that "1 in 4" is affected by a mental illness and that a 'social movement' which encourages talking about mental health issues is a key driver of change against mental health discrimination. GASA presents an interesting window into the emerging global politics of mental health as its narrative merges psychiatric knowledge with the idea of a 'social movement'. Despite the current lack of dedicated funding for the organisation (TTC, 2019), it has stressed that

> eliminating mental health stigma and discrimination is the work of generation and therefore requires long term and sustained activity and investment.
>
> *(TTC, 2019: 3)*

Tweeting anti-stigma

Time to Change, as the leading anti-stigma campaign in the UK, relies heavily on the use of social media to distribute its message, reach, and interaction with the public. In the case of GASA, the most up-to-date information about the campaign can often be found in its social media feeds, particularly Twitter. In the following, we will illustrate, through an engagement with tweets by the *Time to Change Global* twitter account, how 'stigma' is conceptualised within the global agenda of mental health discourse. The notion of 'mental health stigma' as an obstacle to be overcome by countries is invoked through several different narratives that run through *Time to Change*'s online discourse. The key two 'stories' told about mental health by *Time to Change* are summarised in the following two tweets from the *Time to Change Global* Twitter account:

> Mental health problems know no boundaries – it affects all ages, all income groups, and all cultures.
>
> *(Twitter; 10 Oct 2018)*

> Every country in the world can be considered as a developing country when it comes to #mentalhealth.
>
> *(TTC Global Twitter; Vikram Patel; 10 Oct 2018)*

The first tweet mobilises a common statistic ("1 in 4") employed by mental health campaigns in the UK to draw attention to the prevalence and commonality of mental health problems. This idea is now extended to discuss the global phenomenon of rising diagnoses of mental illnesses. Two things are missed in this first tweet. Firstly, mental distress does not affect everyone equally. For example, in the UK, people from Black and minority ethnic backgrounds as well as those living under austerity or harsh economic conditions are much more likely to experience mental distress, to be diagnosed with a mental health condition, and to experience the hard end of mental health services (including force and coercion) (Legraien, 2018; Longhurst, 2017). Moreover, the assertion that "mental health knows no boundaries" seems to suggest that mental illnesses can be diagnosed in any global setting using the same diagnostic logics by which a mind is judged to be 'healthy' or 'unhealthy'. Thereby, the "1 in 4" mentality also aids in the process of 'othering' those who are diagnosed with a mental disorder. Put simply, the idea that mental distress operates without borders puts forward a globalising narrative of mental illness that does not consider the fact that not everyone is affected equally by experiences of mental distress nor, that Western psychiatry may be rejected outside (or even within) its geographical context.

The second tweet exemplifies the problematic narrative of *Time to Change* in two related ways. Firstly, it suggests that there is a relationship between mental health and a country's level of 'development'. This is problematic not only because it leaves unquestioned notions that development is necessary and of who gets to define what counts as development, but also because it posits mental health as an obstacle to development processes (Mills, 2018a). Secondly, since 'every country' is in need of development, it implies that more 'scaling-up' is to be done in terms of tackling mental health stigma. This developmentalist narrative that places 'stigma' at the forefront of mental health issues worldwide forms part of a much broader emerging global mental health assemblage, including calls to 'scale up' access to mental health services worldwide, increase access to the WHO's essential medicines (some of which are psychopharmaceuticals), redistribution of previous clinical tasks to non-specialists through task-sharing, and use of technology to extend reach of mental health services (see Mills and Hilberg, 2018 for a discussion of these processes in India).

Measuring (time to) change

In the last 12 years, a variety of studies and reports have attempted to determine the success of TTC. The results have been mixed. While Sampogna et al (2017) found that active participation with TTC, particularly by mental health service users, can lead to an increased willingness to challenge stigma, the study is limited by the fact that its conceptualisation of 'stigma' corresponds with that of TTC, leading to a one-sided engagement with discrimination. In another study, Henderson and Thornicroft concluded that, while there was an overall reduction of experienced discrimination between 2008–11 there was also a negative shift in public attitudes to some aspects of mental health (2013: 46). Henderson and Thornicroft end their evaluation with a paragraph suggesting that "stigma and discrimination against people with mental illness are global challenges" (2013: 47), which reflects an emergent narrative of scholars concerned with stigma and mental health. An early study of Time to Change (Abraham et al, 2010) found that its logo inspired very little recognition and that its name could be confused with a political message, especially around times of election. A more recent and longer-term investigation into the campaign and attitudes towards mental illness in Britain (Evans-Lacko et al, 2013) concluded that the launch of the Time to Change campaign was successful in offsetting some negative attitudes towards mental illness, but that long-term involvement with the campaign would be needed to bring about more significant change. Despite the diversity in opinion and lack of clarity regarding the evidence of a decrease in population-wide stigma, TTC continues to approach mental health discrimination through stigma in a way that prioritises biomedical understandings of mental illness and places the source of stigma firmly in the individual subject, rather than acknowledging the possibility of systemic causes, or the need for legal redress (the legal ramifications invoked through discrimination do not apply to stigma). This is where mental health anti-stigma campaigns could learn from moves within Disability Studies to work beyond stigma, focusing on discrimination and oppression (Hunt, 1996).

Moreover, the campaign continues to receive millions of pounds in funding annually from the government, which has also made the positioning of the UK as a 'world leader' on mental health a priority.

As will be seen in the following sections, TTC still follows similar logics (educating the public through psychiatric discourse with a specific focus on how prevalent mental illnesses are) to its predecessor campaigns. Although these campaigns only brought about small changes in perceptions of mental illness at a population level, they seem to be treated as a success. While TTC engages the public on a much more direct (and global) level through social media, its basic framework regarding discourses around psychiatric diagnoses and treatment is similar to those followed by campaigns in the 90s and early 2000s. Yet there are some differences. The most interesting shift in narrative has happened on the level of everyday experiences of mental health. There is less of a focus now (certainly in the context of austerity Britain, where mental health services are experiencing drastic cuts in government funding) in increasing access to psychiatric services, and instead more impetus on how to manage one's mental health on an everyday basis that allows one to continue participating in the labour market. Whilst a shift away from traditional psychiatric treatments (e.g. pharmaceutical solutions or therapy) might be welcomed as a challenge to existing psychiatric hegemony, psychiatric logics continue to underpin the concept of 'everyday functioning'. Moreover, a move away from interventionist medical solutions suggests that mental distress becomes normalised as an aspect of everyday life, where treatment takes the form of self-management.

Stories: Performing anti-stigma

Mental health and stigma are 'done' globally in multiple overlapping ways: from campaign materials, and policy documents, to social media presence, and events and performances. Anti-stigma campaigns like TTC rely on the use of personal stories by people diagnosed with a mental illness to communicate a simple message about, for example, the commonality of mental health problems. It is now commonplace for personal stories from service users and/or people who have experienced distress to be used to educate the public and change public attitudes (often through emphasising prevalence and recovery); to raise funds and build brand; and to elicit political support (Costa et al, 2012). Writing about TTC, Crepaz-Keay and Kalathil show how these recovery-oriented developmental narratives follow

> a linear path from illness to wellness where both illness and recovery are re-articulated in terms of bio-medical and social constructions of normality.
>
> *(2013: 13)*

Sharing stories by those who identify as mental health users/survivors, or as psychosocially disabled, "has been central to the history of organizing for change in and outside of the psychiatric system" (Costa et al, 2012: 85) and to questioning unequal power structures and "the medical/psychiatric establishment's role in perpetuating these structures" (Crepaz-Keay and Kalathil, 2013: 4). Yet these stories are now used by organisations and academia to promote personal recovery or individual attitude change rather than as a tool for societal (including, economic and political) transformation. Here personal narratives are reduced to

> another set of data to be analysed and interpreted using existing hierarchical values and criteria or as commodities for marketing institutional or organisational agendas.
>
> *(Crepaz-Keay and Kalathil, 2013: 13)*

Russo has critiqued the academic "re-telling and packaging of individual and collective survivor stories" as highly damaging (Russo, 2012: 28), something which equally applies to organisational re-telling of personal narratives.

Creating spaces to tell stories about mental health and recovery at high-level 'global' events is a key part of how TTC is performed globally. In October 2017, the ninth meeting of the Mental Health Gap Action Programme (mhGAP) Forum took place at the World Health Organization (WHO) in Geneva. The meeting, attended by approx. 225 people (including one of the authors), provides an opportunity for people to network, and to feedback to the WHO about their global mental health products (Mills and Hilberg, 2019). Anti-stigma work played a key part throughout the two-day event. The spaces outside the main plenary session, where people congregate to drink coffee, were festooned with posters (translated into a number of languages) from the WHO's "Let's talk" anti-stigma campaign focused on depression. The Forum fell on World Mental Health day, with a well-attended lunchtime seminar on "Mental health in the workplace", which included presentations from Sue Baker announcing that TTC would be going global, and Adam Spreadbury (co-chair of the Mental Health Network at the Bank of England). The Bank of England signed up to the TTC pledge to tackle mental health in the workplace, in 2013.[1]

A year later, Sue Baker also made an appearance at the Global Ministerial Mental Health Summit, hosted by the UK Government, in 2018. This event aimed to "place a spotlight on mental health at a global level", and build momentum in tackling stigma. TTC had a strong presence at the event, from branded products to hosting a panel about their global work. Speaking about the event, Sue Baker said that

> many of us hope that this first ever global mental health summit will be a tipping point that prioritises more action on mental health. We've made major progress on mental health stigma in England and hope the summit acts as a springboard for change across all countries and cultures, so that there is no shame attached to mental health anywhere in the world.

However, this event and TTC's presence at it didn't pass without critique. Coalitions of mental health activists, psychiatric survivors, and service-users organized open letters detailing their concerns with the global summit and with the Lancet Commission on Global Mental Health and Sustainable Development (Patel et al, 2018), which was launched at the event (Beresford, 2018; NSUN, 2018; TCI Asia Pacific, 2018). One open letter led by the UK's National Survivor and User Network (NSUN) stated that

> [t]he Summit is set to announce the global launch of the anti-stigma programme, Time to Change, with programmes planned in India, Ghana, Nigeria, Uganda and Kenya. Millions of pounds have already been spent on this campaign which claims to

---

1 See video at https://www.youtube.com/watch?v=AQUJ3m_N7e0

have made a positive impact on mental health stigma, while evidence also shows that there has been no improvement in knowledge or behaviour among the general public, nor in user reports of discrimination by mental health professionals.

(National Survivor User Network, 2018)

The letter goes onto raise concerns that while the UK Government funds the TTC programme, it continues to engage in mass stigmatisation of disabled people who claim welfare. NSUN point out that

it is objectionable that the UK government continues to fund a programme that aims to address stigma while carrying on with the most stigmatising and discriminatory policies that affect persons with psycho-social disabilities.

(National Survivor User Network, 2018)

The letter references the work of Alison Faulkner and her critique of anti-stigma campaigns based on social contact and behaviour change. For Faulkner (2017b) the main reason that anti-stigma campaigns have largely failed to have much impact is that they rarely address intersectional and structural discrimination, including the crafting of stigmatisation of certain groups by government. Furthermore, such campaigns largely aim to encourage help-seeking but are not always realistic about what help is actually available to people (Faulkner, 2017b), especially in contexts of austerity, cuts to services, inequality and poverty.

Stigma and anti-stigma and Mad Studies

When thinking about anti-stigma going global, it is worth engaging with how stigma itself is understood in the literature. In literature and practice, stigma tends to be understood as "problems of knowledge (ignorance), attitudes (prejudice) and behaviour (discrimination)" (Thornicroft et al, 2008) that are seen to act as barriers to treatment and to mental health gaining policy traction (Mackenzie, 2014). Public health approaches to stigma have largely relied on public education about illness as prevalent but treatable (Corrigan et al, 2005). In the 2018 Lancet Commission (Patel et al, 2018), reduction of stigma – mentioned alongside discrimination – is explicitly linked to "increasing timely help-seeking" (2018: 1578), and to addressing "demand-side constraints for mental health care caused by stigma and discrimination" (2018: 1553). This approach is modelled on understanding of HIV/AIDS anti-stigma (Patel et al, 2006) where anti-stigma work largely involves educating people about biomedical understanding of disease (Howell et al, 2017).

However, the concept of stigma and the practice of anti-stigma within mental health has been widely critiqued. The majority of research into stigma is individually focused, and based on an interpersonal understanding of one person doing something to another (Hatzenbuehler and Link, 2014). This approach does not acknowledge that models and interventions that conceptualize distress as 'illness' may themselves be stigmatising. This is despite research consistently demonstrating that disease-based and biological explanations for mental distress are more stigmatizing and more likely to increase public desire for distance from those experiencing distress than psychosocial explanations, which have been found to increase empathy and reduce stigma (Corrigan, 2007; Longdon and Read, 2017; Read et al, 2006). A 2012 meta-analysis of data from eight countries over 16 years found that as public belief about the genetics of mental illness at population level increased, stigma also increased (Schomerus et al, 2012). This research suggests that interventions to change public attitudes can actually intensify stigma

(Schomerus et al, 2012), and inhibit collective anti-stigma work (Hatzenbuehler and Link, 2014). Furthermore, anti-stigma campaigns often fail to acknowledge that stigmatization is a structural process shaped by social, political and economic determinants, and that interventions to reduce stigma can also be structural and not only educational (Hansen et al, 2014; and see special issue on structural stigma in *Social Science and Medicine*, 2014).

Instead of assuming stigma is largely in the realm of public attitudes, research shows how structural stigma can be written into state legislation (Corrigan et al, 2005), and that Governments may actively craft stigmatisation of particular groups. For example, since 2008, the UK Government has engaged in the state sanctioned stigmatization of disabled, including psychosocially disabled, people who claim welfare benefits, in order to garner public consent for punitive welfare reform (such as, cuts to public services, welfare conditionality, use of sanctions, and mandatory workfare) (Tyler and Slater, 2018: 727). These policies have been linked to an increase in suicides, worsening mental health, and increases in prescriptions of anti-depressants (Barr et al, 2015; Mills, 2018b). At the same time the UK Government positions itself as a world leader in mental health, exemplified in its recent hosting of the Global Ministerial Mental Health Summit, an event which saw both the launch of the Lancet Commission (Patel et al, 2018), and the launch of GASA.

The sanism and whiteness of anti-stigma campaigns and also of Mad Studies

As anti-stigma work is articulated as global, and as campaigns travel globally, it is important both to draw upon Mad knowledge to understand the potentially sanist practices of anti-stigma campaigns but also grapple with and challenge the whiteness of some Mad Studies scholarship. This chapter brought to bear scholarship from Mad Studies, survivor research and user-controlled research onto a specific anti-stigma campaign in England, and its recent attempts to 'go global'. Using diverse Mad knowledges to rethink stigma and anti-stigma makes visible the ways that anti-stigma work is often constituted by and reproductive of sanism. Furthermore, sanist models of stigma and the anti-stigma campaigns that result from them are being exported globally, while sanism is deeply embedded within and productive of older forms of colonialism and modernity, and continued (settler) coloniality in many parts of the world.

Mad Studies taps into and is a space for the production of ways of knowing that can be used to interrogate "the adultist, disableist, saneist, colonial and racist logics that often underpin the conventional academic imaginary" (Mills and LeFrancois, 2018: 506) and it is thus sometimes described as in/disciplinary in that it disrupts Eurocentric models of knowledge carved into 'disciplines' (Gorman and LeFrançois, 2017; LeFrançois et al, 2013; Russo and Sweeney, 2016). Yet Mad Studies also emerges from a landscape made possible by (settler) colonialism, ableism, racism and more, and has been critiqued for reproducing hierarchies of differentiation which shape all of our lives albeit in very different ways. Like White Disability Studies, Mad Studies also reproduces whiteness, and thus requires an intersectional approach to madness constantly committed to dismantling ableism and sanism (Miles et al, 2017). Crepaz-Keay and Kalathil (2013) illustrate that much can be learned from projects that centre experiences of distressed and/or mad identified people of colour (for example in the UK context) (Atkinsons et al, 2008; Kalathil et al, 2011). For example, they document multiple projects that narrate and use story-telling in ways that, in contrast to many anti-stigma campaigns, make connections between personal narratives and social structures, power, racism, discrimination, and collective action (and that illustrate how narratives are themselves shaped by social and cultural context).

Conclusion

This chapter has drawn upon Mad Studies to contribute an anti-sanist and intersectional analysis of dominant anti-stigma campaigns, with a focus on *Time to Change* as it takes its anti-stigma work globally. We have chosen to highlight our positionality as white, female scholars writing in equally white western universities early on in this chapter as we believe it is essential to reflect on the kind of voices that are being heard (and published) in Mad Studies scholarship. These unavoidable markers of our privileged positionality open up spaces for critical debate about how knowledge in Mad Studies continues to be produced. We are fully aware that people's experiences of anti-stigma initiatives around the world are diverse and might not reflect the analysis put forward in this chapter – all the more important it is to engage discussion on the level of where knowledge about mental health is legitimated through academic discourse. Our contribution to the field of Mad Studies emerged through a critical engagement with the processes of knowledge production in Mad Studies alongside critiques of knowledge production about mental health and stigma on a global scale. Key here is our call to investigate further how structural conditions, including those in academic and research environments, shape our understanding of the intersection between stigma and mental distress.

As researchers in-between disciplines – psychology, global public health, international relations – whose literatures do not always speak to one another in productive ways, we suggest that an interdisciplinary approach that centres diverse forms of Mad knowledge production is necessary to start bringing forward a nuanced critique of global anti-stigma campaigns and to enact alternative collective and structural transformation of the conditions that produce stigma and discrimination. At the centre of any research going forward should be an ethos dedicated to appreciating and revealing the multiple facets in which oppression of those deemed 'mad' manifests – both in psychiatric and anti-psychiatric knowledge production. Finally, we hope that this chapter forms part of an emerging, diverse conversation about the relationships between psychiatry, stigma, and mental illness, which carves out a space for novel challenges to existing regimes of psy power within global politics.

References

Abraham A, Easow J M, Ravichandren P, Mushtaq S, Butterworth L and Luty J (2010). Effectiveness and confusion of the Time to Change anti-stigma campaign. *The Psychiatrist* 34(6): 230–233.

Atkinson A, Douglas C, Francis D, Laville M, Millin S, Pamfield J, Smith P and Smith R (2008). *Lifting Barriers: African and Caribbean people tell stories of struggle, strength and achieving mental health*. London: Mellow, SAFH, THACMHO, East London NHS Trust.

Barr B, Taylor-Robinson D, Stuckler D, Loopstra R, Reeves A and Whitehead M (2015). 'First, do no harm': Are disability assessments associated with adverse trends in mental health? A longitudinal ecological study. *Journal of Epidemiology and Community Health* 70(4): 339–345.

Beresford P (2018). A failure of national mental health policy and the failure of a global summit. *British Journal of Mental Health Nursing*, 7(5): 198–199.

Bhambra G K, Gebrial D and Nişancıoğlu K (2018). Introduction: Decolonising the university? In G K Bhambra, D Gebrial and K Nişancıoğlu (eds). *Decolonising the University*. London: Pluto Press, 1–15.

Corrigan P (2007). How clinical diagnosis might exacerbate the stigma of mental illness. *Social Work* 52(1): 31–39.

Corrigan P W, Watson A C, Byrne P, Davis K E (2005). Mental illness stigma: Problem of public health or social justice? *Social Work* 50(4): 363–368.

Costa L, Voronka J, Landry D, Reid J, McFarlane B, Reville D and Church K (2012). Recovering our stories: A small act of resistance. *Studies in Social Justice* 6(1): 85–101.

Crepaz-Keay D and Kalathil J (2013). Personal narratives of madness: Introduction. companion website to K W Fulford, M Davies, R Gipps, G Graham, J Sadler, G Stanghellini and T Thornton (eds). *The Oxford Handbook of Philosophy and Psychiatry*. Oxford: Oxford University Press. https://global.oup.com/booksites/content/9780199579563/narratives/ Accessed 20 December 2020.

Department of Health and Social Care (DHSC) (2016). Five-Year Forward View for Mental Health. https://www.england.nhs.uk/wp-content/uploads/2016/02/Mental-Health-Taskforce-FYFV-final.pdf. Accessed 06 April 2019.

Evans-Lacko S, Corker E, Williams P, Henderson C and Thornicroft G (2014). Effect of the Time to Change anti-stigma campaign on trends in mental-illness-related public stigma among the English population 2003-13: An analysis of survey data. *The Lancet Psychiatry* 1(2): 121–128.

Faulkner A (2017a). Survivor research and mad studies: The role and value of experiential knowledge in mental health research. *Disability and Society* 32(4): 500–520.

Faulkner A (2017b). Radical change or warm sentiments? A commentary on Gronholm et al (2017) Interventions to reduce discrimination and stigma: The state of the art. *Social Psychiatry and Psychiatric Epidemiology* 52(7): 777–779.

Gorman R and LeFrançois B A (2017). Mad studies. In B M Z Cohen (ed) *Routledge international handbook of critical mental health*. London: Routledge, 107–114.

Gorman R, saini a, Tam L, Udegbe O and Usar O (2013). Mad people of colour: A manifesto. *Asylum* 20(4): 27.

Hansen, H., Bourgois, P. and Drucker, E. (2014). Pathologizing poverty: New forms of diagnosis, disability, and structural stigma under welfare reform. *Social Science & Medicine* 103: 76–83.

Hatzenbuehler M L and Link B G (2014). Introduction to the special issue on structural stigma and health. *Social Science and Medicine* 103: 1–4.

Henderson C and Thornicroft G (2013). Evaluation of the Time to Change programme in England 2008–2011. *The British Journal of Psychiatry* 202(S55): 45–48.

Hunt P (ed). (1966). *Stigma: The experience of disability*. London: Geoffrey Chapman.

Howell A, Mills C and Rushton S (2017). The (mis)appropriation of HIV/AIDS advocacy strategies in global mental health: Towards a more nuanced approach. *Globalization and Health* 13(44): 1–9.

Kadri N and Sartorius N (2005). The global fight against the stigma of schizophrenia. *PLoS Medicine*, 2(7): 0597–0599.

Kalathil J, Collier B, Bhakta R, Daniel O, Joseph D and Trivedi P (2011). *Recovery and Resilience: African, African Caribbean and South Asian women's narratives of recovering from mental distress*. London: Mental Health Foundation and Survivor Research.

Leblanc S and Kinsella E (2016). Toward epistemic justice: A critically reflexive examination of 'sanism' and implications for knowledge generation. *Studies in Social Justice* 10(1): 59–78.

LeFrançois B A, Menzies R and Reaume G (eds). (2013). *Mad Matters: A critical reader in Canadian mad studies*. Toronto: Canadian Scholars' Press.

Legraien L (2018). Mental health detentions four times higher for black or black British people. *Healthcare Leader*. https://healthcareleadernews.com/news/mental-health-detentions-four-times-higher-for-black-or-black-british-people/. Accessed 09 June 2019.

Longdon E and Read J (2017). 'People with problems, not patients with illnesses': Using psychosocial frameworks to reduce the stigma of psychosis. *The Israel Journal of Psychiatry and Related Sciences* 54(1): 24–30.

Longhurst C (2017). Detention figures highlight 'worrying' ethnic disparity. *Mental Health Practice* 21(3): 6.

Luty, J, Rao, H, Arokiadass, S, Easow, J and Sarkhel, A (2008). The repentant sinner: methods to reduce stigmatised attitudes towards mental illness. *Psychiatric Bulletin* 32(9): 327–332, DOI: https://doi.org/10.1192/pb.bp.107.018457.

Mackenzie J (2014). *Global mental health from a policy perspective: A context analysis. Characterising mental health and recommending engagement strategies for the Mental Health Innovation Network*. London: Overseas Development Institute.

McWade B (2019). Madness, violence and media. In A Daley, L Costa and P Beresford (eds) *Madness, violence, and power: A critical collection*. Toronto: University of Toronto Press, 150–163.

Meerai S, Abdillahi I and Poole J M (2016). An introduction to anti-black sanism. *Intersectionalities* 5(3): 18–35.

Miles A L, Nishida A and Forber-Pratt A J (2017). An open letter to white disability studies and ableist institutions of higher education. *Disability Studies Quarterly* 37(3).

Mills C (2018a). From 'invisible problem' to global priority: The inclusion of mental health in the Sustainable Development Goals. *Development and Change* 49(3): 843–866.

Mills C (2018b). 'Dead people don't claim': A psychopolitical autopsy of UK austerity suicides. *Critical Social Policy* 38(2): 302–322.

Mills C and Hilberg E (2018). The construction of mental health as a technological problem in India. *Critical Public Health* 30(1): 41–52, doi:10.1080/09581596.2018.1508823.

Mills, C and Hilberg E (2019). 'Built for expansion': The 'social life' of the WHO's mental health GAP Intervention Guide. *Sociology of Health & Illness* 41(S1): 162–175. doi:10.1111/1467-9566.12870.

Mills C and LeFrançois B A (2018). Child as metaphor: Colonialism, psy-governance, and epistemicide. *World Futures* 74(7–8): 503–524.

Mind (2018). *Annual Review and Financial Statements 2017/18*. London: Mind.

National Survivor User Network (NSUN) (2018). Open Letter to the Organisers, Partners and Delegates of the Global Ministerial Mental Health Summit, London 9th and 10th October, 2018. *Global Ministerial Mental Health Summit – Open Letters*. https://www.nsun.org.uk/news/global-ministerial-mental-health-summit-open-letter. Accessed: 24 October 2018.

Patel V, Saraceno B and Kleinman A (2006). Beyond evidence: The moral case for international mental health. *American Journal of Psychiatry* 163(3): 1312–1315.

Patel V, Saxena S, Lund C, Thornicroft G, Baingana F, Bolton P et al (2018). The Lancet Commission on global mental health and sustainable development. *The Lancet* 392(10157): 1553–1598.

Paykel, E S, Hart, D and Priest, R G (1998). Changes in public attitudes to depression during the Defeat Depression Campaign. *British Journal of Psychiatry* 173: 519–522, DOI: 10.1192/bjp.173.6.519.

Poole J and Jivraj T (2015). Mental health, mentalism and sanism. In J D Wright (ed) *International encyclopedia of the social & behavioral sciences*. London: Elsevier, 200–203.

Priest, R G, Vize, C, Roberts, A, Roberts, M and Tylee, A (1996). Lay people's attitudes to treatment of depression: Results of opinion poll for Defeat Depression Campaign just before its launch. *British Medical Journal* 313(7061): 858–859, DOI: 10.1136/bmj.313.7061.858.

Read J, Haslam N, Sayce L and Davies E (2006). Prejudice and schizophrenia: A review of the 'mental illness is an illness like any other' approach. *Acta Psychiatrica Scandinavica* 114(5): 303–318.

Rimke H and Brock D (2012). The culture of therapy: Psychocentrism in everyday life. In D Brock, R Raby and M Thomas (eds) *Power and Everyday Practices*. Toronto: Nelson, 182–202.

Russo J (2012). 'Give me the stories and I will take care of the rest?' The case of Agnes's Jacket: A psychologist's search for the meaning of madness. *Asylum* Winter: 28–30.

Russo J and Sweeney A (2016). *Searching for a Rose Garden: Challenging Psychiatry, Fostering Mad Studies*. Wyastone Leys, Monmouth: PCCS Books.

Sampogna G, Bakolis I, Robinson E, Corker E, Pinfold V, Thornicroft G and Henderson C (2017). Experience of the Time to Change programme in England as predictor of mental health service users' stigma coping strategies. *Epidemiology and Psychiatric Sciences* 26(5): 517–525.

Schomerus G, Schwahn C, Holzinger A, Corrigan P W, Grabe H J, Carta M and Angermeyer M C (2012). Evolution of public attitudes about mental illness: A systematic review and meta-analysis. *Acta Psychiatrica Scandinavica* 125(6): 440–452.

Sweeney A (2016). Why mad studies needs survivor research and survivor research needs mad studies. *Intersectionalities: A Global Journal of Social Work Analysis, Research, Polity, and Practice* 5(3): 36–61.

Thornicroft G, Brohan E, Kassam A and Lewis-Holmes E (2008). Reducing stigma and discrimination: Candidate interventions. *Int J Ment Health Syst* 2(3): 1–7.

Time to Change (TTC) (n.d.) *About us*. https://www.time-to-change.org.uk/about-us.

Time to Change (TTC) (2017). *Leaflet: Global Anti-Stigma Alliance*. http://www.againststigma2017.com/images/GASA-leaflet.pdf. Accessed: 07 April 2019.

Transforming Communities for Inclusions Asia Pacific (TCI Asia Pacific) (2018). Open Letter to the Organizers and Partners of the Global Ministerial Mental Health Summit 2018, London, 9th and 10th October, 2018. https://tciasiapacific.blogspot.com/2018/10/open-letter-to-organizers-and-partners.html. Accessed: 20 December 2020.

Tyler I and Slater T (2018). Rethinking the sociology of stigma. *The Sociological Review Monographs* 66(4): 721–743.

PART 4

Doing Mad Studies

21

WHY WE MUST TALK ABOUT DE-MEDICALIZATION

María Isabel Cantón

Introduction

I understand de-medicalization as the process of discontinuing psychiatric drugs that were prescribed to treat a theoretical 'disorder', and also, as a perspective, one that recognizes diverse manifestations of psychic and emotional pain as natural to the human experience.

There are many reasons why people choose to go through de-medicalization processes. Some might find the drugs' effects too taxing on their quality of life after some time, some cannot afford them and it might not be possible for them to get the drugs for free through the public health system of their countries, others might not have wanted to take them in the first place and certain life events may require one to be drug-free for better safety, e.g. pregnancy, medical procedures, etc. Regardless of the reasons why one might choose to de-medicalize, de-medicalization has to be taken seriously by 'mental health' professionals, so they are in a better position to assist their 'patient/client' when they choose to de-medicalize, after all, they are the ones who prescribe these drugs to people in the first place, it should be their responsibility to assist discontinuation processes. But I also believe that certain things will not change until the mad community reaches a critical mass, and we are closer now than we have ever been to this. Our lived experience in processes of medicalization and de-medicalization contains valuable knowledge that might serve other persons to be able to make better informed choices about their health in the future.

Starting conversations in our communities about de-medicalization might feel unnerving because of the huge stigma that exists around the topic. Mad people (users, survivors of psychiatry, persons with psychosocial disability) are a collective already heavily stigmatized, and when talking de-medicalization we put ourselves in opposition to a behemoth with immense influence in public opinion.

The Pharmaceutical Industrial Complex dedicates billions of dollars to produce media, advertise to the public and medical journals, fund clinical trials for their own drugs and present biased results, ghost write, miseducate medical professionals (PharmedOut, 2018), fund national 'mental health' and medical associations, lobbying legislation (Open Secrets. Center for Responsive Politics, 2020), and many a time, bury or gag emerging evidence against their products or narratives. There is a tremendous ethical problem when societies allow private corporations, whose main purpose is shareholder wealth maximization, to have such an

DOI: 10.4324/9780429465444-26

influence in fundamental human rights arenas, such as health. How can any person trust that psychiatric drugs are 'safe and effective' when pharmaceutical influence is so pervasive?

My personal perspective and experience with medicalization

Every person has a different history, set of beliefs, circumstances and biology. I consider this diversity of experiences and views to be one of the most enriching qualities we can offer each other as human beings. Regardless of my very radical position in relation to psychiatry and the pharmaceutical industrial complex, I believe that when it comes to deciding to take psychiatric drugs, *informed choice should always be respected and honored.*

I consider it important to share my personal experience because by doing so, it is easier to understand why I hold this perspective and positioning regarding 'mental health' and the de-medicalization of human suffering, but more importantly, because I believe many aspects of our experiences as humans are universal and I know that sharing what I have lived through, provides a great opportunity of reaching and connecting with other humans, which for me, is one of the most important things in life.

I was born in the middle of a civil war in El Salvador and lived there until I was eight years old, but I identify 100% as being Nicaraguan, the country that birthed both my parents and where I have spent most of my life. Nicaragua, which is often referred to as the 'second poorest country in the western hemisphere' has taught me that wealth resides in many and more important planes than just the material/economic. I write this as a white-passing mestiza woman, who grew up and has lived her life in much privilege. Privilege that was afforded in part because I grew up with all my material needs covered and had access to some of the best education available, which is a huge advantage over the majority of my country-humans.

It is precisely because of all the privileges I have enjoyed (white passing, upper middle class, able bodied, cis-gendered, access to great education) that I consider 'mental health' to be above anything else, a social justice issue. If it were not because of these privileges coupled with the fact that I grew up with a psychiatrized father, de-medicalization might have not been an option for me.

I am not sure how much importance one can attribute to personality traits when speaking about de-medicalization. My intuition tells me that being able to consider de-medicalization has way more to do with external factors and experiences than any particular internal 'toolbox' a person is born with.

Before being in touch with the 'mental health' apparatus, I had always been critical of western orthodox medicine and its reductionist views. I have always been suspicious of the 'fix it with a pill' approach, and by choice and privilege, I have always elected the route of tweaking my lifestyle and routines to find sustainable improvements, before I would consider more invasive approaches.

When I became pregnant I found a universe of information that I was not aware of before. By deciding to birth naturally and preparing for it, I learned that in the health system a natural process comes second to hospital policy, risk minimization and your practitioner's schedule, which did nothing to improve my faith in medical approaches to health. The empowerment that came with succeeding at having a natural birth in a medical setting would serve me well in my de-medicalization process. I found myself more open to consider alternatives because my lived experiences prompted me to not regard doctors as an absolute authority, especially because I had discovered by experience the fact that orthodox medicine is inherently patriarchal.

My first personal encounter with the 'mental health' approach to extreme psychic distress happened in 2014, just seven months after the birth of my first child. Even though Nicaragua has universal health care for all, I had a private insurance through my work, which took me to a private hospital instead of the public asylum, so I say confidently that my experience as hellish as it was for me, does not reflect that of the majority of people that go through the public health system.

Private care did not exempt me of the ills that come when confronting the 'mental health' apparatus as a mad woman. Due to life circumstances that can be defined as the 'perfect storm', I ended up disconnecting from consensual reality one morning in July. My husband, who had not been exposed ever in his life to the type of manifestations I was having, did what every person is conditioned to do in western society, he turned to the medical establishment for help.

'Help' turned out to be the most denigrating and horrifying experience of my life. A forced hospital stay where I was physically and chemically restrained in intensive care for one day and injected against my will with no explanation whatsoever. In the proximity of my bed, there was a baby that would start crying desperately and whenever that happened, I would manage to wake up from the stupor the drugs had put me in, with images of my baby being skinned alive over and over again. A whole night spent in absolute panic, where I would call the nurses requesting to see my husband, to see my baby, asking for their help as my breasts were painfully engorged and I feared mastitis, calling them because I needed to pee, and not one of them would engage with me, they were either too busy or afraid, and I was left isolated and ignored.

After four days, I was sent home with a prescription that included an anti-depressive, a neuroleptic/'anti-psychotic' and a benzodiazepine. This all happened while I was still nursing my little baby. When he was born I was determined to breastfeed until he was two years old, this was a very important goal in my experience of motherhood, which is why I decided after a week to stop the neuroleptic and the benzodiazepine, I never took the anti-depressive, as I was not depressed.

The perfect storm I was going through before the hospital, only got worse as a result of my stay there so I ended up disconnecting from consensual reality a second time, fortunately my husband decided not to take me to the hospital after seeing how much suffering the first experience brought upon me, and instead recurred to strong sedation at home while requesting guidance from a psychiatrist he managed to call on the phone.

I found myself in an extremely vulnerable position going through this experience while being the mother of a young baby. People around me would make comments that implied I might be a danger to my baby, even though I never said or did anything to harm him or myself. Quickly I realized I had no other choice but to comply with my husband's demand of going to a psychiatrist and getting on the drugs again if that was the recommendation.

I ended up going to another psychiatrist who prescribed an anti-depressive, a neuroleptic, a benzodiazepine and a mood stabilizer, which I proceeded to ingest as prescribed. Even though I was heavily drugged, I kept having strange ideas and perceptions, which I kept only to myself as I soon realized that the more I shared with the psychiatrist, the more drugs I was prescribed and the more possible labels were brought up in the consultation.

I had never before in my life entered such intense altered states of consciousness so I had no idea what was going on. I felt disempowered and ostracized and ultimately, I had to comply to a narrative that did not resemble in any way, shape or form what I was going through. I surrendered and let my voice be extinguished for a whole year by a stream of pills, mainly because I feared being separated from my baby again.

Coming from a 'mental illness' background

I was born and grew up in a family that embraced without question the 'mental illness' narrative for human suffering. My father was psychiatrized for 58 years. At 17 years of age he was diagnosed with endogenous depression and put on lithium and anti-depressants, thus starting his torment as a 'mental health' patient. After spending two decades on anti-depressants and lithium and receiving several electro-shock 'treatments', he had a 'psychotic episode' when he was 50 years old. This granted him the 'manic-depressive' label and several other drugs added to his regimen.

In my teens and early twenties I observed in his body and through his manifestations the terrible effects of psychiatric drugs: akathisia, tardive dyskinesia, psoriasis, cognitive decline, violent behavior, insomnia and high blood pressure, to name a few. The psychiatrists who attended him throughout the years in three different countries attributed many of these effects to the 'natural' progression of his 'illness'. My father had three strokes as a result of chronic high blood pressure induced by psychiatric drugs, and spent the last 11 years of his life bed ridden with severe cognitive damage. The last decade of his life brought us the realization that drugs had not done much for him, even though they had provided us, his family, with relative peace of mind when he entered altered states. He died psychiatrized in 2013.

Bearing witness to the harm the drugs caused him granted me the determination to do everything possible to get off the drugs I was prescribed. I count this as one of my many privileges, even though a very sad one.

My journey through de-medicalization

Six months after my hospitalization and when my drug 'treatment' had been adjusted in a manner that allowed me to remain awake for most of the day, I started sharing my concerns about the long-term use of the drugs with my husband. By that time I felt safe enough to share more of my real thoughts and feelings with him. He was able to witness how the drugs altered my life, how they affected my ability to mother our son, and I also expressed to him that besides the fear of what prolonged use could bring upon my health, the drugs made me feel dead inside.

The conversation with him lasted for a couple of months, I knew I couldn't push him, it was a very sensitive issue for him, as he was also traumatized by the disruption that my going through this experience had brought upon our family.

Every time that I tried to convey my feelings regarding my experience and how I felt about the drugs to anyone else around me, I was quickly reminded that I was 'doing better' now or was met with silence. So I turned to the internet. I was looking for people who had alternative views on 'mental illness', as my experience felt very spiritual and meaningful to me. After searching for content in Spanish and not finding anything, I started to search for content in English and eventually found the group Shades of Awakening on Facebook. In this group I found a community where I felt heard for the first time in almost a year, and by reading the stories of people who had gone through experiences similar to mine, I started to feel hope and with hope I began to regain my self-confidence.

Eventually, my husband agreed to bring up the topic of discontinuation to the psychiatrist, and with his intervention she agreed to start tapering me off the drugs. I give her full credit for advising that I do the taper very slowly, which after hearing and reading many difficult accounts on discontinuation, I can now appreciate.

The drugs had a very strong effect on me, I was sleepy all the time, it was difficult to find real motivation or excitement about anything, I felt stuck. As I was working full time and being a mother, I did not have the mind or energy to keep a journal of my tapering process, which I now regret. Information about the tapering itself, what percentage of each drug was reduced over what period of time, what manifestations and sensations arose during and after the discontinuation, in sum, all the details of a person's journey that I now realize might be of great value and support to someone considering discontinuation of psychiatric drugs.

After having lost contact with consensual reality in such an extreme way and being labeled by psychiatry as 'extremely mentally ill', even though I leaned towards the opposite path to conventional 'wisdom', it was inevitable for me to internalize part of the narrative my proximity was providing for my experience. I was indeed very afraid of having another 'crisis' for many reasons. I was terrified of being hospitalized again, deep down I feared that having an altered state of consciousness again would swiftly alter my life circumstances and I would lose the right to mother my child and, I was very apprehensive of the possibility of having to take psychiatric drugs the rest of my life.

Two months after having discontinued all drugs, after a night of very little sleep and into a stressful morning at work, I started experiencing an amplification of perceptions and tingling in my limbs, both of these I was familiar with as they had been present before, each time I entered an altered state of consciousness. I decided to go home midday and took some valerian to sleep, as I was concerned if I didn't, I would spiral down and lose control. The following day it happened again, this time I lost all hope, as I was doubting my ability to function in society, I was questioning if I could live a life without the drugs to keep me 'grounded', even though they made me feel zombified. So as the day before, I went home, but instead of going to sleep I called my husband and told him what had been going on, I expressed that I was willing to submit to whatever he deemed appropriate. I told him that if he wanted to call the psychiatrist to call her, and if she said so, I would go on the drugs again.

His reaction was a turning point in my process. He said that none of that was necessary, as he considered I was already doing the things I needed to do to manage myself: taking distance from stress, sleeping, talking about what I was experiencing. With his reaction I realized two things. The first one was how disempowered I had become over my own life in the course of a year, and the second, that he trusted me even when I was incapable of trusting myself. Both of these realizations were important in my healing journey and allowed me to consider other alternatives to managing my diverse psychic manifestations.

Because of all my privileges, I have had time and resources to explore some of my unusual perceptions deeply and as a result, I have been able to find literal and metaphorical meanings in what psychiatrists would have labeled 'delusions' and 'hallucinations', had I shared with them. My lived experience is one of healing and transformation through psychic pain and extreme distress, yes, but I feel more liberated as a human now than I did before experiencing madness. Since I cannot un-liberate me, I do what I can from my imperfections and limitations, to contribute to create a world where most people can be afforded the chance I had when having gone as mad as I went.

The rest of my empowerment and stamina to keep swimming upstream in the waters of activism, has come from meeting so many people who have been as damaged by psychiatry as I have, or family members of persons who were on psych drugs and their 'illness' had not been resolved and now were impaired by the drugs, concerned mothers reluctant to medicate their children, being able to connect with fellow mad activists, etc. I knew then I was not alone, and I felt comfortable publicly sharing my very heretical perspective that psychiatric drugs might not be the best response to human suffering.

Because of this, I have a certain reputation in the minuscule societal group that discusses 'mental health' publicly in my country. When around me, I have heard people use phrases as

'I am pro-science' or 'We have to be responsible when we discuss these matters', which to me only reflects how many layers of the onion still have to be peeled.

Some of the problems with medicalization of human distress

Accepting the pathologization of human distress without a critical view in place is outright dangerous for personal well-being and for social justice struggles in our societies.

Increases oppression of marginalized groups

People belonging to already marginalized groups (race, gender, sexuality, class) are subject to more medicalization than those not marginalized, which not only increases human rights violations but erases social injustices and inequities perpetuating systemic oppression and therefore causing more human suffering (Human Rights Council, 2020: 11).

The science is not there

Having had the privilege of buying and reading some of the books/articles from known whistleblowers in the 'mental health' field, I have come to learn that there is no evidence that supports the popular claim that people presenting manifestations deemed 'mental disorders/ illnesses' have a chemical imbalance on their brains (Moncrieff, 2009: 169) which in its turn makes it sort of a common sense realization that in the lack of a biological marker, psychiatric drugs do not treat illnesses or correct imbalances. So, what do they do?

In Nicaragua, the Diagnostic and Statistics Manual of Mental Disorders (DSM-V) is the guide used to label suffering people with psychiatric diagnosis. What many people still do not know, is that this manual is based on consensus opinions and not on the scientific method. Identifying myself as a radical feminist in construction, it is very hard for me to give credibility to a practice that at one point in time pathologized homosexuality, intended to pathologize domestic violence as 'Masochistic Personality Disorder' on its IV edition, and still pathologizes women's bodies' natural cycle fluctuation and diversity as 'Premenstrual Dysphoric Disorder' (Gøtzsche, 2013: 292).

If one can consider the World Health Organization to provide unbiased literature and data, then what is shown is that medicalization of psychic distress is associated with poorer outcomes in the lives of people that have been labeled and prescribed by psychiatry (Whitaker, 2010: 193).

Absence of informed consent, let alone choice

In Nicaragua, the rule of thumb treatment for extreme manifestations of distress is pharmacologic, no other choice is offered for the general population. Although at least on paper, there have been institutional efforts to promote interculturality when approaching particular manifestations of psychic distress of indigenous communities, the case of Grisi Siknis in Miskitu communities is an example of these efforts; but ultimately, the biomedical narratives are regarded as the correct ones and the health authorities have the final word when information about these experiences is presented to the rest of the country (Martínez-Cruz, 2021).

When I was prescribed psychiatric drugs, I did not give informed consent in the emergency room, and neither was I given all the information about the drugs when I was prescribed by two different psychiatrists. I have yet to hear an account of someone in my country having received all the pertinent information from their psychiatrist regarding the drugs they were being prescribed. This becomes especially problematic when the person does not want to take the drugs in the first place and is coerced or forced to take them. As opposed to other medical specialties the topic of informed consent is approached in a very relaxed manner by psychiatry (Moncrieff, 2009: 213).

If a person feels better while taking psychiatric drugs and is in full knowledge of its effects documented to date, how it was researched, by whom and for how long, how its effectiveness is determined, and they can also read the raw data and not just the abstract published on the clinical trial results, then and only then would I consider someone empowered to make an informed choice in regards as to how little, how much and for how long they want to take a psychiatric drug it.

Decontextualization

The biomedical approach to subjective suffering causes a person's experience in the world to be decontextualized and reduced to the 'clinical picture' they present when they first encounter 'mental health' services. All the possible causes for the person's diverse manifestations, like adverse childhood experiences, traumas, the experience of multiple oppressions, or just a different way of being in the world, are amputated at once and replaced by a supposed mal-function of fancy named neurotransmitters in the brain.

At least at first, people who go to the mental health services to seek help might embrace this theory as the one true cause of their suffering, sometimes with no small measure of relief. The frequent lack of questioning of psychiatric diagnosis and treatments might have multiple factors amongst the Nicaraguan middle to upper class. Some of these factors might include receiving the (dis)information from an authority figure, the medical doctor, not having access to the real science and information that is buried under so much pharmaceutical marketing pitches, and/or a readiness to assume all trends and fads coming from our neighbors from the North as measure of progress and success to ultimately be achieved.

Then, there is the reality of the majority of the population in my country, which might be evenly divided between the group that does not seek help when they are in distress and just ride it out and keep it a secret, due to the social stigma being sky high in a very religious country; and those who are taken by will or by force by their family members to the public health system. For the latter group, the reality of going through the 'apparatus' while mad and underserved is expo-nentially worsened by the dire socio-economic conditions, which in its turn translates into hor-rible conditions in the asylums, staff who are poorly, if at all trained, no availability of psychiatrists on site at all times, which probably means spending as much time physically restrained as it takes the psychiatrist in charge to show up, lack of consistency as far as prescriptions and doctors are concerned, as people are prescribed what is available from the donations received by whoever is available. This adds another layer of complications to an already terrible scenario.

To exemplify how the 'illness' narrative decontextualizes people manifesting distress, I will share an anecdote. Once I was in a radio program promoting the presentation of the docu-mentary 'Crazywise' produced by Phil Borges, which provided a great opportunity to open community conversations where 'mental health' could be discussed from an alternative per-spective. As part of the promotion, I was interviewed and shared part of my personal story. Listeners started calling the show, and they would ask questions and comment about the topic we were discussing. One caller related how his neighbor was 'psychotic' and her family had kept her locked in a room for two years. He criticized, and rightly so, the decision of the family members to keep her locked in, and he questioned why they did not take her to seek help, and asked who could intercede for this woman. During the exchange of comments, he mentioned as a side note, that she had become 'mentally ill' since her father had raped her a couple years ago.

The biomedical approach robs people of their history, their agency and the possibility to bring healing forth. We are complex beings that are very much affected by our environments. Should not it be expected that the cause of our distress be complex and diverse as well?

De-medicalization challenges

The obstacles that a person might face when undergoing de-medicalization are numerous and systemic in nature.

Capitalism

In the current state of the world, where most societies are living under or moving towards a system that seeks only to perpetuate itself by valuing human beings primarily on the basis of their ability to produce and consume, it is no surprise that the suppressing of pain that might distract humans from the main goal (producers/consumers) is the preferred response. Medicalization of distress might prove to be just a nut and bolt within the engine of capitalism.

How can one process and integrate emerging psychic pain when food, housing, safety, nutrition, rest and leisure time, the possibility of finding and connecting with those who extend love and compassion to our suffering, having access to natural spaces, finding time for physical activity and finding time for community building, are all not accessible to the majorities one is part of?

To pathologize people for having natural responses to insane circumstances and make them feel guilty and faulty for not being happy and successful with the 'treatment' provided, is to me, a crime against humanity. And even though I think capitalism has emerged organically through time and space, we now know enough about its destructiveness as societies and individuals to remain complacent, especially those of us who enjoy privileges inaccessible to most.

Lack of alternatives provided in the main discourse

This may vary depending on the country, culture, religion and the different oppressions experienced. In Nicaragua's particular case, other than the biomedical approach that private and government health institutions and professionals provide, people might turn to their churches when experiencing psychic distress, which is not necessarily a safe step to take.

In 2017, a woman from the Nicaraguan Caribbean coast was tied to a tree and set on fire while having an extreme state of consciousness. The pastor of her church deemed her possessed by demons and persuaded parishioners that prayer would expel the demon, when prayer failed they resourced to fire. The criminals stated that the cause of her possession was alleged adultery, her name was Vilma Trujillo (Baker, 2018).

On top of there being a lack of alternatives, I mostly think there is a lack of freedom to explore whichever alternatives one might wish, as the prevalent narrative even pathologizes a person's desire to de-medicalize their own suffering. Non-compliance has become an indicator of how 'ill' a person is, it is now a 'symptom' of 'mental illness' that has been labeled anosognosia (NAMI, 2020).

Withdrawal/discontinuation syndrome

The process of discontinuing one psychiatric drug might prove challenging especially when one has taken it over a long period of time, which is usually the case. When discontinuing more than one drug, things get more complicated as there might be withdrawal effects that can composite and make the process harder to endure.

In the community of ex-users and survivors of psychiatry, it is very common to hear stories full of struggles when it comes to withdrawal experiences. There are those who quit the drugs cold turkey because they lacked information and support, put themselves through an ordeal because of it but eventually make it to the other side. Discontinuation paradoxically can bring even more psychiatrization, as withdrawal effects are frequently attributed to the person's original manifestation of distress, for which psychiatry's response is higher doses, more drugs or a combination of both added to the regimen, almost always causing an inescapable vicious circle (Breggin, 2013: 120–121).

Then there are those people, who even when taking the cautious path of reducing one drug at a time by 10% of the original dose every two–three weeks (Hall 2012: 35) still find themselves struggling for years after first starting to taper.

Psychiatric drugs do create a chemical imbalance in the brain, as the body develops an adaptive response to the drug that causes it to decrease or increase certain neurotransmitters in the brain. When the drug is discontinued, this response no longer finds opposition which brings on what has been labeled withdrawal symptoms. These responses have not been studied in depth and it is unknown if they are reversible in all cases, as well, little is known about how long it can take the body to re-establish its normal operational structure (Moncrieff, 2009).

While tapering psychiatric drugs we swim in the waters of uncertainty. Currently there is no established mechanism by which the persons that have been caused chemical imbalances in their brains for prolonged periods and many times against their will, can hold those responsible accountable for the damage inflicted.

Opposition by prescribers and family members

When I told him that I wanted to come off the drugs that I had been put on, my psychiatrist strongly advised against it. I am inclined to believe that my experience is not the exception, but the rule. Most contemporary psychiatrists have been trained under the biological paradigm and truly believe psychopharmacological treatment is the only avenue to manage manifestations of psychic distress. Many of them might believe that supporting their patient's desire to discontinue drugs is an act of irresponsibility on their part.

So when undertaking discontinuation this might be the first obstacle to overcome. The option to change prescribers is only available to those who can pay private health services, at least in my country. If a person is not a 'consumer', but rather a user of 'mental health' services, they will have to taper behind their prescriber's back, hopefully with the support of family members.

If the person is coerced by their family to follow the psychiatrist's recommendation, thinking about discontinuing might represent a higher risk, as doing it covertly brings its own set of problems. The fear of a crisis, the fear of being put on higher doses and/or more drugs, the fear of being discovered and potentially having certain rights taken away, e.g. parental rights.

Lack of proper support during the process

I wonder if the majority of current professionals that prescribe, whether they are GP or psychiatrists, really know much about the effects that might appear on the body and the behavior of a person and how much these might last when the drugs are discontinued. Their frequent reticence to be associated with drug discontinuation processes makes me suspect they might feel limited by their ignorance on the matter.

The families of people experiencing psychic distress might not be willing or able to offer support to the discontinuation process of their family member for lack of resources and knowledge. Many people struggle for years when tapering psychiatric drugs.

There are few professionals in general and almost none in public healthcare that have a holistic approach towards health. There is no one professional or public service that can provide detailed guidance in lifestyle changes that promote health: such as changes in nutrition, physical activity, non-pharmacological tools that aid sleep like meditation, breath work, etc.

Information on de-medicalization mostly available only in the English language

Most of the information written by professionals and independent researchers originates in the North and takes time to be translated. This causes Spanish speaking countries to have delayed access to the latest scientific information, especially the psychiatric professionals that work both in private practice and public health care. The textbooks are very expensive and very often have to be acquired abroad, which represents another barrier to people from countries of the Global South.

Value of de-medicalization

By having lived a de-medicalization process after being labeled as 'extremely mentally ill' and having met and heard personal accounts of people who like me, have successfully de-medicalized their psychic suffering, I have found some common lessons and learnings.

By not suppressing the manifestations of psychic distress and having a de-medicalized perspective, one has the opportunity to bring to consciousness wounds and traumas that had never been addressed before. Provided one has the proper support, this can be a prime opportunity for healing, integrating and hence, avoiding the cycle of trauma and injustices one has been a victim of.

Living our manifestations of distress fully gives us the opportunity to be able to read our emotional states better, it gives us insight on what triggers us, what our patterns are, through experimentation we can learn which alternative tools help us and which do not. We have the possibility of knowing ourselves better and hopefully accepting ourselves just as we are.

If we begin with the mindset that our pain and suffering are not meaningless, it is more likely that we will be able to find meaning and purpose through it. There is a golden opportunity to get in touch and find out who one really is, to find one's own voice and growth through self-determination, to become one's own person, all in relation to the community one lives in. As an admired brother of mine always says: "What you cannot achieve by yourself, you can achieve with a group".

By being completely in contact with our own suffering, we have the possibility of understanding the suffering of others around us, reconnecting in this way with our own humanity.

Practices that can support de-medicalization processes

Even though the emotional and physical struggles that might appear while de-medicalizing are experienced by the person alone, I believe they can be better processed when shared with a strong network of support, just like any other experience of human suffering.

Peer support groups

Something that can make an enormous difference in a person's life is to have their pain acknowledged. Safe spaces can be found in peer-led support groups for psychic distress and for people discontinuing psychiatric drugs. I have led and participated in peer support groups after my de-medicalization experience. The most important aspects I have observed for a peer support group to be successful are to have the rules disclosed to everyone in the beginning and have the facilitator reinforce the rules throughout the session if need be. I think the most important rules should be horizontality, respect for the other person's point of view and narratives around their pain and respect of the speaking times, as the word is power and thus, should always be passed around. By attending a peer support group one can find a network of support inaccessible in mainstream spaces. Peer support groups represent a very tangible tool for de-medicalization in countries of the Global South, where most types of alternative therapies are only available at a price too high for the majorities to be able to afford.

Activism

Activism provides an excellent platform through which we can build meaning and find motivation to face discontinuation struggles. If we have been harmed by psychiatric drugs, activism provides us with the opportunity to put our suffering at someone else's service by actively sharing our stories, getting involved in our communities and finding a purpose that transcends our individual experiences. If you, the reader, are in Latin America and are a user, ex-user, survivor of psychiatry, mad person or person with psychosocial disability and are in need of a network of peers or just resources in Spanish, look up *Redesfera Latinoamericana de la Diversidad Psicosocial* through social media, reach out and get involved.

Decolonial perspective

Examining the 'mental health' system and its practices from a decolonial perspective served me well, especially when coming from the Global South. Our territories, and us with them, carry colonization pain that has gone unrecognized for generations, and now through globalization, that pain get systematically pathologized and monetized, as institutions of domination that have originated from the very same territories that inflicted such a great wound in the soul of our region (Latin America) are adopted. This collective pain trickles down through families and is manifested individually, sometimes extremely and unusually, like a desperate attempt to free the self and the collective from the insanity of individualism and capitalism. Decolonial perspectives can bring us closer to the wisdom of indigenous peoples, who regard themselves as children of nature and therefore care for it, for they know that her well-being is their good living. Through decolonial reflection one cannot escape the inherent destruction and exploitation that comes along Eurocentric progress.

References

Baker V (2018). The 'exorcism' that turned into murder. Why was Vilma Trujillo killed? *BBC* 28 February. https://www.bbc.co.uk/news/resources/idt-sh/nicaragua_exorcism_vilma_trujillo_murder. Accessed: 28 May 2020.

Breggin P R (2013). *Psychiatric Drug Withdrawal. A Guide for Prescribers, Therapists, Patients and their Families*. New York: Springer.

Hall W (2012). *Harm Reduction Guide to Coming Off Psychiatric Drugs*. 2nd edn. The Icarus Project and Freedom Center.

Human Rights Council (2020). *Report of the Special Rapporteur on the right of everyone to the enjoyment of the highest attainable standard of physical and mental health.* United Nations.

Gøtzsche P (2013) *Deadly Medicines and Organised Crime: How Big Pharma has Corrupted Healthcare.* Oxford: Radcliffe.

Martínez-Cruz J (2021). This knowledge counts! Harmony and spirituality in miskitu critical thought. In M Lugones, Y Espinosa Miñoso and N Maldonado-Torres (eds). *Decolonial Feminism. Caribbean, Latinx, and South American Traditions.* New York: Rowman & Littlefield Publishers.

Moncrieff J (2009). *A Straight Talking Introduction to Psychiatric Drugs.* Monmouth: PCCS Books.

National Alliance on Mental Illness (NAMI) (2020). https://www.nami.org/About-Mental-Illness/Common-with-Mental-Illness/Anosognosia. Accessed: 30 May 2020.

Open Secrets. Center for Responsive Politics (2020). Industry Profile: Pharmaceuticals/Health Products. https://www.opensecrets.org/federal-lobbying/industries/summary?cycle=2019&id=H04. Accessed: 14 May 2020.

PharmedOUT (2018). https://sites.google.com/georgetown.edu/pharmedout. Accessed: 14 May 2020.

Whitaker R (2010). *Anatomy of An Epidemic: Magic Bullets, Psychiatric Drugs, and the Astonishing Rise of Mental Illness in America.* New York: Crown Publishers.

22

IMAGINING NON-CARCERAL FUTURES WITH(IN) MAD STUDIES

Pan Karanikolas

"Free the people, shut all institutions"

Created by a large team of disabled artists and activists in 2017, the Disability Pride mural in Footscray, Melbourne, where the brick wall meets Wurundjeri Woi Wurrung and Bunurong lands, has been called the "first" of its kind in Australia (MacFarlane, 2019). A week after the mural was created, Larissa MacFarlane, local artist, disability activist and organiser of the mural, went to photograph the mural and instead found a blank, brick wall. It so happened that the mural had been removed earlier that morning, the day after International Day of People with Disability. The mural, partially funded by the local council and the building's owners, was intended to remain a permanent fixture on the wall. Subsequently, the local council issued a statement apologising and confirmed the mural was removed by their graffiti removal contractors (Tran, 2017). The Disability Pride mural was then re-made, making the mural you see today as you walk over the bridge across Footscray Station the "second" mural. On her blog, Larisa MacFarlane said:

> "It was a shocking, heartbreaking moment for many of us. For some of the partici-
> pating artists, it was their first time publicly identifying with disability and erasure of
> their stories hit hard. For other more seasoned disability activists, it came as little sur-
> prise to have our voice silenced yet again." […] "This is about identity. This is about
> my identity. This is about Rights [sic]. This is about the lack of respect that disabled
> people have in Australia, the real daily struggle that people face, and the very real fear
> of being marginalised once again. This is stuff that is rarely talked about outside the
> disability community and it is just too easy for the mainstream to dismiss."
>
> *(MacFarlane, 2019)*

Qadri and MacFarlane (2018) locate the mural within a larger tradition of graffiti, street and public art, which provides space for conversation and encounters about disability pride, culture and history (Qadri and MacFarlane, 2018). Part of the wall attests to the mass institutionalisation of disabled people. It reads:

DOI: 10.4324/9780429465444-27

FREE THE PEOPLE. SHUT ALL INSTITUTIONS.

We acknowledge Australia's shameful history of incarcerating tens of thousands of people with disabilities, particularly people with intellectual disabilities and mental illness, in large scale institutions, hidden from view. People lived their entire lives controlled by others, denied choice, privacy, and their civil rights, never knowing freedom. We apologise to those who have suffered from decades of institutional violence and abuse. We honour those advocates and activists that have come before us and fought for freedom. However, institutions for people with disabilities are still operating in Australia today. We ask for your support by speaking up for the closure of all institutions in the name of justice, equality and freedom!

In this section of the mural, as Qadri and MacFarlane (2018) have documented, people have been invited into an active dialogue with the mural's text, where additional graffiti has been added in brown marker. The writer has written:

Disabled ppl [sic] make up a SHAMEFUL percentage of ppl [sic] in prisons! And are often placed in fkn SOLITARY! + the rates are worse for aboriginal disabled ppl!".[1]

(Qadri and MacFarlane, 2018)

Last year, when I lived closer to it, I took photos of this part of the wall; to read and reflect more on what the wall had to say about the historical periods of mass institutionalisation of disabled people, interested in the enduring inheritances of the asylum system. The mural invokes the histories of former institutional sites, including asylums and psychiatric hospitals, many of which in the state of Victoria were closed (quite quickly) in the period known as "deinstitutionalization" in the 1980s and 1990s (Gooding, 2016). In this way, the mural memorialises, but it also contains within it a contemporaneous call to action. In doing so, it also makes the somewhat paradoxical point—in a period we might call "post-deinstitutionalisation"—disabled people, including those who are deemed "mad" or "mentally ill", are still regularly disappeared from public life. The mural's statement gestures towards these enclosures—the aged care facilities, group homes, psychiatric hospitals, residential facilities—all contemporary, interlocking sites of internment which make up what Ben-Moshe, Carey and Chapman call an "institutional archipelago" (Chapman et al., 2014:14). Life within, and shaped by, institutions "has been the forced historical reality, not the exception, for disabled persons" (Russell and Newman, 2001:63). Today, institutional "life" is often justified in the name of care, rehabilitation and "welfare". However, it is the graffiti writer with their brown marker—the wall's interlocutor—who has written explicitly about the hyper-incarceration of Aboriginal and Torres Strait Islander people—making an unambiguous connection to incarceration in prisons and other correctional sites.

A world without prisons: from "cops" to "care"?

A year later, 2020, and the Black Lives Matter movement has again highlighted the crisis of racist violence, inherent within policing and in prisons. In reaction to the killing of George Floyd in Minneapolis, the spotlight in Australia has been on large Black Lives Matter rallies, called for and organised by First Nations activists and on behalf of families and loved ones of those who have died in custody, at the hands of police and in prisons. As so many have pointed out, it was the death of George Floyd in Minneapolis, this event on the other side of the world, which motivated this action, despite the fact that the struggle for justice for so many other

Aboriginal and Torres Strait Islander people who have died in custody remains a constant fight on this continent (Liddle, 2020; Whittaker, 2020). However, with these flashpoint moments have been swelling movements for radical change, including the call to defund, or abolish, police and prisons, heard in places and in ways where they previously may not have been. The prominence of such ideas, of abolitionism and anti-carceral politics, activism and theory is surely due to the tireless activist work of many groups locally, including (but of course not limited to) Sisters Inside, a Queensland-based organisation supporting criminalised women, Sydney's Justice Action, a prison advocacy group and Melbourne's Flat Out, a support and advocacy service for criminalised women leaving prison, which grew out of the anti-carceral feminist activism in Victoria (Carlton and Russell, 2018). Many of these groups have been a part of the prison abolition movement, domestically and internationally, since the late 1980s. Despite informing the ideas of various social movements for some time, the uptake and influence these ideas and political imaginaries in the space of a few years feels rapid, pronounced. In 2017, Ellen O'Brien wrote of a prison abolition event held in Sydney, *Manifesting a World Without Prisons*, by the collective Queer Provocations that "prior to the start of the event, comments were made by the panellists about the number of attendees", much larger groups of people than they had seen at events during the law few years (O'Brien, 2017).

Passing the mural last year, I wondered then about the histories (and ongoing present) of confinement, spatial surveillance and control for those deemed, or who appear to be, mad or "mentally ill", and the vital intersections and connections with struggles committed to ending the racist violence of policing; radical visions of a better society and world. As abolition's influence and demands gain further prominence, there has been increased conversation about the divestment of funds away from police and correctional service portfolios towards investment in health services, in particular "mental health care". A recent online event hosted by the Institute for the Development of Human Arts (IDHA), an organisation based in the United States, interrogated these calls to "replace 'cops' with 'care'" (IDHA, 2020). Despite the seemingly innocuous statements for more funding for mental health services, these suggestions signify a failure to appreciate how, like policing, coercive mental health "care" historically and presently functions as a tool of social control, through legal powers of detention, the use of involuntary interventions and the regulation of those viewed as "mad". There is a real need here for survivor knowledge to be put into much closer conversation with these debates and the politics, scholarship and demands of carceral abolition. It is a timely moment to explore these ideas and contemplate the relationship between Mad Studies and anti-incarceration philosophy, politics and ideas.

Carceral abolition is grounded in anti-segregationist philosophy and ideas, and calls to dismantle and put an end to spaces and modes of incarceration for the violence and social harms they inflict, weaving together the demands of other radical movements for social change. Within a settler-colonial context such as Australia, criminalisation, segregation and imprisonment are (and should be) conceived of as techniques constitutive of settler colonial regimes and their exercise of power. In Australia, under the eliminatory logic of settler colonialism (Wolfe, 2006), police represent and embody "one of the most enduring and deeply entrenched legacies of British colonisation" (Porter, 2016:26), The ongoing genocidal violence of deaths in custody, child removal policies and the over-policing of Aboriginal communities can be traced back to the state's (illegitimate) genesis with the mounted police who fought frontier wars. Many Aboriginal and Torres Strait Islander people who have been criminalised or incarcerated have experienced severe emotional distress and trauma. As Wadjularbinna Nullyarimma, Gungalidda Elder and member of the Aboriginal Tent Embassy puts it: "We cannot flee persecution to another country because we are spiritually connected to our own ancestral lands. So jails and mental institutions are full of our people" (2020). To understand the confinement of those experiencing "madness" today we need this historicisation, locating practices with attentiveness to their contingencies and divergences from confinement in the female factories, in convict labour, orphanages, missions and reserves, the very violent foundational structures of settler colonial states.

Abolitionism itself, expressed by some of the leading figures in the anti-psychiatry movement and those who call for the abolition of mental health law, is not a novel concept for the expansive, inter-disciplinary field of Mad Studies. Since the development of the Convention on the Rights of Persons with Disabilities (CRPD) in 2006, scholars, advocates and human rights groups have supported the position that mental health law is discriminatory and impinges on rights to liberty, autonomy and bodily integrity; and should be abolished, accompanied with moves to integrate supported decision making (Wilson, 2018). While not a mainstream view or demand, the abolition of mental health law has been "clearly and repeatedly articulated as a political goal" by advocates, human rights groups, and scholars; despite states like Australia making interpretative declarations that they do not interpret the CRPD as requiring the abolition of forms of substitute decision-making (Wilson, 2018). Psy-centred knowledge, its connected institutions and the mental health industry are deeply embedded in, and inform, civil legal systems (such as mental health law, disability and guardianship law) *and* criminal legal systems of control. The involuntary detention, involuntary psychiatric "treatment" and legalised use of force against persons experiencing mental and emotional distress is written into the fabric of mental health law, psychiatric practice and substantiated by paternalistic, ableist and "sanist" legal doctrine. Today, in our "post-deinstitutionalisation" period, involuntary "treatment" has moved from psychiatric hospitals and institutions and entered the space of "the community", through the introduction and uptake of community treatment orders (CTOs) enabling forms of "chemical incarceration" (Fabris, 2006, Fabris, 2011, Fabris and Aubrecht, 2014). Despite the prevalence and rates of use of compulsory treatment orders and the rate of involuntary admissions to mental health wards in public hospitals in Victoria, mental health policy and public "mental health" discourses remain incredibly (tellingly) silent on involuntary medico-legal interventions under mental health law (Light et al., 2012).

The extent of police powers under mental health laws mean that police are often the first responders to mental health crises and incidents. In Victoria, where I live, under the *Mental Health Act* (2014) (Vic), legislation grants police the power to detain and transport a person experiencing a mental health crisis for a mental health assessment, if they are satisfied that a person appears to have a mental illness and is at risk of harming themselves or another person.[2] People expressing distress, usually in public are targeted (or as it is more commonly framed, are "over-represented") in incidents that involve fatal and non-fatal police violence. In the state of Victoria, there is an existing record and history of police responses to mental health incidents involving fatal shootings of those experiencing mental distress (McCulloch, 2000). A "mental health crisis" can be thought of as a "criminalisable event", to draw on abolitionist language, as initial contact with police can act as an avenue into the criminal legal system and criminalisation (Stanley and Ebscohost, 2018). Many who face violence and come into contact with the criminal legal system are those who face a myriad of interwoven oppressions, the forces of poverty, systemic racism, ableism, family and domestic violence, deprivation and housing insecurity. None of this is incidental; the management of public "order" and maintenance of social control remains one of the main activities and functions of policing, and those deemed mentally ill are often conceived of as "problem people", who come to the attention of police in public and are presumed to be dangerous and violent.

Critical intersections and imaginaries: Mad Studies and carceral abolition

If policing and the internment of people thought to be mentally ill is one of the main ways madness and mad subjects are managed—how does (or should) Mad Studies approach and understand this? Is it an issue, or subject of inquiry for Mad Studies? How is Mad Studies conceived of broadly as scholarship, epistemology, frameworks and related activism engaging with the problem of policing, especially for those who are also targeted for their location within a dangerous matrix (racism, ableism and sanism)? Conversely, how can carceral abolition activism and theory become more engaged with the critical counter-discourse Mad Studies provides to dominant discourses of "mental illness", sensitive to the violence of psychiatrisation that is often experienced by psychiatric survivors? In attempting to understand and develop a more complete account of our "post-deinstitutionalised" landscapes, where those thought to be "mad" are managed in new ways: trans-institutionalised, or in "community settings", where community care models (whether public or privately run services) retrain their "institutional, medicalized, and individualised modes of care" (Hande and Kelly, 2015), perspectives that draw on the broader context of neoliberal punitiveness, I think should be instructive for Mad Studies. As mad scholars, researchers and activists, I want to make the case for engaging with these flourishing and rich critical discourses for the ways in which they intersect with Mad Studies, with so many other fields of inquiry standing to benefit from incorporating mad ways of knowing and doing.

As Qadri and MacFarlane (2018) reflected, the erasure of the mural and the need for the artists to re-make it raised difficult questions. In her blog, MacFarlane (2019) points out that the mural's removal spoke to ongoing and everyday acts of silencing, the removal of disability and disabled people from public-political space. To this we can also add that when it comes to the memorialising of historical institutionalisation, the "accidental" removal symbolised colonial forgetting, mis-remembering and disappearing of the past. The mural stakes a claim that the various spaces built on segregationist philosophies—both the prison, the asylum, the institution—are not just a part of a "dark history"—but their inheritances reverberate all around us today. I hope to see, and be part of, ways that Mad Studies can chart a course of scholarship, knowledge and practical work towards non-carceral futures, that directly challenges the notion that police will continue to interface with the "mad" and the distressed. The contours of Mad Studies, and its legitimate subject of inquiry should be bold, broad and expansive enough to look at the myriad forms in which madness is managed. I hope to see mad scholarship and activism embrace the broad vision that abolitionist praxis, theory and scholarship offers and is imagining. From Manus to Nauru, where the violence of the Australian border is transmogrified into offshore prison camps, to our psychiatric hospitals, it is the violent, dispossessing act of our founding as penal colony that remains the major underlying dynamic of Australian society today—and such it is impossible to extricate mad people's history from this history.

Notes

1 For images of the mural, see: Qadri, D. & MacFarlane, L. 2018. Disability pride is back. *Public Pedagogies Institute Conference*. Victoria University.
2 Section 351 of the *Mental Health Act 2014* (Vic).

References

Carlton, B. & Russell, E. 2018. *Resisting carceral violence women's imprisonment and the politics of abolition.* Cham: Palgrave Macmillan US.

Chapman, C., Carey, A. C. & Ben-Moshe, L. 2014. *Reconsidering confinement: Interlocking locations and logics of incarceration.* New York: Palgrave Macmillan

Fabris, E. 2006. *Identity, inmates, insight, capacity, consent, coercion: Chemical incarceration in psychiatric survivor experiences of community treatment orders.* ProQuest Dissertations Publishing.

Fabris, E. 2011. *Tranquil prisons: Chemical incarceration under community treatment orders.* Toronto: University of Toronto Press.

Fabris, E. & Aubrecht, K. 2014. Chemical constraint: Experiences of psychiatric coercion, restraint, and detention as carceratory techniques. *Disability incarcerated.* London: Springer.

Gooding, P. 2016. From deinstitutionalisation to consumer empowerment: Mental health policy, neo-liberal restructuring and the closure of the 'Big bins' in Victoria. *Health Sociology Review*, 25, 33–47.

Hande, M. J. & Kelly, C. 2015. Organizing survival and resistance in austere times: Shifting disability activism and care politics in Ontario, Canada. *Disability & Society*, 30, 961–975.

IDHA 2020. Decarcerating care: Taking policing out of mental health crisis response.

Liddle, C. 2020. Australia still turns a blind eye to Aboriginal people dying in police custody. *The Guardian*, 02/06/2020.

Light, E., Kerridge, I., Ryan, C. & Robertson, M. 2012. Community treatment orders in Australia: Rates and patterns of use. *Australasian Psychiatry*, 20, 478–482.

MacFarlene, L. 2019. The Disabilty Pride Mural. *Larissa MacFarlane* [Online].

McCulloch, J. 2000. Policing the mentally ill: An examination of the shootings of individuals with a history of mental illness by Victoria police. *Alternative Law Journal*, 25, 241.

Nullyarimma, W. 2020. [untitled]. *None of us are free until all of us are free: Poems from the inside.* Melbourne: Incendium Radical Library Press.

O'Brien, E. 2017. Beyond prison.

Porter, A. 2016. Reimagining policing. *Human Rights Defender*, 25, 26–28.

Qadri, D. & MacFarlane, L. 2018. Disability Pride is Back. *Public Pedagogies Institute Conference.* Victoria University.

Russell, M. & Newman, M. A. J. 2001. Disablement, Prison, and Historical Segregation. *Monthly Review*, 53, 61.

Stanley, E. & Ebscohost 2018. *Human rights and incarceration: Critical explorations.* Cham, Switzerland: Palgrave Macmillan.

Tran, D. 2017. Maribyrnong Council 'sorry' for accidentally removing disability pride mural it partly paid for. Available: https://www.abc.net.au/news/2017-12-05/maribyrnong-council-apologises-over-mural/9229238 [Accessed 31 October 2020].

Whittaker, A. 2020. Despite 432 Indigenous deaths in custody since 1991, no one has ever been convicted. Racist silence and complicity are to blame.

Wilson, K. 2018. The call for the abolition of mental health law: The challenges of suicide, accidental death and the equal enjoyment of the right to life. *Human Rights Law Review*, 18, 651–688.

Wolfe, P. 2006. Settler colonialism and the elimination of the native. *Journal of Genocide Research*, 8, 387–409.

23

MADNESS IN THE TIME OF WAR

Post-war reflections on practice and research beyond the borders of psychiatry and development

Reima Ana Maglajlić

Introduction

In the 'Milkman' (Burns, 2018), there is a passing reference to a murder that takes place in the midst of The Troubles in an unnamed Northern Irish community where the novel is set. Everyone in the community is aghast – a murder?! A non-Troubles related life-taking?! In our community?! Experiencing and causing death became one of the key experiences of The Troubles. But – outside of it, for no obvious political, or other conflict-related reason? How to make sense of it? While it wasn't the main part of the story's arc, this snippet from the novel really stayed with me. A life-altering event and responses to it shaped so powerfully by the context in which it takes place – one which alters almost all experiences of everyone within it, in that point in time. Relationships with madness during and after the war may be equally shifting, surprising and pause giving.

Experiences which happen during a political conflict impact the people in its midst. One of the sparks for the conflict usually involves some form of othering – how and why I am different than you, not as good, dirtier, barely human. People who start claiming it are not strangers; as the conflict spreads, your neighbours, teachers, colleagues, even your loved ones may express and act upon this view. You flee or are exiled from your home. Before you do, if female (minor or adult), you may be raped – even imprisoned and raped repeatedly until you become pregnant and carry the pregnancy to term. If male, you may be pushed into being a soldier despite still being a minor – or a very scared adult. You can be imprisoned and tortured. You watch your home, your village, your town, your country change and burn. People with a surname very similar to your own are killed just because they have certain religion or a particular background and on such a scale that it is labelled as ethnic cleansing. You flee or you try to stay and survive – in the case of Sarajevo, Bosnia and Herzegovina, through the longest siege in modern warfare (1992–1995). While it all lasts, you don't know when it will end, or how. Once it ends, it doesn't bring peace. For many – regardless of whether they bought into the conflict or not – it doesn't bring resolution, a better tomorrow, nor justice. Anyone who

DOI: 10.4324/9780429465444-28

survives such experiences, directly or indirectly, lives with them from that point on. However, the degree of difficulty and distress they cause to individuals and communities can change, with or without support.

In this chapter, I shall attempt to talk about the relationship between madness and political conflict through the lens of mad studies. I will start by explaining my own experiences and positionality in relation to madness and political conflict, the terminology I use and why I decided to use autoethnography and border thinking to structure my analysis of these experiences. I will also offer a brief explanation of why experiences of political conflict and madness in Bosnia and Herzegovina (BiH, in further text) are relevant for this topic. In the final two sections of this chapter, I will offer evidence for two key conclusions. First, the knowledge on the intersection between mad studies and political conflict through the lens of mad studies is yet to be developed. The hold of the medical – or bio-psycho-social – view of madness still dominates. Second, this is not the only dominant professional knowledge and practice in relation to madness and political conflict – development studies and practice have proven to be equally colonizing in relation to such experiences.

Positionality, terminology and methodology: For the past, present and the future

Part-Bosnian, I have spent a lot of time over the past 20 years working on the reform of health and social care services in Bosnia and Herzegovina through activism, practice and research. This included support for the development of local and national organizations run by people who use(d) mental health services in BiH. I met very few who described their experiences in any other way. Most of those initiatives now no longer exist. The one which remains is 'Fenix' in Tuzla, North-East BiH. The majority of my experiences, in BiH and in general, intertwine with the experiences of people who were considered mad prior to the war or experienced severe distress because of the war. As a result, they frequently experienced prolonged confinement in psychiatric services. All those experiences impact how they engage with others. They struggled to live with their families and within their communities just as much as their families and communities struggled to live with them. I am also a former wife of a former Croatian independence war (1991–1995) soldier who, like many of his peers, struggled to come to terms with his wartime experiences.

I use the term 'mad studies' to refer to 'a project of inquiry, knowledge production, and political action devoted to the critique and transcendence of psy-centred ways of thinking, behaving, relating, and being' (LeFrancois et al., 2013:13). In this chapter, references to psy-centred ways of thinking, behaving, relating and being will include both institutions and community mental health services. When referring to those practices, I shall utilise the terminology utilised by professionals and other people who engage with them (such as mental health practice, community mental health, psychiatric wards and hospitals). I shall refer to the experiences that may lead to contact with psy-centred practices as 'madness', 'distress' or other terms and phrases that describe a relevant experience, particularly if they are used by people who experience them. I emphasise distress because it, together with sadness and feeling strange and surreal, dominates during and after a political conflict compared to the more positive feelings that madness may otherwise cause.

Much like madness, political conflict refers to the complex social phenomena that attracts varied conceptual understandings of it (Skoog, 2015). Schock (1996) offers a so-called conjectural model to understanding and analysing violent political conflict. The model hypothesises that a violent political conflict is generated through the interaction of economic inequality grievances and political opportunities to generate violent conflict. It reconciles the tension observed by Schock between the economic discontent frameworks for understanding conflict and political opportunity ones. This chapter focuses on such, conjectural, violent political conflict and warfare.

Highlighting and clarifying the terms to be used in the text is relevant not only in an attempt to step away from psy-centred thinking, behaving and being or in relation to the complex geographies and histories of violent political conflicts around the world. It is also relevant in relation to the dominance of development practices in the 'war-torn', 'post-war', 'developing' or 'low and middle income' contexts –just some of the labels used to describe countries and contexts that have experienced political conflicts. All those terms have been developed and we share them in English, a frequent medium through which the dominance of psy- and development practices and concepts has been asserted over madness and all other aspects of life in countries experiencing violent political conflicts.

The intersection between the development and the psy-understandings of madness can and should be explored as a form of colonialism (Mills, 2013); hence the relevance of border thinking (Mignolo, 2012). According to Mignolo, effects of colonialism are 'most damaging, far-reaching, and least understood' (Alcoff, 2007:80).

> The modern foundation of knowledge is territorial and imperial ... It was from and in Europe that the classification of the world emerged and not in and from Asia, Africa or America – borders were created therein but of different kinds.
>
> *(Mignolo and Tlostanova, 2006:205, 206)*

In my experience, not all of Europe is allowed to classify itself, either; some parts of the continent are more European than others, in terms of geography, skin colour, passports and the ability to internationally foreground articulations of knowledge of oneself. According to Mignolo (2012), theories and practices already exist which 'sit' at the borders, if not outside of, the colonial matrix of power. Such a border is defined by epistemic difference and geographical stance. Border thinking primarily emerges from the people's anti-imperial epistemic responses to the colonial difference. In relation to madness and war, such an exploration examines what practices and understandings of these two experiences, namely, war and madness – if any – can and do exist outside the dominant psy- and development frameworks.

In order to identify what may sit at the borders, or outside the dominant psy- and development frameworks, I utilised a form of autoethnography, defined by some as critical self-study that enabled me to take 'an active, scientific and systematic view' of my experiences (Hughes et al., 2012:209). I am able to do this as I am privileged with relevant insider knowledge (Chang, 2008). Methodologically, it is in large part reliant on personal memory, which can be unreliable and unpredictable (Chang, 2008:71). This may be remedied by utilizing interviews and other forms of 'text' (photographs, journals and recordings) to help with recall and analysis (Ellis et al., 2011). To prepare this chapter, I first constructed the so-called critical incidence accounts – emic (insider) biographical narratives which are analysed etically (from the outside) (Boufoy-Bastick, 2004) to identify what sits at the borders of psy thinking and doing. I also revisited the results of a rapid review of literature on social work and political conflict I conducted for my other work (details are provided below, as they are relevant). I also conducted an analysis of the four key studies on the reform of mental health services in BiH (Federal MoH and MoH RS, 2009; HNI and SWEBiH, 2000; HNI and SWEBiH, 2003; SIDA, MoH FBiH and MoH RS, 2017). In triangulating the information from these different sources, I hope I avoid one of the key pitfalls of such ethnographies – seeing only what serves one's purpose and providing claims beyond evidence (Thomas, 1993 in Wall, 2008).

This methodology chose me, much more than the other way around. In order to prepare for this chapter, I started writing snippets of memories which were, at first, free associations in relation to the chapter theme, utilizing the lenses of border thinking and mad studies. Which stories do I remember, which stories stand out that talk of these experiences beyond what was already captured or beyond the mainstream? Those that made it into the chapter will appear in italics throughout and, hopefully, offer further insight into the two key points noted in the introduction.

Memory is also important when relevant initiatives fade or disappear from written or other records – particularly if not available in English. One example concerns the memory I have of visiting a four- to six-person group home in Sarajevo, initiated by a German charity immediately after the war in the late 1990s. It provided support for people who have spent most of their lives in long-term institutions, to help them to remember or learn how to live in the community. The local council promised to gradually take over its funding, but this never materialised. The staff there hoped I could help them lobby the local government to ensure its continued work. After initial reservations, all people who lived there started to share their lives with the local community. The charity decided to close it down in the early 2000s. There needs to be some memory, some record that this existed and mattered, shaped someone's life. We need to understand why such practices emerge and why they disappear.

Bosnia and Herzegovina (BiH) matters – and not just to me

I chose not to go into further details of the conflict, the ever-shifting numbers of casualties and numerous atrocities against children and adults during the 1992–1996 conflict across the whole territory of the country of roughly 3.5 million people. I wrote of those details in my other publications. The sources for many of the interpretations and numbers of atrocities are also relevant. Some involve non-BiH authors offering analysis and interpretation of the statistics of war horrors for their own scholarship or for particular 'users' (for example, international or supranational organizations). Others involve BiH authors which regularly get challenged as providing the view of only one (ethnic or other) side of the war.

BiH has wider relevance in relation to madness and political conflict. It is one of the rare post-conflict and middle-income contexts – the latter being a relevant 'identifier' in the sphere of development practice – which introduced a countrywide development of community-based mental health services in the immediate post-war period (Cerić et al., 2001; Račetović et al., 2017). Those experiences are particularly relevant as mental health is now identified as a global development priority (The World Bank, 2016). This translates as follows – unless activists and scholars within the field of Mad Studies establish contact and support their peers in war and post-war contexts, their stories will be co-opted and subsumed within a triangle of psy-centred, traditional (for example, cultural or faith-based) and development practices. And it will all be done with the best of innovative intentions by mental health and development professionals.

Histories, madness, political conflict and the post-war development in the BiH context

Former Yugoslav socialist health care system relied heavily on institutional care, including psychiatric institutions. In BiH, they were initiated immediately after WWII (Cerić et al., 2001). If BiH hospitals didn't have capacity to take people in, they were sent to the larger institutions in

Croatia and Serbia (Pajevic et al., 2010). Some psychiatrists played a particular role in the BiH war and, for example, in the Srebrenica genocide. Dr. Radovan Karadzic, wartime President of Republika Srpska ('Serbian Republic', one of the two BiH entities created during the war) used to be a psychiatrist at the Sarajevo Clinical Hospital. Many other senior figures in the Serbian Democratic Party (a party created by the Bosnian Serbs) were psychiatrists, too (Kaplan and Walter, 2012).

People who were in psychiatric hospitals during the war were, at least on one occasion, used and mistreated for political purposes. On 28 May 1992, Serbian forces 'off-loaded' (Pajevic et al., 2010:308) 164 people who were at the time 'residents' at the nearby Jakeš hospital in Tuzla, NE BiH, which during the war became an area predominately populated by the Bosniaks. All of the 164 people showed signs of neglect, hunger and lack of hygiene (ibid.). Local psychiatrists organized emergency care and housing for all of the people. By the end of the war, some of the 164 people died, while others were either supported to return to their communities or returned to remaining institutions elsewhere (ibid.).

In the aftermath of the war, a common response to the devastated housing and public service infrastructure in the mid-1990s would have been to rebuild mental health institutions. However, several things aligned so that another path unravelled for the BiH mental health services. The local WHO office was staffed by Italian Psychiatrists, who were aware of the importance of deinstitutionalization. Two key figures among BiH psychiatrists, Ismet Cerić and Slobodan Loga, were educated at the Maudsley Hospital in London, UK and also recognised the value of initiating community mental health services. People who were involved in radical practices elsewhere in former Yugoslavia, such as Vito Flaker from the School of Social Work in Ljubljana, Slovenia (who was involved in the Society for the Protection of Madness in Ljubljana in the 1980s) also got involved in supporting the reform. In one of the two main BiH entities (BiH has 14 layers of governance, 13 of which have authority to issue mental health legislation and policy), European funding was used to initiate Community Mental Health Centres (CMHC) within primary health care centres. As of 2014, there are 69 CMHCs across the two entities (Project HOPE, 2014). Services offered by the CMHCs vary, depending on local knowledge and resources; from individual psychotherapy, drop ins, group therapy, occupational therapy, to outreach and community crisis support/crisis prevention.

The hold of the psy-understandings and practices on madness during and after the war

Even if one doesn't directly look for evidence of it, the dominance of psy-frameworks over madness and war is evident. In May 2018, I conducted a rapid review of literature on social work and political conflict. Utilizing the terms 'social work' AND 'political conflict' OR 'war', I searched for relevant articles and dissertations written in English via several search sites, including ASSIA, IBSS, PsycInfo, Scopus, SCIE and Web of Science. I excluded articles published prior to 1990, as well as those which focused on social work education, 'war on drugs', 'war on terror', 'gang war' and the growing US literature on Military social work. Despite the review not being directly related to madness, the majority of identified articles (274 out of 345) stressed the relevance of psy-understandings of people's experiences. Studies focused on the psycho-social understanding of the impact of war on the 'mental wellbeing' of children and young people (e.g. Diab et al., 2015) or on studying these experiences through the PTSD label (e.g. Khamis, 2005). Indeed, the dominance of psy-frameworks and interpretations across all ages has been thoroughly documented (Attanayake et al., 2009; Betancourt et al., 2013; Johnson and Thompson, 2008; Seal et al., 2007). Medical labels, such as the post-traumatic stress disorder (PTSD), tend to dominate the ways that war-induced madness is understood and responded to (Foa et al., 2008).

Such understanding hasn't been without professional criticism (for a summary, see Kienzler, 2008). In his overview of war and mental health literature, Summerfield (2000:232) stresses that the reframing of war-related distress as 'psychological disturbance is a serious distortion' of those experiences. Even interdisciplinary fields like global mental health have been criticised for over-reliance on the psy-frameworks (Mills and Fernando, 2014; Whitley, 2015). Critics have stressed that the individualization of the experiences of madness during political conflict and their processing through a psy-lens usually ignores their relational and social dimensions (Summerfield, 2000; Richters, 2001). Instead, they call for 'social healing' (Richters, 2001) through community and group-based mutual support, storytelling, as well as employment of social justice instruments, such as local and international war tribunals.

However, law is not necessarily an instrument of healing. Conceptions and mechanisms of ensuring social justice remain divided at the borders of different countries, societies and cultures, as well as across genders and social classes (Amadiume and An-Na'im, 2000). For example, Doucet and Denov (2012) note that in Sierra Leone, forgetting may be a culturally preferred way to ensure reconciliation and collective healing after the war. On the other hand, Amadiume (2000:41), citing both the South African Truth Commission and the tribunals for the genocides in BiH and Rowanda, condemns the policy of silence and denial of memory about Biafra, which, according to Amadiume, denied the Biafrans 'the right to tell their truth and expose the wounds of the past'.

Attempts at alternative understandings tend to be framed by professionals – whether local or international – and remain within the dominant professional frameworks. For all intents and purposes, a commendably collaborative effort between international scholars (including a lead author from the US, as well as those from Palestine) recently resulted in a mixed-methods exploratory study which 'develop[ed] and validat[ed] a quantitative measure of a new construct of mental suffering in the occupied Palestinian territories' (Barber et al., 2016: e0156216). The theme and category they use to sum up the experiences of 68 Palestinians in the West Bank, East Jerusalem and the Gaza Strip is powerful – they call it 'feeling broken or destroyed' (ibid.). This phrase is likely to resonate with anyone who experienced war or other forms of prolonged political conflict. And yet, the article and the category remain bound by both positivist and psy- frameworks. While Palestinians who took part in the study emphasised that the political context plays the central role on how they felt, the authors still refer to it as one of the 'domains of functioning'. Later in the article, authors describe how they measured 'trauma–related stress' using the PTSD Symptom Scale.

The construct of feeling broken and destroyed emerged through the interviews and an attentive exploration of local characterizations of suffering. The article can be commended for aiming to present local cultural understandings of own experiences, captured by and expressed through Arabic language. The authors do note that people who expressed such feelings did not 'specifically elicit reports of mental suffering' (ibid). Nonetheless, the authors ambition for future work rests in a perceived need and value in 'elaborat[ing] and quantify[ing] the correlates or predictors of this type of mental suffering' (ibid). Politicians and professionals remain central to the interpretation and processing of war experiences among the civilians and soldiers. Making mental health a global development priority just gave such interpretation a first-class seat to travel across the globe, as opposed to opening a space to develop new ways to address the impact of war on people who experience it.

Professional control over how experiences are framed, explored, interpreted and labelled is also evident in the four key studies on the reform of BiH. Table 23.1 provides an overview of the study methodologies, key findings, and the role that people who use mental health services

Table 23.1 Review of methodology and findings from the four key studies on the reform of mental health services in BiH

Study reference	HNI and SWEBiH (2000)	HNI and SWEBiH (2003)	Federal MoH and MoH RS (2009)	SIDA et al. (2017) – focus on the availability of mental health services
Number of people who use mental health services who took part in the study	50 people, contacted via 5 CMHCs in the Federation of BiH (FBiH)	67 people contacted via 13 CMHCs across BiH	213 people contacted via 50 CMHCs across BiH	486 people, contacted via 13 CMHCs (356 people), 3 Hospitals/Clinics (92) and 1 Institute for Substance Misuse across BiH (28)
Study methods	Semi-structured interview	Semi-structured interview	An international client satisfaction questionnaire (103) Structured interviews (110)	Questionnaire from the WHO Study on Pathways to Care
Other engagement in the study?	No	One person with the experience of using mental health services was a member of the overall research team of 7). She helped create the interview guides, conducted the interviews with her peers, analysed the findings and helped promote the results.	The same person with the experience of using mental health services as in the previous study was one of the 15 interviewers. Only professionals were part of the research team.	No
Key findings	Most people would prefer to receive psychotherapy as opposed to medication. 'Some' (p. 22) indicate that the 'care should focus on war-related trauma and trauma in general' (ibid.)	Both people who use CMHC services and professionals working there noted the prevalence of problems due to the war, especially poverty and social issues (lack of stable housing options, unemployment and poverty, in particular). People who contact the CMHCs are those directly affected by the war – refugees, internally displaced, former soldiers, civil war victims. Issues that led them to contact CMHCs include sleeplessness, nightmares, loss of family members. This also frequently leads to family problems. The most important method of work in the CMHC is 'conversation' (p. 18). People mentioned being hospitalized as refugees while abroad.	When asked why they visit the CMHC, people answered by using their psychiatric label. PTSD or war was noted by 15.5% (17). Two-thirds (65%) noted that they were hospitalised in the past and 'some' (p. 29) people noted that this was a bad experience for them, as they were beaten, tied, had food withdrawn from them. Advantages of the CMHC are the warmth and humanity of the staff (59.1%), contact with people who have similar experiences (11.8%) and group activities (11.8%). A lack of peer support organizations is noted as the least favourable thing about the CMHCs.	The study and the results focus on where and from whom people seek mental health support. Nearly half (46.8%) of people first sought help from their GP. 6.5 percent noted that their first source of support was a religious healer, 1.5% that it was a herbalist and 0.6% relied on homeopathic support first and foremost. 18.5 percent had secondary psychiatric services as their first point of call.

played in each study. No people who have personal experience of using mental health services were members of the research team in the first and the last study.

All but one study uses the established medical language and terminology to seek people's views and share the results. In the HNI and SWEBiH (2003) study, I was the main researcher and, hence, was able to include Halida Vejzagić, one of the members of the National Association of people who use services (which existed at the time) in the research team. She took part in all parts of the research process – creation of the methodology, data gathering, as well as data analysis and promotion of the results. It remains the only study that mentions any other aspect of people's lives, particularly the impact that the war had on housing, employment opportunities and poverty.

All studies concluded that people appreciated the support provided within the community-based services, particularly when compared to hospitalization and institutionalization. However, from the mid-2000s, external funding for the reform was slowly coming to an end, increasing the on-going pressures on both people who use and people who worked in the community-based services:

> *I met the staff of one of the Sarajevan CMHCs during the data gathering for the 2002 Assessment of all BiH CMHCs. An all-female professional team, including a psychiatrist, psychologist and several nurses loved their work and felt passionate about their CMHC and people who visit it. They were plagued by the lack of resources they had and a lack of understanding among other services housed within the same primary health care centre. As they saw the value in offering a variety of support, they worked extra hours. Many people who visited the CMHC lived in extreme poverty; the staff would use their salaries to feed people who came to the Centre, as well as to buy toiletries and other supplies that people needed. Many knew that they can't continue to work this way. They faced challenges by their own families and colleagues from other Health Centre services. When I visited the CMHC again, several months later, most of the staff were on a long-term sick leave.*

> *Nermin (pseudonym) is in his early twenties. He has spent his teenage years as a refugee in the UK, on his own. He is clever, ambitious and eloquent in several languages. He also looks and presents much more as a geezer, than a young Bosnian. He misses his life in the UK. The reason he came back is painful and unraveled slowly. He became mad and was carted off home, to Bosnia, against his wishes. Another kick follows only a year later. Nermin was convinced that, if only he had a job, if only he was able to work, all would be better. He'd feel better, if only there was a job. And now he has found a job – and he is definitely not better, not only according to other people's opinions.*
>
> *Cut to low simmering anger, pain and loss, threaded at the floor of every conversation … What was lost, what was warped. Things that cannot be repaired, for which no justice can be found. Helplessness and pain running as a current at the core of everything, peppered with clever and warped humour. Can't move for it. 'Šuti, dobro je' (Hush now, s'alright – a difficult to translate universal Bosnian response to majority of life's joys, problems and outright disasters).*

The Centres still exist, as do collaborative practices between mental health practitioners and people who use services, although only one Association remains of the original seven (including the National Association) run by people who have used or use mental health services. Nonetheless, the psy-understanding and practices still have a hold and it's due to get even stronger. In mid-2018, BiH signed a Memorandum of Understanding with the Council of Europe to fund the reconstruction and equipping of six psychiatric hospitals across BiH (Vijesti, 2018).

The trouble with development

How did we come full circle? In part, it is due to the dominance of psy-understandings of madness and political conflict. However, it is also due to the fact that the reform was primarily a development 'project'. Implementation of all development reforms in BiH and research on them have been rightfully criticized as driven by donor priorities and agendas (Papić, 2001; Sampson, 2004). BiH is not an exception; this is common in wider development practices (Mosse, 2011). Reforms in post-war contexts tend to focus on a specific theme, implemented through short-term projects, lasting one–two years. Frequently, major support is withdrawn after this period, or significantly reshaped. Such changes are set in a top-down manner, rather than based on increased knowledge of the local contexts and people's actual needs.

> *One of the key international organisations which supported the reform created a local organiza-tion in 2002 'to ensure sustainability' of their work during (organising and providing counselling support) and after the war (support for the development of community mental health services). Within the next year, post-war mental health was no longer 'sexy.' There were other conflicts and more pressing needs elsewhere. Under new, local, management, and due to a lack of available funding, the organization followed the money and, from 2003, started a project which provided repairs and equipment for children's hospitals.*

Furthermore, mental health reform wasn't joined up with other reforms. Social care reforms focused almost exclusively on child and family services. Long-stay social care institutions for people with learning difficulties and people with mental health issues provided continued options for institutionalization in this sector (BiH Ombudsman, 2018). Politicization of benefits, particularly for former soldiers, results in further inequalities when it comes to pov-erty alleviation and in-kind benefits (Hronesova, 2016).

> *Mirjana (pseudonym) is a local poet in her early thirties who I met at the Day Centre at the Psychiatric Ward of the Clinical Hospital in Sarajevo. People remember how cool Mirjana was in her early youth, prior to the war and first experiences of the local psychiatric clinic. They remember her poetry and her presence around town. She still lives in her own flat, but it has burnt to the ground – not during the war, but because Mirjana managed to burn it down using a makeshift stove. She doesn't trust anyone who tries to visit her but loves to visit the Day Centre. When a newly established drop-in shares its space with an office of the community mental health reform project, she likes to pop by the office and to diagnose the staff working there with a variety of DSM labels. They are not fans of her expertise. Professionals describe her as non-engaging, and other people who use services don't want to spend time with her as she talks too much and doesn't wash regularly. With all the reforms, no one manages to establish a relationship with Mirjana, until she is carted off to a social care institution where she later dies. This is possible as, despite the reform of mental health services, long-stay institutions still exist in social care.*

In the chasm between the psy- and other professional understandings of madness and those caused by development practice agendas, people's own experiences remain out of sight, unless telling a narrowly defined 'success story' of a particular reform intervention. While many of the reform initiatives provided valuable support and changed the ways in which (some) professionals in BiH engage with and understand madness, there are also people who either fall prey to religious 'exorcism' of madness (see Table 23.1) or whose experiences are institutionalized or otherwise marginalized, yet again.

I leave you at the borders

In hindsight, I realize that I have lost a valuable chance to do two things. First, I lost an opportunity to record and archive some of the experiences and practices that existed only for a brief while, details of which are lost to my memory, my existing documentation of the reform, within online repositories, or to the memories and archives of people I shared these experiences with. I already provided one such example earlier in the chapter. Second, any archives of people's stories I have helped to create were always processed for a particular funder and a particular, professional, political and/or donor, audience. Hence, by necessity, the ones I share here rely on my memory and those reports. While they are memories of how people shared their stories with me, they weren't committed to my memory or shared with others on people's own terms, how they want their stories to be remembered.

Stories of war and madness within the discipline of mad studies are yet to be written, related practices are yet to be created. While any blueprints need to be avoided, there are certain ingredients:

- They need to start and remain devoted to the experiences and needs of people who experienced political conflict and madness, at a minimum through co-production.
- Stories of war and madness will have to find a way to stitch across political divisions and manipulations, present in all conflict and post-conflict settings.
- At least some will have to focus on supporting people in distress within their communities – even at the times of severe distress – as well as poverty alleviation and mutual support within the community.
- All those stories and practices will have to carefully circumnavigate psy-understandings and practices, as well as the development 'project' format, as funding for such initiatives is likely to stay exclusively based in Western and Northern Europe, North America and Australia. They will also have to carefully navigate collaborative and co-produced practices between people who use mental health services and mental health professionals. In many contexts, including BiH, mental health professionals are 'a given', and coproduction is enacted solely through the acceptance of psy-frameworks.
- Understanding of international collaboration will have to be redefined, making it mutual, equitable, inclusive and co-productive, rather than colonial. Collaboration has to be led and initiated 'from within', but supported from the 'outside'. The international aspect of collaboration should focus on amplifying 'insider' experiences and voices, so they can be understood and supported more widely.
- Any such collaboration also needs to be intersectional, not least to consider the gendered experiences of both political conflict and its impact on the post-war livelihoods.

Finally, stories of war and madness may not be readily available for immediate sharing, particularly not though words. They will require relationship-building, trust and numerous stumbling attempts (of which this truly is one) over a prolonged period of time. Hence, it will also require new ways of exploring our own experiences through practice and research. Autoethnography was my current choice – but not an easy one, or one I'd settle for. While some authors (Ellis et al., 2011:273) see it 'as a political, socially-just and socially conscious act', in both practice and research, I think mad studies has potential to become much more creative. So – to be continued.

References

Alcoff L M (2007). Mignolo's epistemology of coloniality. *The New Centennial Review*, 7(3), 79–101.

Amadiume I (2000). The politics of memory: Biafra and intellectual responsibility. In I Amadiume and A An-Na'im, (eds.). *The Politics of Memory: Truth, Healing and Social Justice*. London: Zed Books, 38–55.

Amadiume I and An-Na'im A (2000). Introduction: Facing truth, voicing justice. In I Amadiume and A An-Na'im, (eds.). *The Politics of Memory: Truth, Healing and Social Justice*. London: Zed Books, 1–20.

Attanayake V, McKay R, Joffres M, Singh S, Burkle Jr F and Mills E (2009). Prevalence of mental disorders among children exposed to war: A systematic review of 7,920 children. *Medicine Conflict and Survival*, 25(1), 4–19.

Barber B K, McNeely C A, El Sarraj E, Daher M, Giacaman R, Arafat C, Barnes W and Mallouh M A (2016). Mental suffering in protracted political conflict: Feeling broken or destroyed. *PloS one*, 11(5), e0156216.

Betancourt T S, Borisova I, Williams T P, Meyers-Ohki S E, Rubin-Smith J E, Annan J and Kohrt B A (2013). Research Review: Psychosocial adjustment and mental health in former child soldiers–a systematic review of the literature and recommendations for future research. *Journal of Child Psychology and Psychiatry*, 54(1), 17–36.

BiH Ombudsman (2018). *Specijalni izvjestaj o stanju prava osoba sa intelektualnim I mentalnim teskocama u Bosni I Herzegovini*. https://www.ombudsmen.gov.ba/Dokumenti.aspx?id=28&tip=4&lang=BS Accessed: 2 February 2019.

Boufoy-Bastick B (2004). Auto-interviewing, auto-ethnography and critical incident methodology for eliciting a self-conceptualised worldview. *Forum: Qualitative Social Research*, 5(1), 37.

Burns A (2018). *Milkman*. London: Faber & Faber.

Cerić I, Loga S, Sinanović O, Cardaklija Z, Cerkez G, Jacobson L, Jensen S, Reali M, Toresini L, Oruc L, Danes V, Mikovic M, Mehic-Basara N, Hasanbegovic M, Lagerquist B, Flaker V, Mollica R, Pavkovic I, Skobic H, Lavele J, Horvat D, Nakas B, Kapetanovic A, Bradvica L, Weine S, Masic I, Puratic V and Dancevic M (2001). Reconstruction of mental health services in Bosnia and Herzegovina. *Medicinski arhiv*, 55(1 Suppl 1), 5–23.

Chang H (2008). *Autoethnography as a Method*. Walnut Creek, CA: Left Coast Press.

Diab M, Peltonen K, Qouta S R, Palosaari E and Punamäki R L (2015). Effectiveness of psychosocial intervention enhancing resilience among war-affected children and the moderating role of family factors. *Child Abuse & Neglect*, 40, 24–35.

Doucet D and Denov M (2012). The power of sweet words: Local forms of intervention with war-affected women in rural Sierra Leone. *International Social Work*, 55(5), 612–628.

Ellis C, Adams T E and Bochner A P (2011). Autoethnography: An overview. *Historical Social Research/Historische Sozialforschung*, 36(4), 273–290.

Federal MoH and MoH RS (2009). Analiza situacije i procjena usluga mentalnog zdravlja u zajednici u Bosni i Hercegovini. http://www.mentalnozdravlje.ba/uimages/pdf/izvjestaj.pdf Accessed: 24 April 2019.

Foa E B, Keane T M, Friedman M. J and Cohen J A (eds.) (2008). *Effective Treatments for PTSD: Practice Guidelines from the International Society for Traumatic Stress Studies*. London: The Guilford Press.

HNI and SWEBiH (2000). *Assessment: Community Mental Health Care in the Federation of Bosnia & Herzegovina*. Sarajevo: HNI.

HNI and SWEBIH (2003). *Situation Analysis and Needs Assessment in the Community Mental Health Centres in Bosnia and Herzegovina*. Sarajevo: HNI.

Hronesova J (2016). Might makes right: War-related payments in Bosnia and Herzegovina. *Journal of Intervention and Statebuilding*, 10(3), 339–360.

Hughes S, Pennington J L and Makris S (2012). Translating autoethnography across the AERA standards: Toward understanding autoethnographic scholarship as empirical research. *Educational Researcher*, 41(6), 209–219.

Johnson H and Thompson A (2008). The development and maintenance of post-traumatic stress disorder (PTSD) in civilian adult survivors of war trauma and torture: A review. *Clinical Psychology Review*, *28*(1), 36–47.

Kaplan R M and Walter G (2012). From Kraeplin to Karadzic: Psychiatry's long road to genocide. In C Tatz (ed.). *Genocide Perspectives IV: Essays on Holocaust and Genocide*. UTS ePress, 122–165.

Kienzler H (2008). Debating war-trauma and post-traumatic stress disorder (PTSD) in an interdisciplinary arena. *Social Science & Medicine*, *67*(2), 218–227.

Khamis V (2005). Post-traumatic stress disorder among school age Palestinian children. *Child Abuse & Neglect*, *29*(1), 81–95.

LeFrancois B A, Menzies R and Reaume G (2013). *Mad Matters: A Critical Reader in Canadian Mad Studies*. Toronto: Canadian Scholars' Press Inc.

Mignolo W D (2012). *Local Histories/Global Designs: Coloniality, Subaltern Knowledges, and Border Thinking*. Princeton: Princeton University Press.

Mignolo W D and Tlostanova M V (2006). Theorizing from the borders: Shifting to geo- and body-politics of knowledge. *European Journal of Social Theory*, *9*(2), 205–221.

Mills C (2013). *Decolonising Global Mental Health: The Psychiatrisation of the Majority World*. Hove: Routledge.

Mills C and Fernando S (2014). Globalising mental health or pathologising the Global South? Mapping the ethics, theory and practice of global mental health. *Disability and the Global South*, *1*(2), 188–202.

Mosse D (ed.) (2011). *Adventures in Aidland: The Anthropology of Professionals in International Development*. New York: Berghahn Books.

Pajevic I, Hasanovic M and Kopric A (2010). Psychiatry in a battle zone. *Bioethics*, *24*(6), 304–308.

Papić Ž (ed.) (2001). *Policies of International Support to Southeast European Countries: Lessons (Not) Learnt in Bosnia-Herzegovina*. Sarajevo: Open Society Fund Bosnia-Herzegovina.

Project HOPE (2014). *Mapiranje stanja pruzanja usluga u oblasti mentalnog zdravlja u Bosni I Herzegovini*. https://bih.iom.int/sites/default/files/downloads/publications/A5_mentalhealth_BOS.nove%20ispravke.pdf Accessed: 2 February 2019.

Račetović G, Slavica P, Rosic B and Grujic-Timarac S (2017). Community based mental health care in Bosnia and Herzegovina – an overview of the last six years. *European Psychiatry*, 41, S613–S614.

Richters A (2001). Trauma as a permanent indictment of injustice: a socio-cultural critique of DSM-III and DSM-IV. In M Vewey (ed.). *Trauma und Ressourcen*. Berlin: Verlag für Wissenschaft und Bildung, 53–75.

Sampson S (2004). Too much civil society? Donor-driven NGOs in the Balkans. In L Dhundale and E A Andersen (eds.). *Revisiting the Role of Civil Society in the Promotion of Human Rights*. Copenhagen: Danish Institute for Human Rights, 197–220.

Schock K (1996). A Conjectural Model of Political Conflict. *Journal of Conflict Resolution*, *40*, 98–133.

Seal K H, Bertenthal D, Miner C R, Sen S and Marmar C (2007). Bringing the war back home: Mental health disorders among 103 788 US veterans returning from Iraq and Afghanistan seen at Department of Veterans Affairs Facilities. *Archives of Internal Medicine*, *167*(5), 476–482.

SIDA, MoH FBiH and MoH RS (2017). *Ispitivanje dostupnosti usluga mentalnog zdravlja u Bosni i Hercegovini*. http://www.mentalnozdravlje.ba/uimages/biblioteka/izvestaj.pdf Accessed: 24 April 2019.

Skoog L (2015). Political conflicts and the mechanisms behind the concept. *XXIV Nordic conference on Local Government Research*. Gothenburg November 26–28. https://spa.gu.se/digitalAssets/1552/1552372_skoog--political-conflicts-and-the-mechanisms-behind-the-concept--norkom-xxiv-2015.pdf Accessed: 23 January 2019.

Summerfield D (2000). War and mental health: a brief overview. *BMJ*, *321*:232–235.

The World Bank (2016). *Out of the Shadows: Making Mental Health a Global Development Priority*. http://documents.worldbank.org/curated/en/270131468187759113/Out-of-the-shadows-making-mental-health-a-global-development-priority Accessed: 28 January 2019.

Vijesti (2018). *Za obnovu sest psihijatrijskih bolnica I ustanova u BiH osigurano 23 miliona KM*. https://vijesti.ba/clanak/414472/za-obnovu-sest-psihijatrijskih-bolnica-i-ustanova-u-bih-osigurano-23-miliona-km Accessed: 2 February 2018.

Wall S (2008). Easier said than done: Writing an autoethnography. *International Journal of Qualitative Methods*, *7*(1), 38–53.

Whitley R (2015). Global mental health: concepts, conflicts and controversies. *Epidemiology and Psychiatric Sciences*, *24*(4), 285–291.

24

THE ARCHITECTURE OF MY MADNESS

Caroline Yeo

The architect designs the physical spaces where life takes place. They construct the world within which we live, study, work and die. In our homes, schools, offices and hospitals the scripts of our lives play out surrounded by glass, bricks, timber or steel.

Architecture has the power to control. It contains space and people within walls. Whether by choice or against our will the building is a container of life. The architect designs both the home and the prison, the university and the hospital.

Architecture has always played a large part in the madness of my life. I studied Architecture at University and never wanted anything to do with working in the world of "mental health" research or activism, however this is where I have found myself. I would like to tell the story of my madness through the buildings and spaces which tried to contain it.

The house

The architect Le Corbusier claimed that the "house is a machine for living in" (Corbusier, 2013: 4). The machine I grew up in was a nice, unassuming detached house, sitting at the top of an ordinary cul-de-sac, on an ordinary road in a little town.

Nothing special.

The house was a place of kindness and love. I was greatly loved by my mum, brother, grand-mother and our cat Angel. I remember lovely times in our garden playing cricket. I remember playing computer games with my brother and the delicious Sunday dinners my mum used to cook.

The house was also a place of cruelty, abuse and tyranny. My father was abusive. He ruled over the house with his anger and his threats. He said he would kill himself, he would kill us, he would kill our Angel.

I was afraid of our ruler.

The house was not a place of safety for myself.

My madness was born in that house.

I was lucky that my home was in a good state of repair, had a nice garden and was in a "nice" neighbourhood. The house or as Cameron rightly points out, more importantly the home plays such an important role in recovery. Safe housing played such a large part in my own story.

DOI: 10.4324/9780429465444-29

Choice has also played another key role. As a person who has been abused, a person who has been hospitalised against my will and has had forced treatment, choosing a place to live and creating a home for myself was vital to me regaining power over my life and personal freedom.

The University

When I was 14 I wanted to be an architect. My art teacher flying around the classroom telling me about Frank Lloyd Wright and other great architects inspiring me to choose that particular career path.

I went to University and loved studying architecture, making models, drawing and travelling the world. I fell in love with the concepts of sustainability and the beauty of green buildings. I started teaching at the University, inspiring students with their designs, lecturing on climate change and environmental design.

I would go out with friends, drink wine and talk about art, philosophy, politics or gossip about boys. I had many friends, many laughs, tears, and discussions of both depth and superficiality. I was on the road to a career as a lecturer in architecture, my dream job. On the road to marrying a nice man and living the middle-class dream of barbeques and intelligent, polite conversation.

It was a beautiful dream.

Sometimes I wish I could fall asleep again.

Unsee what I have seen.

Unknow what I know.

It is at the University on its beautiful green campus with its grand buildings where I went mad.

My mind was my place of freedom whilst I grew up. Within my imagination I constructed worlds to live in.

When I started living freedom, whilst at University, I remembered my trauma and I went mad in the tiny room of my student accommodation.

I saw beyond.

I saw beautiful things.

I saw painful things.

I saw meaning.

I saw truth.

The University was not a place of safety for myself.

My madness exploded free.

And I ended up in a mental hospital.

The hospital

I went to hospital for help.

What I found there was more pain and abuse.

I witnessed horrific human rights abuses and treatment. I experienced them myself.

And I met the most extraordinary, kind and wise people I have ever met.

Not doctors or nurses but the patients in the "asylum".

The clinical world did not accept my madness nor even try to understand. My freedom was lost along with the opportunity to heal my wounds of trauma.

The hospital was not a place of safety for myself.

Righteous anger brewed.

My madness grew more and more.

The streets

On the streets I searched for truth, in the heart of my madness I wandered the streets, at night, alone. Friends and family were worried, said I was unsafe. The quiet of the night, the cold air, the homeless sleeping in shop doorways, a 24-hour fast food restaurant for sustenance. Nothing happened to me on the streets. I was not attacked, not abused, not sexually assaulted as people feared I may have been. Perhaps I was just lucky, but for me the streets were safer than the hospital wards where I was abused in every way possible.

The city streets are different in the day. There is a strange peace at 3am. Hardly a car, a quietness as the lucky people sleep.

Those who can sleep, how lucky they are? Sleep evades me, my trauma keeps me awake at night. The ideas, fears, anxieties dancing in my mind. The walk a way to evade the thoughts. Call the crisis team and that is what they suggest. Go for a walk, have a bath, call a friend. At 3am when the trauma arrives and the possibility to sleep disappears what choice do I have? A friend at 3am?

I find my friend in the written word. Stay in my bed and I write, my trauma flowing, hoping someone will read it, connect, believe me, accept me and respond.

This year I found someone to write to at 3am.

A friend, a fellow survivor, a peer.

She knows who she is.

I thank you from the bottom of my heart.

We wrote, wrote and wrote in emails on any day, at any time.

My stories of pain, abuse, laughter, songs, art, poetry and spiders flowed into emails, emails to a friend.

And she replied.

Those emails were filled with humour, sadness, anxiety, fears, paranoia, joy and pain, so much pain.

The emails heal me.

Within the architecture of the internet I found my saving grace.

Sharing and being responded to.

Being accepted.

Being believed.

She has saved my life this year.

This year is the year I accepted my madness and I recovered what I lost or rather what was stolen from me, in the childhood and then by the mental health system.

My freedom.

The cafe

The place I come to write. The act of writing, the way to solidify my thoughts, to make the stream of consciousness possibly understandable. My madness is like all the connections of everything all at once and the inability to share with others, to connect. The act of writing slows the pace and offers the possibility of making sense of the stories and thoughts dancing like a dervish in my mind.

So the cafe. So many kinds. My favourite places are quiet, not empty, not silent but where my thoughts can slow. The lighting gentle, the furnishings dark, beautiful adornments on the walls, softness and style.

I love to try different ones most times, in different cities of the world. Sitting outside can be a preference if the weather is right, the air pure, the view worthwhile and again the quietness.

Quiet but not silent as I like the hum of a little life, a little of the world to connect with. As the words flow, not on a piece of paper but my phone, my act of writing on a phone in an email, like writing to a friend, to connect with someone in the world. Writing to myself or writing to another, a way to express the madness and stories of my life.

The cafe is a place of both solitude and the possibility for connection. The architecture of the interior or connection with the exterior needs to inspire.

And it needs to have good coffee, there needs to be good coffee.

I will avoid the chains, with their lack of personality, all the same or at least they try to be, like people trying to fit in, be the same, be normal.

Fuck normal. I want different, I want music, poetry, art and originality. I want madness. Do not fix me.

The coffee is also disappointing like sadly many people.

I just wish people were kinder to one another.

I heard of an initiative called kindness cafes, which are a "pop-up movement in the spirit of giftivism. To encourage human connection and kind acts around the world" (Kindness Cafes, n.d.).

I think I would like to have a coffee in one of those cafes.

With a peer.

With a friend.

I have with my email pen pal.

We have sat eye to eye a few times and drank coffee and ate avocados on toast.

Together in person.

Me and my internet pen peer.

The park

Sitting on a bench in meditation or thought, alone or with company.

In the connection to nature and the universe can the silent mind reside. At one with the sounds of birds, the bark of a dog, the drop of a leaf, the subtle or loud conversations of lovers, families or one man and his dog.

Most days I go for a walk in the humble park near my home to try to still my mind, to forget the horrors of the past and be at one with nature and the moment. Again the crisis team suggestions go for a walk, have a bath, call a friend.

Can you go to the park and scream or howl to the moon?

Not if there are others there.

Is it possible in company to scream, howl or even laugh too loudly?

Is it acceptable to truly feel and to express joy, sadness or distress?

Must our emotions always be suppressed, through physical restraint or medication?

What if we had places to set or emotions free?

Is the hospital the only venue for the screams of the soul to be released?

Can there be architecture to contain madness?

Is madness too wild?

Can people handle wildness?

Nick Totton in "Wild Therapy – Undomesticating inner and outer worlds" argues that wildness of the human psyche and the landscapes that surround us is vital to our sanity. His approach to working with people is to be open to the spontaneous and the unexpected (Totton, 2011).

The office

The office box of academia has hard, solid walls, locks and keys.

They use swipe cards there, like in hospital.

Once whilst working in a survivor-led organisation with a fellow mad woman and allies we did a take-over of the building and transformed it into a locked ward. We stuck up signs like on hospital wards forbidding people to use the toilet or leave the building for a cigarette unless at certain allotted times as an act of taking away a human's most basic needs and desires. This was a celebration in honour of Creative Malajustment week and Dr Martin Luther King Jr's call that one cannot be sane in an insane world. It was a Mad Carnival celebration of colour, pride and chaorder.

Chaos and order is how I describe my madness.

The inbetween.

For a day the University building became a place of madness, play, joy, sharing, honesty and the holding of deep pain. The office plain, white walls covered in the art of anarchy, rebellion or revolution. To me I class the office as a place of the slow evolution of thought or at least that is my hope. For a person who has an interesting relationship with time, one might say I live in a beautiful and difficult trauma time, the pace makes an activist both frustrated and righteously angry. It can be a place of ignorance and fear. Within the clear glass windows the academics wish to keep their secrets hidden. I as the survivor researcher, as the peer opening up the most painful of traumatic wounds as part of my job faced by silence, pitying eyes or empty words.

How brave, how sad, how different her experiences are to our nice lives of middle class privilege with our nice homes and comfortable lives?

I have joined the ranks of middle class privilege and I am glad. Should I feel guilty after I spent years living on pitiful Personal Independence Payments in and out of hospital? Sometimes I do and sometimes I don't.

The building a symbol of silence and the hidden. A place of possibility of uncovering truth. Slowly.

The white walls of formality make it look like a prison.

It is the people within that makes this place at times a prison to me as a mad woman. A prison of mind, where only evidence-base's, RCT's or gentle, careful words are tolerated. No tears or anger just smiles and niceties.

How false?

I sit in the toilets and cry at the injustice in the world and the powerlessness I feel. The toilet becomes a safe place, a place of refuge, solitude and feeling. In this multi-million pound architectural statement, I find comfort in the toilet, the least considered of architectural spaces.

In Hong Kong there is a golden toilet, in Japan the toilets squirt water to clean your most intimate of parts, there is the sustainable composting toilet and there is the hole in the ground. A place of evacuation, a place to dump your shit, your pain, your tears and your trauma. If only we could talk in the white walls of the office rooms our truths and share like peers our pain.

Can we sort through our shit together and come to some kind of solidarity?

I write about challenging things, I become righteously angry and I upset my colleagues and myself.

The office is not a place of safety for others.

My madness is disliked.

I am a disliked mad woman in the academy. I work in the academy, but I do not want to be an academic. I want to be a researcher, a mentor, an activist and a reflector. I guess I have to publish some papers as well.

A nice pay cheque does feel very nice.

I now have a nice life of middle-class privilege. I have a nice house, finally a home to make my own and a comfortable life.

Am I a hypocrite?

Am I a sell out?

Probably.

I am unfair to them.

Can they understand?

Can they know madness?

Can they know abuse?

Can they know injustice?

Can they know what it is like?

I have lived it.

If they do not understand, who will, where do I go?

To my emails. She is also a survivor and she understands.

I can write.

The theatre

I feel like an actress most days. Wearing different masks as I go to work each day.

Survivor. Token. Researcher. Joker. Fool. Great Pretender.

It feels like a pantomime at times. A conference, a workshop, a lecture. As Shakespeare wrote "All the world's a stage, and all the men and women merely players: they have their exits and their entrances; and one man in his time plays many parts, his acts being seven ages" (Shakespeare, 2009); I play my life each day. I am a recovery ninja battling in the shadows and in the light to reclaim the grassroots values of recovery and peer support in sometimes hostile and toxic environments. At least I am trying to be. Perhaps that is a grandiose scheme. I have never been called that before.

I am an activist, acting most days in a theatre of the oppressed (Boal, 2000).

Sometimes I wonder if it is only me.

So I send her another email.

And she understands.

The guest house

My godparents owned a guesthouse in Kent by the sea. I loved going there. It was a place of love. It was a place where I felt safe. It felt like home.

When I think of my godparents guest house I think of a place of retreat and a place of salvation. In the recovery movement the Soteria houses of "salvation" were set up to aid the recovery of people who had received a diagnosis of schizophrenia with minimal use of neuroleptic medication. The first house had 12 rooms for up to 6 people, 2 non-professional staff members and volunteers, who were chosen for their ability to create a safe, supportive, warm and relaxed environment (Thomas, 2014). The Hearing Voices Network in Australia co-produced a list of ways people who hear voices have said have helped them cope with distressing voices, many of which are very simple – visit a friend, draw, meditate, cry, dance, diary, sing, eat healthily, have a cup of tea with someone (Baker and Romme, 2009). The Leeds Survivor Led Crisis Service Dial House open during the nights and over weekends offer visitors a place to relax in a homely environment, get some crisis support, be with others (Coles and Diamond, 2013). Have a cup of tea with someone.

My own madness can be a place of distress, a yearning for connection to others, a need for a place to find some kind of peer support.

This year I went to two residential workshops, which I found difficult, healing and profound. One of them was organised by Katie Mottram of Emerging Proud in the beautiful setting of a guesthouse in Norwich, surrounded by a garden with a pond and wildlife. In a circle we shared deep pains as human beings. Not all of us were survivors but we were all people willing to open up trauma and share. We were peers sharing a human experience without labels or "diagnoses".

I swam in the sea, I laughed loudly, I howled to the moon and cried.

A lot.

About 6 months later I went to Port Ness on the Isle of Lewis, Scotland. Again, beautiful nature and a remarkable silence. The workshop was organised by Ron Coleman and his wife Karen Taylor and all 9 of us shared a human experience of "peer-ness". Everyone was part of the journey and I offer them all my gratitude.

I swam in the sea, I laughed loudly, I howled to the moon and cried.

A lot.

When I went to Norwich, I forgave my father.

When I went to Port Ness, I forgave myself.

This is the power of peer support.

The city

The City and the Architecture of my Madness.

I have found unsafety in the buildings and places architects have designed.

I have found unsafety in my own mind.

What is safety?

What is a place of safety?

I needed a place to howl and scream and cry and my trauma to pour out.

I found that place.

In the peer retreats and in my emails to my friend.

Thank you to the architecture of the internet, which connected me to a person who is helping to heal incredibly deep wounds.

Thank you to the survivors and the peers.

Thank you to us.

Finally back to the guesthouse, the safe space of my childhood.

The physical architectural space.

And, the madness that which lives within me, yes that is like a guesthouse.

I welcome you in.

The guest house

My own experiences of psychiatric abuse and forced treatment have made me sure that there needs to be a better way to treat people than hospitals, restraints and treatment against the will of the patient.

I advocate the idea of the guest-house, the retreat and the asylum in the truest sense of the word. A place to find safety. I did not find safety on the wards, only trauma.

I advocate for beautiful spaces filled with kind and caring people.

I advocate for green spaces, for light and for fresh air.

I advocate for spaces where emotions can be held, explored and released.

I want a place of love not abuse.

I want home.

Home is kind.

We can be architects and design environments through our actions and ways of being which help not harm, love not hurt, heal not abuse.

Home is in the heart.

References

Aalto A and Fleig K 1970. *Alvar Aalto: Complete Works*. Editions d'architecture Artemis.

Beresford P 2010. *A straight talking introduction to being a mental health service user*. PCCS Books.

Beresford P 2018. *Social policy first hand: an international introduction to participatory social welfare*. Policy Press.

Day C 2017. *Places of the soul: Architecture and environmental design as a healing art*. Routledge.

Dickens C 1859. *A tale of two cities*. Gawthorn.

Goodyear D 2014. *The New Yorker*. Paper Palaces: The architect of the dispossessed meets the one per cent. https://www.newyorker.com/magazine/2014/08/11/paper-palaces. Accessed: 09.07.2020.

Guimapang K 2019. *Archinect News*. Shaping an architectural legend: what inspired I.M. Pei? https://archinect.com/news/article/150137086/shaping-an-architectural-legend-what-inspired-i-m-pei. Accessed: 09.07.2020.

Hattaway M 2009. *As you like it (The New Cambridge Shakespeare)*. Cambridge University Press.

Kahn L I 2003. *Louis Kahn: essential texts*. WW Norton & Company.

Kindness Cafes n.d. http://www.kindnesscafes.com/. Accessed 09.07.2020.

Lin Z 2010. *Kenzo Tange and the Metabolist movement: urban utopias of modern Japan*. Routledge.

Rumi J 1995. The guest house. In C Barks, J Moyne, A J Arberry and R Nicholson. *The essential Rumi*. San Francisco: Harper, 109.

Shakespeare W 2009. *As You Like It*, Act II, Scene 7.

Sweeney A, Beresford P, Faulkner A, Nettle M and Rose D 2009. *This is survivor research*. PCCS Books.

TM 2016. *Toer Magazine*. Zaha Hadid / Architecture, A Special Experience. https://toermagazine.wordpress.com/2016/04/09/zaha-hadid-architecture-a-special-experience/. Accessed: 09.07.2020.

Wright F L 2010. *The essential Frank Lloyd Wright: critical writings on architecture*. Princeton University Press.

25

RE-CONCEPTUALISING SUICIDALITY

Towards collective intersubjective responses

David Webb

Editors' intro

After his own "four years of madness" in the late 1990s, David Webb looked into the literature on suicide and was alarmed to find that the first-person voice of attempt survivors was
almost completely absent. Even more lacking from the literature was any mention of spirituality, which was the key to David's recovery and survival. This enquiry became a PhD at
Victoria University, completed in 2005, which is thought to be the world's first PhD on suicide
by a survivor. In 2010 David published a book *Thinking About Suicide* based on his PhD research
into suicidality. For more than a decade, he argued, advocated and campaigned for the inclusion
of attempt survivors in the public discourse on suicide – in academia, in public discussions on
suicide and, importantly, in disability human rights forums. This included time on the board
of the World Network of Users and Survivors of Psychiatry (WNUSP) and working for the
Australian Federation of Disability Organisations (AFDO). David has represented both these
organisations at numerous United Nations disability forums. He had to retire from active work
in 2012 when he was diagnosed with a rare auto-immune disorder.

We are pleased to present the slightly edited closing chapter of David's PhD thesis in this
collection. Originally entitled "Epilogue: Who are we?" this part of the thesis was not included
in his book "Thinking about Suicide". In strong connection with that book this text also
stands on its own and offers important ideas about how we could re-think suicidality and turn
prevention into a collective, community endeavour. David's text is also offered as a reminder
of efforts to make sense of our collective experiences that existed long before the term Mad
Studies was coined.

Suicidality as a crisis of the self

Thinking about suicide – that is, contemplating suicide for yourself – is an intimately personal,
private and often secret feeling that many people struggle with. The story of my book[1] tells
something of this struggle for one individual. It tells of the pain of struggling to live in your own
skin. It tells of the anguish of feeling an utter misfit in the world you find yourself living in. It
tells of the agonising crisis of the self, where life as you experience it has lost all meaning and
purpose. It tells of the dark, inner loneliness and isolation, the hopelessness and helplessness, of

DOI: 10.4324/9780429465444-30

nowhere to go with these feelings. The story there also tells of attempts to overcome or perhaps deny these feelings, sometimes through a noble search to find meaning in life, at other times through the less noble escape into self-medication. It also tells of seeking help but only finding more hopelessness and helplessness. And at the end of this story, unlike many other similar stories, there is a happy ending, when peace was finally found where it was least expected but where it had been all along – in the silent, spiritual heart of my being.

The motivation to tell this story of one individual's thinking about suicide is to offer it as my contribution to our collective thinking about suicide – that is, our efforts to comprehend suicide so that we might help prevent it. Some people may think that we can learn little from one individual story, especially, according to one school of thought, when that story does not end in a 'completed' suicide. I obviously disagree with this view, although I do not attempt to make any generalisations from a single story, particularly when that story is my own. On the contrary, I regard suicide and suicidality as mysterious as life itself. But this does not mean that we cannot understand it much better than we currently do. Along with my personal story in the narratives of my book, which I regard as the most valuable contribution that I have to offer, I have also reflected on the various aspects of this story in the commentaries. The aim here is to encourage, stimulate and provoke critical thinking and discussion about these issues. But the emphasis throughout the book is on understanding the individual experience of suicidality. In this epilogue I feel obliged to consider and make some comment on how the stories in this book might help us find a way forward in our suicide prevention strategies and campaigns.

My experience, and my subsequent research and 'making sense' of it, has shown me that the greatest flaw in our current thinking about suicide is that we don't understand it at all well. In particular, current thinking about suicide prevention does not appreciate or give enough attention to what suicidal feelings mean to those who experience them. Enormous effort and expense are being expended on identifying risk and protective factors, medical explanations and treatments, and ways to encourage the suicidal to come forward and seek help. But remarkably little effort has been made to comprehend the actual lived experience of suicidality – the silent, invisible meaning of it to those who live it. On the contrary, there has been a distinct lack of attention to the subjective meaning of contemplating suicide, so much so that it seems like a determined effort to look the other way.

In the prologue of my PhD thesis I spoke to my suicidal soul-mates and urged them first and foremost to respect and honour their suicidal thoughts and feelings as real, legitimate and important. I now make the same call to the experts of suicidology, but also to all concerned about suicidality in our communities. Any attempt to reduce the incidence of suicide and other self-harming behaviour must include – and should be based on – an understanding of suicidal feelings and what they mean to those who live them. This cannot and does not happen while we continue to pathologise these feelings as symptoms of some (dubious) mental illness. It is these feelings that are central to understanding suicidality because it is our feelings, not some notional illness, that cause us to deliberately choose death. Current 'expert' thinking about suicide largely disregards subjective feelings as irrelevant to understanding suicidality. This arises partly from medical prejudices against subjective knowledge, but also from prejudices found in the wider community that see suicidal feelings as mad, bad or somehow 'broken' feelings for a person to have.

These prejudices tell us more about our fears around suicide than they do about the lived experience of feeling suicidal. Behind these prejudices we find two of our most potent fears, which come together in our fear of suicide – the fear of death and the fear of madness. As a society we still tend to have more fear of death than respect for it as a part of life. Our fear and denial of madness as also a part of life are perhaps even stronger. In some ways this is under-standable, for death and madness can be painful or ugly to experience or witness, so that we want to look away and not see them. But they also go to the very heart of the mystery of what it is to be human. To deny death, or madness, is to deny life. We can, and indeed must, acknow-ledge our fears as part of respecting and engaging fully with life. But not to allow these fears, which become prejudices when we deny them, to poison our efforts to understand suicidal feelings. If we hope to make progress in suicide prevention, we must all recognise these fears but not allow them to become prejudices that deny the real, legitimate and important feelings of those contemplating suicide for themselves.

The denial by suicidal people themselves of the legitimacy of suicidal feelings only complicates and undermines their struggle to stay alive. So I urge my suicidal soul-mates to respect and honour these sacred feelings. Equally, the denial of the legitimacy of suicidal feelings by those we seek help from, and by the general community, complicates and undermines our efforts at suicide prevention. So I call upon the experts of suicidology, and the wider commu-nity of everyone concerned about suicide, to also respect and honour suicidal feelings as part of the sacred mystery of life. Without this the toxic taboo that surrounds suicide, fed by ignorance and shame, fear and prejudice, will continue to dominate and thwart our efforts at suicide pre-vention. The first and most important message that I hope might be taken from my work is the need to change our thinking about suicide from one of fear and denial of suicidal feelings to one of respect and honour for them. This applies equally to the expert thinking about suicide prevention as it does to the personal thinking about suicide of my suicidal soul-mates.

In the Interlude section of my book that asked, 'Who Am I?', I argued for our thinking about suicide to shift from a medical, mental illness way of thinking to a more whole-of-person approach that sees it as a crisis of the self. I argued that reconceiving suicidality as a crisis of the self raises important and useful questions, in particular around the lived experience of suicidality and the personal, subjective meaning of suicidal feelings to those who live them. This would by itself go a long way towards promoting a healthier, more respectful attitude to suicidal feelings – and to those who have them. Thinking about suicidality as a crisis of the self also prompts useful questions about the *social* self, or the relationship between self and community. This important aspect of our sense of self for many people has not been emphasised in the stories in my book because my particular journey into and out of suicidality was very much a private, personal and spiritual journey. This is not the case for everyone though (another reason why I do not try to make generalisations from my own story). When we look at the current, expert collective thinking about suicide we find that the social aspects of our sense of self are almost as neglected as our personal, subjective feelings. Once again it can be seen that this exclusion of the social self is due to the excessive influence of medical ways of thinking.

Some experts in suicidology would argue that this is unfair of me. They would say that suicidology, reflecting its roots in sociology, is much more aware of the social dimension of sui-cide than is found in the broader mental health field. While I would agree with this, I would interpret this as a sad reflection on our approach to mental health rather than something for suicidology to be too boastful about. I have said throughout my book that suicidology, under the dominant influence of psychiatry and the medical 'treatment' of suicidality, still sees suicidality very much in terms of a medical pathology that is located within the individual. There is some competition between psychiatry and psychology whether this pathology is located in the mind or the brain, but little serious discussion about the possible social origins of suicidality. With these underlying medical assumptions, most of the social analysis that suicidology does pursue is primarily the ubiquitous epidemiological study that searches for risk and/or protective factors for preventing or alleviating this pathology. The sociology of suicidology is largely the demographic analysis of sub-populations. It gives almost as little attention to the social self and our sense of social wellbeing as it does to our individual sense of subjective wellbeing.

In the broader mental health field, there is also some competition between the medical model of mental illness and what is sometimes called a 'social model' of mental health. The *psychosocial* approach of this model gives more consideration to a person's social environment and emphasises recovery and rehabilitation rather than the 'diagnose and treat' approach of the medical model. Although there is quite a bit of talk of integrating these various models into a *biopsychosocial* approach, the reality is that the 'bio' of the medical model continues to dominate, consuming the vast bulk of limited resources available for mental health. I strongly support the move towards a genuine biopsychosocial approach, but even this does not really address the 'social self' that I am referring to.

The critical weakness of many of the more social approaches to suicidology (and mental health) is the same weakness that we find in the models that focus on the individual. As they strive for the same scientific credibility that psychiatry and psychology claim for themselves, they use essentially similar, and equally flawed, criteria for their notion of 'evidence based' practice and research, with similar consequences. The invisible, subjective, lived experience of the social self fails to register on their objective, scientific radars that see only visible, third-person 'data'. And just like the subjective, individual self that the medical model fails to see so that it ignores, dismisses or denies it, social models that work only with third-person perspectives will be similarly blind to the vital *intersubjective* lived experience of the self as a social being.

Suicidality as intersubjective experience

The term 'intersubjective' is not a familiar one for many people (it's only appeared for me as a result of my research), so it is worth being clear and careful with our language here. As with the excursion into postmodern thinking in the Interlude, I am particularly indebted to the American philosopher Ken Wilber (2000) for his clarity on this topic and, in general, follow his terminology. We are all familiar with the notion of the personal, subjective, invisible world of our own inner lived experience, which has been the emphasis in my research. Sometimes this is called the first-person perspective of *felt experience*, as opposed to the third-person perspective of *observable behaviour*. As social creatures, we also have *mutually shared* subjective – that is, intersubjective – experiences. Our intersubjective world is every bit as important as our subjective world, and is similarly neglected by objective science, including much of the social sciences.

Let's make this clear with an example or two. I used the example of love as a significant and meaningful subjective experience that a strictly third-person science simply fails to detect at all. Love is an equally good example of a mutually shared intersubjective experience. Along with the *individual* subjective feeling of love, which can occur with or without the loved one present, there are also those precious moments when we feel a sense of mutually shared union, or communion, with a loved one – the intersubjective experience of love. Anyone who has experienced this knows that love exists, is real and that it is often shared. And just like the individual, personal feeling of love, these shared moments are of enormous meaning and significance to those who experience them. And in exactly the same way that the subjective experience of love is invisible to medical science, so too is the intersubjective experience of it.

Love is perhaps a particularly powerful example, but there are many more everyday, intersubjective experiences. The individual, subjective experience is sometimes described as that 'Ah-hah' moment when we recognise something to be true – when we *live* the truth of that moment. Intersubjective experience is then sometimes called a collective 'Ah-hah' moment when we experience and live a mutually shared recognition of the truth of that moment. A common example of such collective 'Ah-hah' moments is humour or comedy when laughter spontaneously rises up within us as we collectively recognise and delight in the wit and humour of a good joke or a funny moment. There are also those times when we bear witness to someone's pain and suffering and recognise it as our own, whether through some similar experience we've had or because of a natural empathy for the other. This can occur between two people or in groups of thousands – indeed 'mob hysteria' is another example of shared, intersubjective experience, this time of fear.

Intersubjectivity refers to collective, first-person experiences, in the same way that subjectivity refers to individual, first-person ones. Ken Wilber (2000) highlights this by describing the language of subjectivity as 'I' language while the language of intersubjectivity is 'We' language, or the first-person plural – in contrast to the 'It' language of third-person, objective knowledge. The significance of the first-person domains of knowledge (both the singular 'I' and the plural 'We') is that they are the domains of *value* and *meaning*. Wilber calls the singular, subjective 'I' knowledge *aesthetic* knowledge, which is characterised by values of sincerity, integrity and truthfulness. Collective, intersubjective 'We' knowledge, is *cultural* knowledge characterised by a sense of morality based on shared values. Objective, third-person knowledge, on the other hand, is almost by definition value neutral. A clear example of this is that the science of the brain is totally value-neutral – knowledge about the brain's neurotransmitters, for instance, tells us nothing about the value and meaning of what we experience.

Yet what is most significant and important in any human experience is the value and meaning of that experience to those who live it *as it is lived*. And value and meaning can only ever be found in the first-person knowledge of subjective and intersubjective lived experience. Put another way, value and meaning can never be found in objective, third-person knowledge. Despite this, the traditional sciences of third-person, objective knowledge have become privileged above first-person, subjective and intersubjective knowledge. Moreover, the ideology of the traditional 'hard' sciences is *exclusively* third-person so that first-person knowledge is deliberately and systematically excluded by its criteria for what constitutes valid evidence that can only be met by third-person forms of knowledge. Nowhere is this more evident than in mental health where we see the medical colonisation of what it is to be human by the narrow and shallow evidence criteria of biological psychiatry.

Returning to suicide, suicidality and mental health in general, we can see that collective, intersubjective, first-person knowledge is every bit as neglected as individual, subjective, first-person knowledge. An immediate consequence of this is the widespread individual and collective failure to recognise and appreciate suicidal feelings as real, legitimate and important. But there are other, equally significant consequences. The first of these is that excluding vital first-person knowledge and expertise inevitably leads to an impoverished understanding of suicide and suicidality (and mental health in general). We see the most extreme expression of this in modern psychiatry with its almost total denial of first-person knowledge and experience in the pseudo-science of the DSM (American Psychiatric Association, 1994) and the meaningless, value-neutral science of biological psychiatry.

Despite frequent claims by all branches of mental health that 'consumer participation' is now a priority, the reality remains that the unique expertise of those who know about suicidality 'from the inside' is still largely excluded. Engaging meaningfully with the first-person expertise of mental health consumers is impossible under the constraints of exclusively third-person science. Even with the best of intentions, the current collective thinking about mental health is intellectually crippled by its ideological commitment to an obsolete notion of what is good science.

There are other reasons why the first-person data, knowledge and expertise, and in particular the collective, intersubjective kind, are necessary for suicide prevention (and mental health promotion). The stories of my book have focussed mainly on the individual, subjective experience of suicidality. I have only touched on some other stories where the collective meaning-making of shared, intersubjective experiences have been part of this larger story, such as family and friends, my time with Alcoholics Anonymous (AA) and Narcotics Anonymous (NA), and the spiritual community of the ashram. I could have acknowledged these more than I have, but my own sense remains that my own spiritual journey was very personal, very individual and also very lonely. This is not at all a complaint, and may be a reflection of my personality as perhaps a bit of a 'loner'. Besides, today I feel very fortunate and one of the lucky ones, not only because I have survived but also because I am very happy to be where (and who) I am today, which includes being grateful for all of my history, including my suicidality. Despite this, despite my own 'solo' journey of recovery, I am quite certain that the real hope for preventing suicide lies in a collective, intersubjective response to it.

When discussing suicide prevention it is necessary to distinguish between preventing suicidality and preventing 'completed' suicides. I repeat again that the emphasis of suicide prevention needs to shift to preventing suicidality, not just 'completed' suicides. But before looking at the importance of the collective, intersubjective response to preventing suicide, I want to return to another major theme of this book.

Making safe-spaces to share our stories

Story-telling is essentially an intersubjective experience where we tell our stories and hear the stories of others. We humans have been described as 'meaning-making' creatures and story-telling is such a central feature of this that we could call ourselves story-telling creatures. It is through our stories that we not only come to know others but also come to know ourselves. And the stories that contribute most to this meaning-making are those that resonate for us where something in someone else's story 'connects' with something in our own lives in a significant way. Sometimes this might be a private, personal 'Ah-hah' moment when we recognise a truth that we hadn't seen previously – and we learn and grow with this new, first-person knowledge. At other times, story-telling triggers a collective, shared 'Ah-hah' moment and we feel intimately connected with some others. Again, we learn and grow from this. We are all familiar with these occasions and we all recognise them as significant – *and they are all first-person, subjective or intersubjective, occasions*.

Story-telling is the primary means we humans use to find and create meaning in our lives and also to connect with others. Touch is also very important – both touching and being touched – as is doing things, the various tasks and activities where we learn through the doing, both by ourselves and with others. But it is mainly through story-telling that we make sense of our lives, of others, and of the world we live in. In this sense we might think of the theories of science as stories we humans tell ourselves to help make sense of our world. We also tell our stories through art, dance and theatre – there are many ways that we tell our stories. And always, what gives any story its significance is the *value* we find in it and the *meaning* we are able to create from it. This is equally true for the theories or stories of science as it is for the stories of Shakespeare. And *always*, these significant, value-laden, meaning-making occasions are subjective or intersubjective experiences, sometimes both. First-person knowledge is the knowledge of lived experience and the source of all our meaning-making and all that we value.

We need to resurrect story-telling as vital for both suicidality prevention and suicide prevention. We need to do this to restore subjective and intersubjective values to our suicide prevention efforts. First of all we need to hear the stories of those who know suicidality from the inside in order to understand it much better than we currently do. This individual, subjective knowledge is vital but will only become available if we are able to enter into meaningful, intersubjective engagement with those who have the first-person expertise. We need to create spaces where, first of all, these stories can be told, but then we also need to be able to be in these spaces so that they can be heard.

This is perhaps the most critical and urgent need in mental health today. For people struggling with mental health difficulties, whether suicidality or any other expression of mental, emotional, social or spiritual distress, what we most need is *a safe space to tell our stories*. Telling your story is the beginning of any healing or therapeutic encounter. Indeed, by itself, or perhaps together with hearing the stories of others, the telling of your story may be all the healing or 'therapy' that you need. But this can only occur if we feel safe. The calamity of mental health today is that in our current mental health system we have the exact opposite of a safe space where we can tell our stories.

Returning to suicide prevention, a safe space to tell your story is necessary if we are to overcome the biggest obstacle to helping the suicidal. How often do we hear that the first and most urgent task of suicide prevention is to encourage people to seek help – to come forward and tell their story? But psychiatric wards and the psychiatrist's office are not safe spaces to tell stories of suicidal feelings. Nor, in many cases, is your doctor's office. It is also probably difficult, if not impossible, to share your story with family or friends. For a whole host of reasons, not the least of which is the fear and taboo that surrounds suicide making almost anywhere in the community difficult, often impossible, and sometimes dangerous to tell your story. Once upon a time we might have 'confessed' our story to the priest, but this is also out of bounds for many people today. No, there are very few safe spaces to tell a story about feeling suicidal. This reflects very poorly on the so-called experts in mental health, but it also reflects poorly on all of us. As a society, we have lost the capacity to create spaces – intersubjective spaces – where these distressing stories can safely be told.

But these safe, intersubjective spaces are needed for more than just helping us to first come forward with our stories. The opportunity to tell your story, and to have it heard respectfully, can by itself be very healing. The intersubjective experience of sharing stories – telling yours and hearing those of others – can make a vital, life-saving, contribution to your own making sense of your struggles, which in turn can lead to a pathway out of and beyond them. By sharing our stories, we learn that we are not quite as alone and unique in our despair as we usually feel when we are suicidal. We also learn from those who have been there before us and can find comfort and solidarity among those who, like us, might still be struggling. We might also learn to our surprise that our story becomes part of the precious gift of healing to others who struggle alongside us. Sharing your story, in a safe space, alongside your peers, can at least make a vital contribution to your recovery, and may even be all that you need to move beyond your current story of pain.

In my story, the outstanding example of just such a safe space for story-telling is Alcoholics Anonymous (and related 'fellowships' like Narcotics Anonymous). However, the foundation of AA is not the 12-Step program that many people first think of when AA is mentioned. The foundation of AA is the regular meetings where you are invited to 'share' your story among a group of your peers, fellow alcoholics, and to hear their stories. And what makes AA a safe space for this sharing is first that you are among your peers so that your own struggles will be respected as real, legitimate and important, without negative judgement. And second, there is the cardinal rule of AA that enshrines anonymity as both permitted and protected, one of the key ingredients of the safe space created by AA for sharing what are often shameful and difficult stories.

In mental health and other health and disability fields, groups similar to AA are typically called 'peer support' groups. They are greatly valued by participants or 'consumers' and some groups do it very well. But they all have a lot to learn, I believe, from the 'experts' in peer support, the drunks of AA. And as a society we also have a lot to learn from these drunks about how to support each other when we experience times of difficulty in our lives. And governments and health departments have a great deal to learn about the healing power of such communities that are so much more effective, and also cost-effective, than the current expensive medicalising of human difficulties and distress.

This brings us to how these safe, intersubjective, story-telling spaces are vital for the even bigger task of preventing suicidality – that is, of preventing suicidality from arising in the first place. I am sceptical whether we can achieve significant reductions in the suicide toll if we just focus on trying to prevent the already suicidal from killing themselves. It seems to me that surviving suicidality is often a matter of grim determination by the individual, combined with a fair bit of pot luck, as in my own story. First there is the problem already mentioned that we tend to go underground and can be very hard to reach. Then there is the luck or otherwise, it seems, of whether you survive your initial attempts to kill yourself. Next is how problematic it can be, should you reach out for help, to find someone who you can safely talk to and who can maybe help. Although we still need to do all we can to help the actively suicidal, it all seems a very perilous journey. The real hope for suicide prevention is preventing suicidality.

Who are we?

For me, the key to preventing suicidality is to promote and create healthy communities. This is a slow process and a long-term goal but one that will be more effective (including cost-effective) in the long run. Suicidality is just one of many symptoms in our society of not only high levels of distress in the community but of our collective failure as a society to prevent and respond to this distress. We need to include with suicidality things like our widespread drug abuse and drug addiction (especially with alcohol and prescribed drugs), the high levels of crime and homelessness, and I would include other public health issues such as obesity, asthma and diabetes. And most of all, and often not unrelated to these other issues, we need to re-think what we mean by mental health. We need to ask what would a mentally healthy *community* look like and how might we proceed towards creating that?

I think a few critical issues leap to our attention when we ask these questions. First, despite our material abundance, we are not a particularly healthy society. We are overweight, the incidence of asthma and diabetes seem to be rising, and we are seriously drug-addicted (of all kinds – alcohol, coffee and especially prescription drugs). We are also not a very happy or contented society with widespread anger, sadness, social stress and emotional distress, and massive consumption of anti-depressant medications. Despite these widespread difficult personal and social issues, and despite our material abundance, economic and material values still dominate our thinking and the political agenda. We are not very generous or compassionate to our neighbours, whether they are within or outside our national borders. We are in fact not very compassionate to ourselves. Everyone seems to be working harder just to stay where they are, with stress and distress a constant feature of most people's lives. Many people are dropping out of the rat-race, either by deliberately choosing less affluent but more peaceful lifestyles, or by escaping into drugs, madness and suicide. As one wit observed, the real problem with the rat-race is that even when you win you're still a rat.

Instead of responding to this as a medical epidemic of 'depression' and getting people back to work with the help of their 'happy pills', we need to re-focus on creating and promoting wellbeing. We have the material wealth these days to make wellbeing and *quality* of life a national priority, if we choose. If we choose this rather than the current self-destructive madness, then we would find that what we need is not that dissimilar to what the suicidal, the mad, the addicted, and other 'drop-outs' so desperately need. We need to connect or re-connect with what is most important to us. We need to discover or rediscover what really gives life value and meaning. We need to listen to our pain and suffering, and to the pain and suffering of others. We need to care – truly and deeply care – for ourselves and for each other. For this we need to tell our stories, and to hear the stories of others.

We need safe spaces where we can tell our stories. In families, in the schools, in local neighbourhood community centres, in the workplace, in sporting clubs, in churches, mosques and temples. We need to discover how to trust each other again. We need to create time simply to be with each other, as well as time for quiet, private solitude where we can reflect on and tell ourselves our own most intimate stories. We need to ask the same question that I discovered was behind my suicidality: 'What does it mean to me that I exist?'.

You might find it odd that I've not mentioned spirituality in this epilogue, given that it is so central to the story of my book. But I believe that the challenge we face as a society that wishes to reduce the suicide toll is exactly the same challenge I faced when I was struggling with my suicidal feelings. At the core of suicidality is a crisis of the self and the key to my recovery was a deep, personal enquiry into who or what I was and am. For me, this led me into spiritual territory and, frankly, I don't see how it could ever be otherwise. But I might be wrong. For others, self-enquiry might take them into reconnecting with family and community, or to a new relationship with their working life. Others might turn to the creative arts to give expression to a renewed, reinvigorated and re-enchanted sense of self. All of these possibilities, and others such as joining a church, are for me full of spiritual value and spiritual wisdom. If we attend to what is *really* most important and re-connect with what our souls are really crying out for, then it seems to me that suicidal feelings and many other forms of madness are much less likely to arise. And as social creatures, to do this we need to touch and feel and hear each other. We need to share and communicate who we are and what we need to live life fully. And to do this … we need safe spaces where we can tell our stories.

Having painted this somewhat optimistic and thoroughly idyllic dream of the future, it is necessary to remind ourselves that suffering and madness are probably always going to be part of our lives and our communities. The challenge then is still much the same. We need to respect and honour suffering and madness as a rich and vital, if difficult, part of life's mystery. Suffering and madness have so much to teach us about what it is to be human. We need to hear these stories so that we can learn from them. Again, to do this … we need safe spaces where we can tell our stories.

The final, perhaps obvious, observation that needs to be made as we look at the broader issues around suicide prevention is that societies and communities can also be suicidal. Once more we find that the emphasis on suicide as a pathology of the individual distracts us from our collective suicidality, which may indeed be a major contributing factor in individual suicidality. Even if we take a simplistic symptomatic approach to suicidality, as psychiatry does, then we can see many symptoms in our societies that could be called suicidal symptoms. Some have been mentioned above – crime, drugs, the madness 'epidemic'. We can add to these the environmental crisis where we are destroying the biosphere on which we depend. This is surely collective suicidality. We demonise and lash out against the 'other', failing to recognise that in doing so we are harming ourselves, and the current globalisation of economics as almost the sole measure of our wellbeing diminishes us and will perhaps destroy us. And spirituality, which lies at the heart of the mystery of our being, has been reduced to a fashion statement as another optional lifestyle choice.

If we are serious about reducing the suicide toll then we must also get serious about our collective sense of self. In the same way that my personal suicidality forced me to confront the fundamental spiritual question of 'Who am I?', our collective suicidality obliges us to ask an equally spiritual question – 'Who are we?'.

Note

1 All mentioning of 'book' throughout this chapter relates to Webb, D. (2010) *Thinking about Suicide: Contemplating and Comprehending the Urge to Die*. Ross-on-Wye: PCCS Books.

References

American Psychiatric Association (1994) *Diagnostic and Statistical Manual of Mental Disorders: DSM-IV*. Washington: American Psychiatric Association.

Wilber, K (2000) *Integral Psychology: Consciousness, Spirit, Psychology, Therapy*. Boston: Shambhala.

Webb, D (2010) *Thinking about Suicide: Contemplating and Comprehending the Urge to Die*. Ross-on-Wye: PCCS Books.

26

DE-COUPLING AND RE-COUPLING VIOLENCE AND MADNESS

Andrea Daley and Trish Van Katwyk

Introduction

In this chapter, we critically engage with the problematic coupling of violence with madness. We begin by first exploring what is meant by, "the coupling of violence with madness", underscoring the perpetrator–victim binary that characterizes the research literature and media representations of violence and madness. We argue that while an ideal liberatory goal might be the de-coupling of violence from madness, we also raise concern that existing attempts to de-couple violence from madness further entrench the perpetrator–victim binary, along with individualized and medicalized accounts of violence. In response to this concern, we explore the re-coupling of violence and madness as an intervention, of a sort, which serves to relocate violence away from Mad people and to political and social structures and processes that govern social institutions, including those that are charged with managing madness. We suspend the dichotomy by using Judith Butler's (2016) conceptualizations about vulnerability and resistance. In doing so, we centre Mad Studies as a necessary intervention, yet recognize critiques and concerns related to its presence in academe. We conclude by considering the ways in which Mad Studies has always/already lived in community, and how its birth as an academic field of study/discipline might continue to be informed by grassroots organizing, community dialogue, mad narratives and critically reflexive actions.

Responsibility and accountability

Before moving forward, however, it is first necessary to engage with the important issues of responsibility and accountability from our respective locations as academic researchers, educators, and practitioners in social work, community members, and activists.

Andrea: My thinking about violence and madness is most immediately informed by recent collaborative work with Lucy Costa and Peter Beresford on the edited book titled, *Madness, Violence, and Power: A Critical Collection* (Daley et al., 2019). The collection of interdisciplinary writings that form the book constitutes critical scholarship that makes visible and addresses violence and madness by broadening the violence lens and offering new perspectives, evidence, and calls for action to address violence as manifest in the lives of mental health service users. I was drawn to the questions of which the book engages because of my understanding of the

DOI: 10.4324/9780429465444-31

ways in which I have participated in the operation of power and violence as a social worker with a community assertive treatment (ACT) team in Toronto, Canada. Most notably, in this role I participated in practices that promoted epistemic violence (Spivak, 1994) through the psychocentric authoring of people's experiences of distress and the surveillance of behaviours to determine or establish "abnormality" and "normality"; the former often established by assessing the potential for violence (to self and others) and the latter often established by enacting processes of forced/coerced hospitalizations and treatments (including community treatment orders). I was also drawn to the questions of which the book engages because of the ways in which, as a social work practitioner, I understood and witnessed gross acts of oppression and injustice, recognizing that while my work was guided by critical feminist, queer, anti-racist, anti-oppressive and social justice principles and practices that my participation in institutionalized violence compromised my adherence to these principles and practices. In both these ways, I acknowledge that I have participated in the harm and suffering of others. This critical engagement with violence, madness, and power, and related academic work (eg. Daley et al., 2012; Daley and Ross, 2018; Pilling et al., 2018), offers one way for me to take responsibility for my involvement in violence and to be accountable to those who I have harmed.

Trish: While my practice, research and teaching have been shaped both by critical perspectives about madness and by academic and clinical contexts within which I all too easily reproduce oppression and inequity, I find myself considering my family. My younger brother, who is black, used mental health services from an early age. Race significantly influenced the care he received. Over time, I witnessed the deepening furrow of the child welfare, psychiatric and prison systems' trajectory of his life that extends to the current day. A cross-generational history of suicide and institutionalization significantly shape the contours of our family's constellation, impacting how we celebrate new life and grieve lost lives.

When I became a social worker, I began in the women's and family shelter system of Toronto, and then moved into a psychiatric crisis response team guided by the principles of the consumer-survivor movement. Half of my co-workers as well as the board of directors identified as psychiatric service users. One of my mentors was Pat Capponi, a leading activist for the consumer-survivor movement in Toronto, who taught me how psychiatric responses that disregard the human rights of people reveal how many services and policies carry an underlying assumption about the incomplete humanity of Mad people. I began to reconsider my brother's experience, as well as those of the women I had encountered in the shelters and those of the people I worked with at the crisis centre. I became keenly aware of the ways gender, class, sexual orientation, and race intersect with the experience of madness.

I have gone on to become a professor of social work. Time and again, I see evidence in this discipline of a propensity to disempower and dehumanize. My own privileges are bolstered by an inadequate comprehension of the ways I disempower in my teaching, my research, my writing, and my practice. My privileges across the matrix of domination that Collins (1990) described obscure my view, so that I can become entitled about a sense of ubiquitous belonging.

Not long ago, I sought support for my son when he became afraid of harming himself. We saw doctors, nurses and social workers who treated him as dangerous to others. I, as a woman and mother, was treated as complicit to and even blameworthy of his dangerousness. Eventually, we changed tactics, and now I work closely with my son and our trusted community, alongside friends, family, and colleagues who are committed to conducting themselves in liberatory ways. I see the impact that critical reflexivity can have in revealing insidious debilitating constructions about madness. I see the significance of centring voices that are not professionalized, that do not serve a neoliberal agenda of conformity and effective citizenship, in order to begin to imagine a larger and more human truth.

Our intention

In approaching the important topic of violence and madness we emphasize that our intention is not to engage debate that exists in the literature and public sphere about whether or not people with "mental illness" are more likely to be violent or experience violence when compared to the general population. We also acknowledge that there is violence in all communities that is the outcome of complex intersecting factors, and that for some communities talking about this violence is (more) risky given already existing myths, stereotypes, and stigma, along with sensationalized media accounts of community violence. This may be the case for Mad communities. In response, we note that given our respective positionalities it would be irresponsible to focus our discussion on community violence in relation to madness. Rather, our responsibility is to contest and challenge individualizing and medicalizing discourses, shifting the focus on violence and madness to violent social institutions.

Madness and violence coupled

We start this chapter by asking, if we are exploring the de-coupling of violence and madness, then what exactly do we understand as constituting the coupling of violence and madness? To this end, we identify dominant discourses on violence and madness that either construct Mad people as inherently unpredictable and dangerous or alternatively, as especially vulnerable to danger (LeFrançois et al., 2016; Shimrat, 2013). We note that it is not our intent to argue the validity or truth-value of either discourse, but rather to establish the perpetrator-victim binary as an outcome of dominant discourses on the association between violence and madness. In terms of the former, the Mad perpetrator of violence – or the 'madman' – is firmly embedded in the public imaginary (Metzl and MacLeish, 2015); as such, the association between violence and 'mental illness' continues to be a point of perverted or dangerously misguided curiosity and interrogation in both research and the media. Research has explored, and continues to explore, associations between madness and violence, attempting to identify clinical characteristics (e.g., 'paranoia') associated with violent behaviours, and relatedly, how to 'treat' these characteristics in an attempt to prevent violent behaviours (Van Dorn et al., 2017; Link et al., 2016; Varshney et al., 2016; Coverdale et al., 2013; Maniglio, 2009; Choe et al., 2008). More recently, and more prominently in the U.S. context, research has focused on the relationship between madness and gun violence and mass shootings, including the media's role in perpetuating myths and stereotypes related to the dangerousness of mental health service users (Metzl and MacLeish, 2015; Coverdale et al., 2013). In this regard, Coverdale et al. implicate the media in circular reasoning that couples violence with madness,

> … if a person is identified as belonging to the category "mad" or "mentally ill" (Nairn, 2007) it is anticipated that they will act in violent, criminal, and unpredictable ways and, as a corollary of that categorization, a person who acts in violent, criminal, and unpredict-able ways is readily seen as mad (Eglin and Hester, 1999b; Rapley et al., 2003) (2013:202)

Some of the existing research serves to challenge this troubling association between violence and madness, citing statistics that challenge the overrepresentation of Mad people as violent (Metzl and MacLeish, 2015) and exploring alternative explanations for violence beyond 'mental illness', such as general stress strain (Link et al., 2016). Other scholarship examines the coupling of violence and madness through an intersectional lens by interrogating, for example, how particular diagnoses and Mad people are more likely to be implicated in mad violence. For example, Keating (2016), citing Marie and Miles (2008) states that "[D]angerousness is [also] more likely to be associated with men and a diagnosis of schizophrenia", (2016:177) while underscoring the ways in which the constructs of "black, dangerous, and mad" (2016:179) operate together to position racialized men as particularly prone to enacting violence against others. In fact, citing Jackson, Kanini remarks that "violence was listed as a form of mental illness for many African Americans who were incarcerated in the late 19th and early 20th centuries" (2011:9). In addition, Metzl and MacLeish note that "[A]nxieties about insanity and gun violence are [also] imbued with oft-unspoken anxieties about race, politics, and the unequal distribution of violence in US society" (2015:241).

In terms of the latter, violence and madness has been coupled in research literature that explores the ways in which mental health service users may be more likely to experience violence. The association of violence and madness in this way includes both the querying of violence, such as childhood physical and sexual abuse as a cause of madness (Link et al., 2016; de Mooij et al., 2015) and the role of madness in creating "vulnerability" to violence including intimate partner violence, property crimes, and vandalism (Khalifeh et al., 2015).

Undoubtedly, these discourses couple violence and madness in a simplistic non-critical perpetrator–victim binary that relies on individualized and medicalized accounts of interpersonal violence. These accounts of violence position both the perpetration of violence and victimization as the result of irrationality, lack of capacity, and lack of agency. Park, for example, notes that individualized and medicalized accounts of violence – either in relation to perpetrators or victims – assign violence to "the choices of delinquent and disordered people" (2017:268). To this point, understandings of, or explanations for, violence in the context of madness often attribute violence to clinical characteristics, or rather promote psychocentric (Rimke and Brock, 2012) configurations of violence. For example, Khalifeh et al. state, "[V]iolence experienced by people with severe mental illness (SMI) is associated with poor symptomatic and functional recovery, high rates of comorbid post-traumatic stress disorder and poor treatment adherence" (2015:275). These individualizing and medicalizing accounts of violence serve to further pathologize mental health service users.

It is important to note that the perpetrator–victim binary is influenced by intersections between madness and gender, race, class, and sexuality, among other social identities and locations. That is, intersections between madness and social identities often determine which side of the binary Mad people are located – whether Mad people are more likely to be seen as perpetrators of violence or victims of violence. Relatedly, sometimes for some people intersecting identities complexify assessments of rationality, capacity, and agency, and thus, clinical assessments of responsibility and deviance. For example, Pilling et al. interrogate the role of gender, sexuality, race, and class in psychiatric assessments of insight, and relatedly, rationality, capacity and agency stating that,

> [F]eminist and anti-racist scholarship, [which] has shown how knowledge production about madness and mental illness have long been gendered and racialized. Psychiatry has positioned women as less rational than men, people of colour as less 'civilized' and 'evolved' than white people, and gender and sexual dissidence as pathological.
>
> *(2018:200)*

If we accept as a conceptualization of the coupling of violence and madness a perpetrator–victim binary that relies on individualized and medicalized accounts of interpersonal violence that are firmly embedded in gendered, racialized, and classed assumptions underlying notions of irrationality, capacity, and agency, then how do we begin to resist the coupling of violence and madness? In other words, are there effective strategies for de-coupling or un-yoking violence from madness? One might argue that statistical analyses in research are used to challenge per-petrator of violence associations with madness; however, this seems an impotent stigma-busting strategy given the remoteness of academic and scientific research from the "every day" and as muted by the potency of sensationalized media stories about the 'madman'. Similarly, stat-istical analyses of the association between childhood physical and sexual abuse and madness and the likelihood of adult victimization that are often used to inform calls for individualized trauma-informed services seem limited in their ability to de-couple violence and madness by undoing complex operations of power that produce interpersonal violence. As an approach to de-coupling violence from madness it constitutes a reactive strategy rather than preventa-tive strategy. After all, it constitutes a response to the coupling of violence and madness rather than a destabilization of this coupling. Quite the opposite, we argue that the approaches briefly described above are, indeed, informed by the perpetrator–victim binary; that is, the research literature largely represents siloed accounts of and responses to the likelihood of Mad people being either a perpetrator *or* victim of violence. In this way, the research reflects and reproduces the perpetrator-victim binary. We suggest, then, that an effective strategy to de-coupling vio-lence from madness is to challenge the perpetrator–victim binary itself; a strategy that is well-aligned with Mad Studies' critiques of binaries (Spandler and Barker, 2016).

Challenging the perpetrator–victim binary requires that narratives of violence and madness move beyond individualized and medicalized accounts of interpersonal violence and the notion that violence in the lives of Mad people is nothing more than "the choices of delinquent and disordered people" (Park, 2017:268). We conceptualize this strategy as a *re-coupling* of violence and madness, which serves to relocate violence away from Mad people and over to political and social structures and processes. In making this assertion, we suggest that the re-coupling of violence and madness is a necessary intervention to destabilize the perpetrator–victim binary, and that central to this intervention is Mad Studies. It is our intention that re-coupling violence and madness in this way widens its analytical framing so that violence is understood within the broader context in which it is produced.

Challenging the perpetrator-victim binary

We have seen that a perpetrator–victim binary emerges out of individualized accounts of madness that serve to limit agency for those bound to a discourse that in the end pronounces the worth of one's experience and narrative according to which side of the binary they find themselves on. Butler (2004) describes the effect of the perpetrator–victim binary as a failure of recognition of the humanness of the individual. Brenner (2013) considers the legal ramifications of conferring full humanity on one person and depriving another person of theirs, which, she asserts, is the effect of the perpetrator–victim binary.

The denial of full humanity is social injustice. Social justice is concerned with equal access and opportunity for all human beings, so that unequal access and oppression constitutes dehumaniza-tion. The biomedical model depoliticizes health and madness, holding the individual accountable for their wellbeing, without meaningful consideration of social, political and economic factors, so that the individual becomes disconnected from the society and its institutions (Ashcroft and Van Katwyk, 2016). Neoliberal ideologies support such individualized/individualizing accounts in order to sustain a series of reproducing practices that differentiate human beings from one another to such an extent as to sap humanity out of one and attribute extreme humanity to the other. It is in the capacity to deprive a human being of their humanity that social injustice, the viola-tion of human rights, becomes possible. In fact, it is with diminished humanity that the inequity necessary for a thriving capitalist psychiatric industry can occur (LeFrançois et al., 2013). The perpetrator–victim binary necessitates a psychiatric response that serves to control and protect, as is asserted by Foucault (2003) when he suggested that psychiatry is premised upon a "pathologization of crime and a criminalization of the pathological" (Koivisto, 2018), where it becomes difficult to differentiate between treatment and punishment (Foucault, 2003).

In our critique of the violence/madness bind, we have seen how the structures of a neoliberal system lose their opacity in our questions about the intersections of oppression that get lost in this binded narrative. What begins to come into clear view is how gender, race, class, sexuality, religion, and even first language are relevant, emerging out of the fog that the violence/madness bind has placed upon them. In our deconstruction of the violence/madness association, we see the multiple impacts that diverse identities, knowledges, and social experiences can have on the experience of madness, and we are able to consider a carefully constructed, socially and politically immersed account that relinquishes the individual from blame, shame, and failure (Brenner, 2013; Butler, 2004; McCarthy, 1993).

A critical examination of the impact of a dominant biomedical model that depoliticizes madness and creates self-serving binaries such as perpetrator–victim constitutes a deconstruction that is necessary in order to contemplate reconstructing creative alternatives. We disassociate violence from madness with a clear intention of re-associating in order to create possibilities for change. But first, in accordance with Fook (2015) and McCarthy (1993) who describe the social justice work of deconstructing in order to reconstruct, we must suspend the perpetrator-victim dichotomy in order to return to a more just position.

Butler (2016) offers a means of suspending the dichotomy in her considerations of vulnerability and resistance. Butler describes the ways in which one is acted upon, named and defined by the discourse of the social and political environment. We are named, and we name ourselves, in accordance with this discourse. When we explore the ways in which Mad people are named (Ingram, 2016; Koivisto, 2018), how the knowledge and experience of Mad people is treated as invalid (LeBlanc and Kinsella, 2016; LeFrançois et al. 2013; Liegghio, 2013; Russo and Beresford, 2015), when the perpetrator–victim binary is imposed upon Mad people, we are encountering the ways in which Mad people are named within and outside of the psychiatric system. The naming is stigmatizing, and when that stigma is internalized, it is a way in which Mad people name themselves in accordance with an oppressive discourse. Koivisto (2018) offers a compelling metaphor for the self-naming process:

> Obviously, the mechanics of objectification carried out by means of cultural representations is too multifaceted and nuanced to be reduced to an encounter between a lobster and a lobster trap. However, we can try another metaphor that might reflect more poignantly the nature of this intertwinement. We can keep the lobster if we want (and I do want, because I happen to like lobsters), but substitute the trap for something else: plastic microfiber. Like many other marine animals, lobsters ingest microplastic, which accumulates in their bodies … The microplastic dwelling in the oceans are components of an infrastructure; an artificial construction. In addition to the infrastructures that surround us, there are infrastructures that can enter us, permeate us, access us. And remain in us.

The process is one of performativity, whereby we are told who we can be, how to think, how to behave, and in this way, we act and we are acted upon (Butler, 2004). However, it is not inevitable. We can choose not to perform according to how we are being called upon to perform. Butler considers the agency that is a refusal to perform according to the norms being imposed upon a person. To not act in accordance with that which is imposed upon us requires a vulnerability to the pressures of those norms and a vulnerability that comes with performing in a way that is not in accordance with those norms.

While Arendt (1958) also describes the ways in which vulnerability as exposure becomes a political agency, Butler suggests that Arendt, by presuming a fixed infrastructure for that exposure to occur in, delimits the interactive, fluid and relational field that is the site of agentic vulnerability. There is no need for a preordained infrastructure, rather, the resistance that is a part of the vulnerability creates an infrastructure by claiming a space in which the vulnerability can occur. In so doing, the resistance is the complex accomplishment of telling your story even as there exists no infrastructure where such a story can be platformed. The fact that there is no infrastructure indicates that the norms of the structures that have neglected to create the necessary infrastructure are also being resisted; by creating a site of vulnerability, a claim to vulnerability, exposure, agency, and identity has been made.

LeBlanc and Kinsella (2016) consider the power of vulnerability in their discussion about epistemic injustices that are leveled against Mad people. They describe the testimonial injustice that occurs when powerful knowledge sharing by Mad people is responded to with invalidating, erasing, and objectifying gestures. While the responses are dehumanizing, this is no reflection upon the validity of the knowledge and the strength of the vulnerability that is being demonstrated (Butler, 2016).

This is where the relationship to infrastructure becomes very important, and is found in other madness discussions as well. Butler writes:

> [W]hat I am suggesting is that it is not just that this or that body is bound up in a network of relations, but that the body, despite its clear boundaries, or perhaps precisely by virtue of those very boundaries, is defined by the relations that makes its own life and action possible … . we cannot understand bodily vulnerability outside of this conception of relations.
>
> *(2016:5)*

Relations feature in LeBlanc and Kinsella's (2016) description of the role of the hearer. In discussing epistemic injustices against Mad people, they identify two reciprocal processes: testimonial injustice and hermeneutic injustice; how testimonies are responded to in ways that invalidate and dehumanize, and how hearing is contaminated by presumptions about the capacities to understand and interpret the speaker. Likewise, LeFrançois et al. (2013) describe relationships to the infrastructure when they define Mad Studies' focus on the dialectic relations between "self and society, between private and public, between subjectivities and social relations, between human agency and social structure, and … between the politics of Mad identity and the imperatives of collective struggle against sanism in all its forms" (p. 16). We suggest that it is through vulnerability as resistance that we are able to transcend the perpetrator–victim binary through a deep acknowledgement of the multiple, complex, and immersed ways in which we are situated interactively within a larger infrastructure, and that vulnerability is both agency and resistance. We also suggest that Mad Studies' focus on the relationship between Mad people and their infrastructures is most impactful in its goal of social justice when Mad people remain at the centre of this focus, located within their communities.

Re-coupling violence and madness

The re-coupling of violence and madness in ways that destabilize the perpetrator–victim binary includes two considerations; each characterizes Mad Studies. First is a consideration of how violence is conceptualized to refuse the notion of interpersonal violence and structural vio-lence as discrete categories. Drawing from Park (2017), we underscore the capacity of Mad Studies to provide an analytical framework that promotes an understanding of a "violence con-tinuum" (Scheper-Hughes and Bourgois, 2004:1) whereby forms of violence are recognized as "overlapping and simultaneously occurring", that is, as necessarily interconnected (Park, 2017:271). Following this is a consideration of the ways in which the recognition of over-lapping and simultaneously occurring forms of violence can serve to contest and re-author psychocentric (individualized and medicalized) understandings of violence as "social and psy-chological deviance" (Park, 2017:270) that undergird the perpetrator–victim binary. These interrelated considerations may serve to relocate violence away from Mad people, as either perpetrators or victims, to reveal the violence of the infrastructure, those political and social structures and processes that govern social institutions, including those charged with managing madness. This counter discourse to the perverted curiosity and interrogation of Mad people as either perpetrators or victims of violence, vis-à-vis Mad Studies, unequivocally implicates violent social institutions in both.

Indeed, critical interrogations of madness by Mad scholars and allies working in parallel critical spaces in social sciences, humanities and cultural studies (including disability studies, equity studies, gender studies, law, public policy, medicine, and social work) are doing just this – revealing the blurring of interpersonal and structural violence, while challenging long held beliefs that violence is a consequence of "the choices of delinquent and disordered" (ibid, 2017:268) individuals and making visible the violence of system and sector legislation, policy, and practices. In these ways, Mad Studies scholarship challenges the normative ways in which colonial violence, racial violence, gender violence, the violence of heteronormativity – the list goes on – is foundational to and reproduced in social institutions through the dominance of psy discourses and related practices (Spandler and Barker, 2016). Similarly, community-based interrogations offer socially and politically immersed accounts of violence in the lives of Mad people and communities (Psychiatric Disabilities Anti-violence Coalition, 2015).

The challenge that Mad Studies is up against is the fact that Mad Studies, as an aca-demic entity, is located in an institution that is being increasingly critiqued as a corporatized neoliberal entity (Bhattacharyya, 2013; Chomsky, 2015; Paleariet al., 2015). By asserting a monopoly on knowledge and truth (Van Katwyk and Case, 2016), the academy erases the cap-acities, knowledges, and lived experiences of diverse communities that constitute the centre of community-engaged and democratic knowledge production and mobilization (Kelley, 2016). For Mad Studies to attend to the challenge of their position and the potential of a justice-oriented relationship with the Mad community, Mad Studies as an academic entity must strive for mutuality rather than elitism, as well as sharing equitably its expertise in an authentic acknowledgement of the equal value of the knowledge and experience that is held in the com-munity (Kecskes and Foster, 2013) by Mad people. Mad Studies can heed the call of academic and activist Robin Kelley, who admires those who are able to "be *in* the university, but not *of* the university" (2016).

Centring Mad Studies in the re-coupling of violence and madness as a necessary interven-tion to destabilize the perpetrator–victim binary requires that we attend to its critiques and concerns. On one hand, Mad Studies is critiqued as elitist and inaccessible, given its status as an emerging discipline "pioneered by Mad people *within* academia" (as supported by "the user/survivor/mad movements, which has encouraged people to be 'out' about their madness") and as being overly reliant and/or committed to the academy (Spandler and Barker, 2016). On the other hand, concern has been raised about whether or not Mad Studies will survive the academy. In this regard, Ingram, referencing Mills (2013, 2014) states that, "[I]n order to enter the university, Mad Studies would have to practise 'sly normality,' and the people comprising Mad Studies would have to take this approach" (Ingram, 2016, p.13).

In order to survive the academy, the important work of Mad Studies cannot lose its place in the community and in the hands of service users. Spandler and Barker (2016) describes Mad scholarship as "going back at least to the early 1970s with the birth of the Mad movement and Mad liberation, and then in the 2000s with the development of Mad Pride". Miller (2018) points to other important connections between the Mad Studies and grassroots social movements,

> The theory and practice of madness may involve such diverse perspectives as: civil rights (e.g. Minkowitz, 2014); anti-psychiatric abolitionism (e.g. Burstow, 2014); feminism (e.g. Diamond, 2014); trades unionism (e.g. McKeown et al., 2014); revolutionary politics (e.g. Burstow and LeFrançois, 2014); post-colonial indigenism (e.g. Tam, 2013); disability rights (e.g. Beresford and Menzies, 2014); neurodiversity (e.g. McWade et al., 2015); and contemporary spirituality (e.g. Farber, 2012) – and no doubt others as well.
>
> *(Miller, 2018:305–306)*

Remaining embedded in grassroots social movements is a necessary response to critiques of and concerns for Mad Studies as they have been, and continue to be, the places and spaces in which agentic vulnerability and political agency can be/is enacted and validated – where choice to not perform according to how Mad people are called upon to perform can be realized; where challenges to being told who to be, how to think, and how to behave are imagined; and, where humanity is restored. One might argue that it is, indeed, *collective* resistance that is part of a *collective* vulnerability that constitutes the space of a social movement. In this regard, the collective vulnerability that constitutes the Mad movement and intersecting social movements are critically necessary spaces to perform agentic vulnerability given the risks inherent to declaring vulnerability for people who have always/already been named as 'vulnerable' by psychiatry and associated disciplines.

In this regard, Beresford writes, "the most influential and radical analyses of mental health … have come not from professional commentators and radicals, but from service users themselves" (2016:6). The centre position of service users in the Mad movement is a defining feature, a feature that cannot be lost to the academy. Costa (2014) reiterates that while Mad Studies bring together scholars, community members, and service users, it is the service users who must remain leaders so that their experience, knowledges, and ideas continue to impact the direction of this field of study. Beresford (2016) conjures Freire and the concepts of 'praxis' and 'conscientization' where theory, practice, and dialogue come together to become a site for change, a site that is ideologically aligned with the people and not the institutions that construct practices and truths that primarily accommodate the most privileged. LeFrançois et al. similarly refer to the work of Freire as they articulate the achievements and aims of Mad Studies as enacting a critical pedagogy "in the radical co-production, circulation, and consumption of knowledge" (2013:14). It is in and through relations – the collective voice and agentic vulnerability of service users in community – that experiences of violence and madness are politicized towards the re-imagining of ways that unbind and re-couple the perpetrator–victim binary.

Concluding thoughts

Some time has passed since writing the first and last words of this chapter; events in between have inevitably been interpreted through its ideas – perpetrator–victim, binaries, vulnerability, agentic vulnerability, and political agency, among others. And, the interpretation of these events brings us into different or (re)new(ed) spaces of self-understanding and being. As such, it seems important to revisit our earlier discussion of responsibility and accountability with respect to writing about violence and madness from our respective locations as academic researchers, educators, and practitioners in social work, and as community members and activists.

Andrea: In my earlier statement on responsibility and accountability I started by saying that my thinking about violence and madness is most immediately informed by recent collaborative work with Lucy Costa and Peter Beresford on the edited book titled, *Madness, Violence, and Power: A Critical Collection*. However, this isn't entirely accurate. It was through a discussion with my mother about *Madness, Violence, and Power*, towards the end of writing this chapter, that I came to understand my commitment to interrogating the binding of violence and madness, as a social injustice, in a different way. More specifically, I began to think about the professional/personal binary and how I've always located my responsibility and accountability in my professional work as a social worker; being in the position of 'expert', one committed to critical and social justice-oriented social work but nonetheless complicit in oppression and violence … perhaps an act of redemption, of sorts. But, my responsibility and accountability to this work is informed by the 'personal' – my personal. My discussion with my mother reminded me of this; it reminded me that one of our family narratives is of violence and madness – a narrative of distress, 'disorder', and violent ends across generations. Since this discussion I have become curious about how I came to lose this narrative. I suppose my most immediate response is that it was subsumed by the dehumanization inherent in the colonial and heterocispatriarchal space of academe – the academic world where the personal is invalidated in the making of a 'scholar' (a form of violence in and of itself). However, I think the loss of the narrative is more complex and nuanced. While I have not yet fully figured it out (and likely, may never), I think the narrative of distress, 'disorder', and violent ends is obscured by another family narrative – a narrative of immigration. This narrative includes the inevitable normalization of hardship and suffering in life and the need to 'fit in' or to be 'seen' in just the right way (not 'making waves' and being seen as 'normal'). Perhaps rather than being a narrative of immigration, it is more truthfully a narrative of vulnerability as risk. As I remain committed to this reflexive stance, I am intrigued with the possibility of expanding understanding of my responsibility and accountability to the work of interrogating violence and madness through a critically conscious engagement of the narrative of distress, 'disorder', and violent ends – this, of course, requires a shift from the professional to the personal; from vulnerability as risk to vulnerability as resistance.

Trish: Last year, I spend a day with my cousin, a quiet, private, and pleasant man, and his young daughter. She was thrilled because we were going to be making zines. She persistently coaxed her father to join in the art making. He eventually sat down with us at the kitchen table. We each made a zine about something we wanted to say of our lives and our family. Then we told each other about the little booklets we had created. As my cousin described his pages, his daughter put her hand on his shoulder, riveted by his words. When he finished, she said, "But there is such sadness!" Her expression was one of gratitude, relief, and respect. She listened for his full human experience, which includes the suicide of his only sibling, and responded with empathy and with gratitude for having been included in his authentic sharing of self. This moment became significant as both deeply personal and profoundly political. I see in this moment, as we sat around the table creating personal narrative art, how it is that vulnerability as resistance is about the active relationship between the story told and the story heard; that profound encounter between the teller and the listener. I think about the communities and their infrastructures, the fortifications and the pushing back that would enact such encounters, so that vulnerability as resistance can combat stigma and responses that ultimately serve to violate rights and humanity. I think about a kitchen table that brings communities together, a kitchen table that is located within community rather than outside of it.

As we explore the possibilities of relationship, collective response, and community immersed knowledges and leadership, we pause in order to consider critical reflexivity. Fook (2015) refers to a capacity to look both outward and inward in order to make connections between the social, the cultural and the personal. LeBlanc and Kinsella (2016) also refer to critical reflexivity as they identify an ongoing need to "correct identity-prejudiced belief systems" that interfere with the ability to validate the knowledges presented by service users. Such belief systems are sustained by inequitable power dynamics that determine the production of knowledge and, at the same time, reproduce these power dynamics by narrowly defining knowledge systems as valid/invalid (Fricker, 2007). Listening to and speaking alternative knowledge requires courage: vulnerability as/and resistance through which change becomes possible.

References

Arendt H (1958). *The Human Condition*. Chicago: The University of Chicago Press.

Ashcroft R and Van Katwyk T (2016). An examination of the biomedical paradigm: A view of social work. *Social Work in Public Health*, *31*(3), 140–152.

Bhattacharyya B (2013). How can we live with ourselves? Universities and the attempt to reconcile learning and doing. *Ethnic and Racial Studies*, *36*(9), 1411–1428.

Beresford P (2016). From psycho-politics to mad studies: Learning from the legacy of Peter Sedgwick. *Critical and Radical Social Work*, *4*(3), 1–13.

Brenner A (2013). Resisting simple dichotomies: Critiquing narratives of victims, perpetrators, and harm in Feminist theories of rape. *Harvard Journal of Law and Gender*, *36*, 503–568.

Butler J (2016). Rethinking vulnerability and resistance. In J Butler, Z Gambetti, and L Sabsay (eds.). *Vulnerability in Resistance*. Durham: Duke University Press, 12–27. DOI: https://doi.org/10.1215/9780822373490-002.

Butler J (2004). *Undoing Gender*. New York and Oxfordshire: Routledge.

Choe J Y, Teplin L A, and Abram K M (2008). Perpetration of violence, violent victimization, and severe mental illness: Balancing public health concerns. *Psychiatric Services*, *59*, 153–164.

Chomsky N (2015). Neo-liberalism and higher education/society. Interview: *Public Engagement and the Politics of Evidence Symposium*, 22–25 July 2015 [Video file]. https://youtu.be/OE56bEhx8b8. Accessed: 27.06.2020.

Collins P H (1990). Black feminist thought in the matrix of domination. *Black Feminist Thought: Knowledge, Consciousness, and the Politics of Empowerment*, *138*, 221–238.

Costa L (2014). Mad Studies–what it is and why you should care. *Mad Studies Network [blog]*. https://madstudies2014.wordpress.com/2014/10/15/mad-studies-what-it-is-and-why-you-should-care-2/#_ftn1 (dostęp: 20.02. 2017). Accessed: 25.04.2019.

Coverdale J H, Coverdale S M and Nairn R (2013). "Behind the mug shot grin": Uses of madness-talk in reports of Loughner's mass killing. *Journal of Communication Inquiry*, *37*(3), 200–216.

Daley A and Ross L E (2018). Uncovering the heteronormative order of the psychiatric institution: A queer reading of chart documentation and language use. In: J Kilty, E Dej (eds). *Containing Madness*. Palgrave Macmillan, Cham, 169–190.

Daley A, Costa L and Ross L (2012). (W)righting women: Constructions of gender, sexuality & disorder through psychiatric documentation practices. *Culture, Health and Sexuality: An International Journal for Research, Intervention and Care*, *14*(8), 955–969.

Daley A, Costa L and Beresford P (2019). *Madness, Violence, and Power: A Critical Collection*. Toronto: University of Toronto Press.

De Mooij L D, Kikkert M, Lommerse N M, Peen J, Meijwaard S C, Theunissen J, Duurkoop P W R A, Goudriaan A E, Van H L, Beekman A T T and Dekker J J M (2015). Victimisation in adults with severe mental illness: Prevalence and risk factors. *The British Journal of Psychiatry*, *207*, 515–522.

Fook J (2015). Reflective practice and critical reflection. In J Lishman, (ed). *Handbook for Practice Learning in Social Work and Social Care: Knowledge and Theory*. Chicago: Jessica Kingsley Publishers, 440–454.

Foucault M (2003). *Madness and Civilization*. London and New York: Routledge.

Fricker, M. (2007). *Epistemic Injustice: Power and the Ethics of Knowing.* Oxford: Oxford University Press.

Ingram R A (2016). Doing mad studies: Making (non)sense together. *Intersectionalities: A Global Journal of Social Work Analysis, Research, Polity, and Practice, 5*(3), 11–17.

Jackson V (2005). *Separate and Unequal: The Legacy of Racially Segregated Psychiatric Hospitals. A Cultural Competence Training Tool.* https://www.academia.edu/1312868/Separate_and_Unequal_The_Legacy_of_Racially_Segregated_Hospitals?auto=download. Accessed: 15.04.2019.

Kanani N (2011). Race and madness: Locating the experiences of racialized people with psychiatric histories in Canada and the United States. *Critical Disability Discourses, 3.* https://cdd.journals.yorku.ca/index.php/cdd/article/view/31564. Accessed: 15.04.2019.

Keating F (2016). Racialized communities, producing madness and dangerousness. *Intersectionalities: A Global Journal of Social Work Analysis, Research, Polity, and Practice, 5*(3). https://journals.library.mun.ca/ojs/index.php/IJ/article/view/1664. Accessed: 05.05.2019.

Kecskes K and Foster K M (2013). Three questions for community engagement at the crossroads. *The Journal of Public Scholarship in Higher Education, 3,* 7–17.

Kelley R D (2016). Black study, Black struggle. *The Boston Review.* http://bostonreview.net/forum/robin-d-g-kelley-black-study-black-struggle. Accessed: 06.07.2020.

Khalifeh H, Johnson S, Howard L M, Borschmann R, Osborn D, Dean K, Hart C, Hogg J, & Moran P (2015). Violent and non-violent crime against adults with severe mental illness. *The British Journal of Psychiatry, 206,* 275–282. DOI:10.1192/bjp.bp.114.147843.

Koivisto M O (2018). "I know you think I'm crazy": Post-horrorcore rap approaches to disability, violence, and psychotherapy. *Disability Studies Quarterly, 38*(2).

LeBlanc S and Kinsella E A (2016). Toward epistemic justice: A critically reflexive examination of 'sanism' and implications for knowledge generation. *Studies in Social Justice, 10*(1), 59–78.

LeFrançois B A, Beresford P and Russo J (2016). Editorial: Destination Mad Studies. *Intersectionalities: A Global Journal of Social Work Analysis, Research, Polity, and Practice, 5*(3). https://journals.library.mun.ca/ojs/index.php/IJ/article/view/1690. Accessed: 05.05.2019.

LeFrançois B A, Menzies R and Reaume G (eds.) (2013). *Mad Matters: A Critical Reader in Canadian Mad Studies.* Toronto: Canadian Scholars' Press.

Liegghio M (2013). A denial of being: Psychiatrization as epistemic violence. In B A LeFrançois, R Menzies and G Reaume (eds.). *Mad Matters: A Critical Reader in Canadian Mad Studies.* Toronto: Canadian Scholars' Press, 122–129.

Link N W, Cullen F T, Agnew R and Link B G (2016). Can general strain theory help us understand violent behaviors among people with mental illnesses? *Justice Quarterly, 33*(4), 729–754, DOI: 10.1080/07418825.2015.1005656.

Maniglio R (2009). Severe mental illness and criminal victimization: A systematic review. *Acta Psychiatrica Scandinavica, 119,* 180–191.

Marie D and Miles B (2008). Social distance and perceived dangerousness across four diagnostic categories of mental disorder. *Australian and New Zealand Journal of Psychiatry, 42,* 126–133.

McCarthy T (1993). Deconstruction and reconstruction in contemporary critical theory, *Canadian Journal of Philosophy, 23*(supp1), 247–264, DOI: 10.1080/00455091.1993.10717350.

Metzl J M and MacLeish K T (2015). Mental illness, mass shootings, and the politics of American Firearms. *American Journal of Public Health, 105*(2), 240–249.

Miller G (2018). Madness decolonized? Madness as transnational identity in Gail Hornstein's Agnes's Jacket. *Journal of Medical Humanities, 39,* 303–323, DOI 10.1007/s10912-017-9434-8

Mills C (2013). *Decolonizing Global Mental Health: The Psychiatrization of the Majority World.* London, UK: Routledge.

Mills C (2014). Sly normality: Between quiescence and revolt. In B Burstow, B A LeFrançois and S Diamond (Eds.). *Psychiatry Disrupted: Theorizing Resistance and Crafting the (R)evolution.* Montréal, QC: McGill/Queen's University Press, 208–224.

Park H (2017). Racialized women, the law and the violence of white settler colonialism. *Feminist Legal Studies, 25,* 267–290.

Paleari S, Donina D and Meoli M (2015). The role of the university in twenty-first century European society. *Journal of Technology Transfer, 40*(3), 369–379.

Pilling M D, Daley A, Gibson M F, Ross L E, and Zaheer J (2018). Assessing 'insight', determining agency and autonomy: Implicating social identities. In J Kilty, E Dej (eds) *Containing Madness.* Cham: Palgrave Macmillan, 191–214.

Psychiatric Disabilities Anti-violence Coalition (2015). Clearing a path: A psychiatric survivor anti-violence framework. Toronto. https://torontoantiviolencecoalition.files.wordpress.com/2016/02/clearing-a-path-dec-2015.pdf. Accessed: 04.07.2019.

Rimke H and Brock D (2012). The culture of therapy: Psychocentrism in everyday life. In M Thomas, R Raby and D Brock (eds). *Power and Everyday Practices*. Toronto: Nelson, 182–202.

Russo J and Beresford P (2015). Between exclusion and colonisation: Seeking a place for mad people's knowledge in academia. *Disability & Society*, *30*(1), 153–157.

Scheper-Hughes N and Bourgois P (2004). Introduction: making sense of violence. In, N. Scheper-Hughes and P. Bourgois (eds), *Violence in War and Peace: An Anthology*. Malden: Blackwell Publishing Inc., 1–31.

Shimrat, I (2013). The tragic farce of "community mental health care". In B A LeFrançois, R Menzies and G Reaume (Eds.). *Mad Matters: A Critical Reader in Canadian Mad Studies*. Toronto, ON: Canadian Scholars' Press, 38–48.

Spandler H and Barker M (2016). *Mad and Queer Studies: Interconnections and Tensions*. https://madstudies2014.wordpress.com/2016/07/01/mad-and-queer-studies-interconnections-and-tensions/. Accessed: 25.04.2019.

Spivak G C (1994). Can the subaltern speak? In P Williams and L Chrisman (Eds.). *Colonial Discourse and Post-Colonial Theory: A Reader*. New York: Columbia University Press, 66–111.

Van Dorn R A, Grimm K J, Desmarais S L, Tueller S J, Johnson K L and Swartz M S (2017). Leading indicators of community-based violent events among adults with mental illness. *Psychological Medicine*, *47*, 1179–1191.

Van Katwyk T and Case R A (2016). From suspicion and accommodation to structural transformation: Enhanced scholarship through enhanced community-university relations. *Engaged Scholar Journal: Community-Engaged Research, Teaching, and Learning*, *2*(2), 25–43.

Varshney M, Mahapatra A, Krishnan V, Gupta R and Sinha Deb K (2016). Violence and mental illness: What is the true story? *Journal of Epidemiology and Community Health*, *70*(3), 223–225.

27

UPCYCLING RECOVERY

Potential alliances of recovery, inequality and Mad Studies

Lynn Tang

Introduction

Originating in the US in the late 1980s and early 1990s, the recovery movement started as a progressive grassroots movement in which we, as survivors, assert our right to control our own lives in the face of dominant psychiatric power. Contrary to the notion of chronicity and deficit often found in Western bio-medical models, recovery-oriented mental health services emphasise the hope of living a valued and decent life with or without the limitations caused by distress and ill-health (Anthony, 1993). Over the years, recovery as a concept has become a frequent discursive feature in mental health policies in various Anglophone countries such as the UK, New Zealand and Australia. In other places, such as Hong Kong and mainland China, where there is a lack of national mental health policy, the recovery approach is often perceived as a welcomed and relevant concept which requires local adaptation (Tse et al., 2013a; Tse et al., 2013b).

Despite the seeming 'success' of the mainstreaming of recovery, its implementation has been criticised (Spandler and Calton, 2009; Morrow, 2013; Slade et al., 2014; McWade, 2016). Some service-user groups even argue for jettisoning the concept altogether. They see it as being co-opted into the current mental health system and becoming a disciplinary force that limits users' autonomy rather than championing it (Recovery in the Bin, 2016). Mad studies has been one of the important spaces in which the recovery concept has been critiqued (Morrow, 2013; McWade, 2016). In this chapter, I will discuss whether we should reclaim the concept of recovery and the possibility of reconceptualising it as a project of community that puts social justice at the core and tackles multi-levelled inequalities. Drawing on my research and observation in the UK, as well as in Chinese-speaking worlds, I will discuss the controversies of recovery and argue for reclaiming rather than jettisoning it. Then I will illustrate how, by throwing light on inequalities and oppression, including those within the psychiatric system, can reveal what can limits service-users' life chances and constrain their pursuit of valued lives (Tang, 2017). I argue that seeing recovery as a project of community would require challenging these inequalities collectively with cross-sectional movements. Following this I propose Göran Therborn's (2013) conceptualisation of three killing fields of inequality, namely, vital, existential and resource inequalities, as a means of envisioning potential alliances of recovery, inequality and mad studies.

DOI: 10.4324/9780429465444-32

Shall we jettison recovery?

In its original emphasis, the recovery movement foregrounds lived experience and the experiential knowledge of service-users as well as advocating a shift of power from professional dominance to users' self-determination. It proposes a change from a notion of deficit in illness model to therapeutic optimism. Patricia Deegan, a disability-rights advocate with lived experience, wrote in the early days of the recovery movement that recovery is not a linear process. In her work 'Recovery as a Journey of the Heart' (1996), she wrote that the goal of recovery is not for individuals to get mainstreamed or become 'normal'. Rather, the aim is to transform the mainstream so that there are rooms for everyone to be themselves and to pursue a life they want. What Deegan conveyed is the agency for us to exist and grow with full potential as human beings. The recovery movement gained momentum and mental health professionals, often co-producing with service-users, have built on research from the recovery movement to produce knowledge on how to change the mental health system itself. For example, Slade (2009) delineates the difference between 'clinical recovery' and 'personal recovery' and argues for the mental health system to change its focus from the former to latter. 'Clinical recovery' is understood as professionals prescribing what recovery is and such prescription is often preoccupied with symptom remission and the use of medication to eliminate symptoms, while 'personal recovery' goes beyond a narrow medicalised understanding of mental distress and respects recovery goals and processes defined and valued by individual service-users. Elements that promote personal recovery, such as connectedness, hope, positive sense of identity, finding meanings in life and empowerment, are also articulated (Leamy et al., 2011).

The uptake of recovery discourse in policy in Anglophone countries can be due to the fact that recovery is a polyvalent and ambiguous concept that can mean recovery from illness which resonates with the traditional bio-medical model, or recovery from the invalidation of lived experience which service-user movements strive for (Pilgrim, 2008). Thus no one will disagree with 'recovery'. Yet, once mainstreamed, despite the efforts of proponents to propose a paradigm shift in understanding recovery, it lost its original progressiveness as a liberatory discourse in challenging bio-medical dominance. The dominant ideas about what people have recovery from are left unchallenged (Spandler and Calton, 2009). Societies remain intolerant of differences and thus only permit recovery goals that are aligned with socially sanctioned definitions of what a 'normal' functioning person should do (Rose, 2014). Morrow (2013) and McWade (2016) argue that neoliberal discourses shape mental health policies which absorb but also co-opt the recovery movement. Drawing on Foucault's concept of 'bio-power' (1980), Morrow (2013) argue that neoliberalism prompts us to take charge of and manage our individual bodies and minds. Policies under neoliberalism favour welfare entrenchment and individual responsibilities. Biopsychiatry, she argues, is tied to neoliberalism through promoting an individualistic understanding and solutions to collective social problems that cause distress in the first place. Public issues become medicalised personal troubles and individual 'health' issues that require biomedical intervention. In this context, recovery is co-opted to promote self-management that emphasises individual responsibility to 'recover' in a way sanctioned by the neoliberal society.

Morrow's critique can be exemplified by McWade (2016)'s detailed account of the New Labour government's reform of the NHS during the 2000s in the UK. On the one hand the government promoted 'recovery' as policy vision. On the other hand it increased coercion through introducing community treatment orders and reducing welfare support to service-users. McWade (2016) argues that the mental health promotion discourse that 'mental illness is like other physical illness' shifted attention from social problems that cause suffering to medicalising suffering that legitimises bio-medical intervention. Individuals are to be self-responsible for their success or failure in recovering into an employable 'functioning' citizen. Thus some service-user groups argue for jettisoning recovery as it turns against them and becomes a disciplining discourse that puts the blame on people who 'don't recover', denies them the disability benefits they need for survival and pushes people out of services (Recovery in the Bin, 2016). Recovery, originated as a 'protest' narrative that challenges bio-medical dominance and paternalism, which became a 'role model' narrative against individuals who do not live up to societal expectations. The neoliberal policy context outlined above reduces well-intended efforts to transform the mental health system 'from within' into limited changes as the unequal power within the mental health system remains intact. Similar observation can be seen in the peer support movement. In the US, Penney and Prescott (2016) observed that peer workers are encouraged to acculturate into, rather than transform, the existing culture of the institutions they work in. Both recovery and peer support movements share a similar fate of co-option. It is in this context that mad studies emerges as a potential space for protecting and asserting the distinctiveness of experiential knowledge in enlightening our understandings of mental health and madness, as well as ways to alleviate people's suffering (LeFrancois et al., 2013; Ingram, 2016; Russo and Sweeney, 2016).

Shall we jettison recovery or reclaim it? I would argue for the latter. First, critiques that argue for jettisoning recovery emerge in countries where recovery is incorporated in national policy and operating as an oppressive discourse. In places like Hong Kong where there is a lack of national mental health policy and recovery discourse remains marginal, recovery does not have the same powerful disciplining effect as in the UK. In Hong Kong, while the mainstream discourse is blatantly based on the Western bio-medical model and paternalism that asks service-users to obey professional knowledge also prevails, in the non-profit sector the recovery movement seems to open up space for alternatives. In one major mental health non-governmental organisation (NGO) that promotes recovery-oriented services, a hearing voices group was founded by a survivor social worker. Such alternatives are still important in impacting cultural changes albeit in small ways. Second, the notions of recovery still resonate with the experiences of many service-users. For example, people suffering from acute anxiety, depression, suicidal ideation, penalising voices do want to recover from the torment of their mental distress and regain a sense of control in their lives. I concur with Morrow's (2013) view that dialogues about recovery in which individuals share their lived experience of negotiating or resisting psychiatry and exploring ways to regain control from sufferings have transformative potential.

In sum, rather than seeing the recovery concept as in itself problematic, I see recovery approaches and the way proponents are attempting to change the system 'from within' as insufficient in changing the status quo of the mental health system. Mad studies' positioning as an in/discipline 'from outside' the knowledge production of the mainstream psy-professions, is crucial in retaining the critical edge of grassroots mad politics and survivor movements (LeFrançois et al., 2016). The current development of mad studies seems to focus on articulating and establishing its epistemological and methodological differences to protect and reinvigorate the production of experiential knowledge as protest narratives. Yet it is less clear about how advocates of mad studies would want to influence the system. In this regard, I see recovery as a concept/approach that needs to be critically interrogated and its meaning reclaimed rather than leaving professionals inside the system to define it.

Upcycling recovery into a project of communities

The above critiques of recovery point to the need to not just change mental health services but for the wider society to respect and assert the rights of individuals in order for meaningful recovery to take place. I suggest 'upcycling' recovery – a shift from seeing recovery as a project of individuals to one of communities in order to create the social conditions conducive to recovery. My research project in UK was one that identified such social conditions for Chinese people who lived in the UK, having received a psychiatric diagnosis (Tang, 2017). I took a bottom-up approach and asked what recovery means for individuals in this minority ethnic group. As this group is subjected to an intersection of different inequalities such as ethnicity, class and gender, this study illustrates how recovery as a project of communities should tackle multi-level inequalities.

To discover arenas that recovery as a community project should work on, I used the capabilities approach to explore the enabling and deleterious social conditions Chinese service-users faced. Similar to the spirit of recovery approach, the capabilities approach is not concerned with what a person ultimately chooses to do, but whether they have the substantive freedom to be and do what they value (Sen, 1999; Nussbaum, 2000; Hopper, 2007). Capabilities here refers to substantive freedom rather than the abilities they possess. Substantive freedom has two dimensions. One is the process of exercising choice. The other is the opportunities available to an individual, for choice is not real choice if there are no real opportunities, such as a variety of treatment options or employment opportunities, available. Another useful concept in the capabilities approach is adaptive preference. Individuals' preferences and aspirational for life choices can be unknowingly shaped and conditioned by the barriers and disadvantages they face. The capabilities approach has been adapted in recovery research in various ways to explore and define what capabilities service-user value (Ware et al., 2007) and their experiences in different capabilities domains, such as living in physical security and engaging in productive and valued activities (Brunner, 2017). Wallcraft (2011) used adaptive preference to explain why service-users tend to underrate decreases in their quality of life as they might have minimised how good their life can be. I used the capabilities approach as a heuristic framework to explore what enables and constrains the capability development of Chinese service-users along their recovery journey.

The findings provide pointers for what recovery as a collective project could work on for this group. I found that the inequalities that contributed to their distress and ill-health in the first place shaped the extent they could recover or redevelop the capabilities. Their marginalisation in the labour market, the harsh working conditions in Chinese catering businesses, the pressure of parental expectation of high educational achievement on young people, as well as the isolation faced by overseas brides and the elderly are common issues faced in this group (Tang and Pilgrim, 2017). Language difficulties, stigma and disempowerment related to diagnosis and treatment, as well as grievances during involuntary hospitalisations were also found in the experience of service users. For some, this constrained their ability to use services to their full benefit. Others, felt acute power inequality with professionals and hesitated to seek help from services again. This results in further isolation, especially as they did not have other alternative sources of help available (Tang, 2017). Self-determination in living arrangements, community participation and economic participation were found to be crucial capabilities for building a life they valued after crisis. Yet disempowering attitudes of frontline practitioners, insufficient opportunities for them to participate in the community due to cuts in services and lack of employment opportunities due to racial and disability discrimination limited their life chances to realise their potentials (Tang, 2018a). My point about putting social inequalities into focus is more apparent if we consider how hope is experienced. Hope, an important element in recovery, but can be problematic in some circumstances. The ideology of achieving a perfect life and body image through consumerism can perpetuate a false hope that creates more anxiety in an unequal society and is thus capability diminishing. The diminished opportunities some face due to discrimination, ageism and racism can also dampen hope. This results in some people not wanting to embrace hope as it can bring vulnerability and disappointment when encountering barriers in the community (Tang, 2018b).

Recovery as a project of community means identifying and challenging multi-level inequalities and oppressions that limit people's life chances, make them ill in the first place and hinder recovery later on. The above discussion highlights the collective capabilities we need to recover and develop at the community level in order for Chinese people in the UK to thrive and feel hopeful. Individuals' recovery progress can't be forced, but we can create favourable social conditions for recovery and capability development to take place.

The need for broad and cross-sectional movements

What is the implication of upcycling recovery as a project of community? For Chinese communities, there is a need to open up a space to facilitate experiential knowledge production to challenge dominant recovery discourses. In my fieldwork, I found that some participants would present 'standard scripts' of bio-medical models on the necessity to take medicines when asked what advice they would give to other service-users, even though in the same interview they reported grievances and ambivalence about the usefulness of medicine. This discrepancy reflects the need to empower service-users to reflect and articulate experiences that may be dissonant with mainstream discourses (Tang, 2017). Yet, recovery as a project of community wouldn't necessarily entail collaborations beyond a particular community. The class, gender, ethnic and other inequalities mentioned above do not just adversely affect UK Chinese service users. The various inequalities may intersect in a particular way to shape the social conditions that this minority ethnic group live in, but inequalities have a deleterious effect on health across the whole population. Take income inequality as an example. Wilkinson and Pickett (2018) provide evidence to show that countries with larger income disparities have higher rates of people with psychological suffering such as stress, anxiety and depression. They argue that the link is evaluation anxiety, as judging each other's social position and status exacerbates fear and sense of insecurity. Thus I agree with Ferguson's proposal to build 'a broad, rather than a narrow, movement to challenge the causes of mental distress, defend existing services and put forward alternative visions of the kind of mental health services we need' (2017:117).

The political strategy against neoliberal mental health and welfare policy in the UK suggested by Moth and McKeown (2016) provides an example of what such broad movement can be. Two dimensions of the neoliberal political project are restructuring the welfare state and intensification of work. Policies which cut welfare provision and push people to move away from mental health services and 'return to work' (often in the name of 'recovery') create stress for mentally distressed welfare claimants. What they are asked to reengage in is toxic working conditions characterised by an intensification of work which is common nowadays. Thus Moth and McKeown (2016) point out that a shared insecurity towards income and job stability can be found across welfare claimants, temporary workers and those in more stable employment. Solidarity across these groups, they argue, can be built not just because of their shared material interest, but the potential for a new consciousness of collectivities against neoliberal policies. They show that such possibility of broad cross-sectional movement is evidenced in anti-austerity activism. For example, service-user activists and mental health workers working together to campaign against pathologising unemployed individuals, as well as service-user activists and trade unionists joining forces in campaigns against service closures.

Such broad cross-sectional movements need to acknowledge the internal diversities and tensions. The potential for solidarity requires 'a fundamentally democratic ethos to ensure that unequal and oppressive social relations are not reproduced within cross-sectional mobilisations' (Moth and McKeown, 2016:385). Unequal social relations within a movement should be addressed. This can be illustrated with the story of a participant in my study. Young, with his English-speaking skills, was able to find a job in the mainstream labour market and disclosed his mental health history to his employer. Yet, rather than having reasonable adjustments in his work tasks, his disclosure seemed to work against him as his colleagues often blamed him for being slow. He admitted that because of his mental health conditions sometimes he might feel that his body had stopped moving and he did not know how long he had stopped. But often he felt that his colleagues exaggerated the length of time he had stopped and he did not receive help when this happened. Eventually he was fired being told that he was 'lazy'. I asked if he had ever considered seeking help from a trade union so that there could be a third party assessing whether he was unfairly treated. Yet, he had no idea how to approach a trade union representative and also assumed that they could not help. (Tang, 2017). Young's perception revealed possible barriers for minority ethnic groups and disabled people in seeking help from the trade union. Chinese people are under-represented in union membership (TUC, 2014). This under-representation raises questions about whether trade unions proactively reach out to this group, the consciousness of labour rights among Chinese communities and whether Chinese people anticipate discrimination in the trade union. Young also felt that the trade union would only act on a worker's behalf if a strong case could be put together. This suggests that trade unions need to proactively provide information and support to under-represented groups and address diversity and equality among their members. The story of Young may also suggest that Chinese communities in the UK are inward looking and rarely join mainstream movements to address issues such as labour rights, which is a shared concern of both mainstream and minority ethnic groups (Tang, 2018c). Thus this story illustrates the need for cross-sectional movements that address inequalities and diversities within them.

Recovery, inequality and mad studies: potential alliances

As for cross-sectional movements among recovery, inequality and mad studies, I propose that Göran Therborn's (2013) conceptualisation of the three kinds of inequality may be able to provide a framework to envision potential alliances. These three kinds of inequality, namely vital inequality, existential inequality and resource inequality, also impact upon each other. Among the three, existential inequality is of particular relevance to this edited book on mad studies. Investigation of vital and resource inequalities can be found in conventional studies of health inequity, social determinants of health and social inequalities. Vital inequality refers to the 'socially constructed unequal life chances of human organisms', such as morbidity rates, mortality rates and life expectancies (Therborn, 2013:49). Therborn links psycho-somatic consequences of the class and status system as one reason for vital inequality which is evidenced by Wilkinson and Pickett (2018). People who have received a psychiatric diagnosis have a mortality rate and life expectancy notoriously lower than that of the general population (Brown, 1997; Laursen, 2011). Resource inequality refers to resources for human action, such as income, intergenerational mobility, educational opportunities, social network, and power (Therborn, 2013). Discrimination faced by service-users in the workplace and the community limits their opportunities for earning a decent income and connecting with other members in the community. Robust equal opportunity legislation (for example, the inclusion and proper implementation of reasonable accommodation in disability discrimination ordinance) has the potential to rectify this inequality and increase employment opportunities for people with psychosocial disabilities.

Therborn defines existential inequality, as 'the unequal allocation of personhood, i.e., of autonomy, dignity, degrees of freedom, and of rights to respect and self-development' (2013:49). Examples he quotes include sexism, racism and caste system. The concept of existential inequality can be linked to our advocacy of experiential knowledge in the recovery movement and mad studies, for its emphasis on 'personal autonomy, recognition and respect' (ibid:50). Newbigging and Ridley's (2018) application of Fricker's concept of 'epistemic injustice' (2007) in evaluating the effectiveness of independent mental health advocacy services in the UK can help us further elaborate the existential inequality experienced by service users and how this can be challenged. Epistemic injustice takes place when a person is 'wronged specifically in her capacity as a knower' (Fricker, 2007:18, in Newbigging and Ridley, 2018:37). This prevents certain groups of people from contesting distorted understandings of their lived experience. There are two forms of epistemic injustice. Firstly, testimonial injustice happens when one's account is considered less credible or invalidated. Secondly, hermeneutic injustice arises when a marginalised group lacks shared conceptual resources to make sense of their experiences in ways that feel are comfortable or appropriate. In Newbigging and Ridley's study (2018), testimonial injustice was found as participants felt that their voices were not respected by the doctors and their concerns were dismissed as irrelevant. Their findings show that independent advocates can in some way promote testimonial justice by acting as an epistemic witness to balance the power asymmetry between the service-user and the professionals in the context of detention under the mental health legislation. Hermeneutic injustice was also found as bio-medical discourse was dominant over other possible ways of framing such as trauma or other social perspectives. Yet, this seems to be more difficult to challenge. This, as Newbigging and Ridley argue, was possibly due to the fact that in face of compulsion, advocates focus on safeguarding rights rather than negotiating alternative understandings (2018). The potentials and limitations of statutory independent advocacy service in rectifying existential inequality illustrated in this study can be a learning point for places where the problematics of compulsory detention are less discussed, such as Hong Kong.

These three kinds of inequality impact on each other. This can be illustrated by the tragic story of the suicide of a young novelist in Taiwan (BBC, 2018). Lin Yi-han published a novel on sexual assaults which was later revealed to be drawn from her own experience. Before her death, she was open about her experience of mental health problems and had pledged to fight for destigmatisation of mental illness. It was after her suicide that her parents revealed the causes of her suffering was rape by a private tutor when she was a young girl. Rape as an existential inequality, i.e. sexual assault as a violation of personhood predominately imposed by men against women, results in vital inequality (e.g. the high rate of sexual assault and harassment survivors receiving a diagnosis of post-traumatic stress disorder). According to the news report, Lin, because of depressive symptoms and several suicide attempts, could not finish the university degrees that she had started. This shows how vital inequality results in resource inequality as incompletion of university degree adversely impacted on her further education and employment inequality.

Two learning points can be taken from this sad story as an example of possible cross-fertilisation of recovery, inequality and mad studies/movements. First, tackling mental health symptoms and stigma faced by people receiving a psychiatric diagnosis are not enough to recover one's personhood. Therapies, be it in the form of medicine or psychological intervention to heal from the trauma, could help, but we need to collectively challenge the patriarchy so that no one will experience sexual assault and harassment in the first place. Also, rectifying existential injustice can bring healing and empowerment at a collective level. The tragedy of Lin and the subsequent #metoo movement originating from the West have fostered the development of #metoo movement in Greater China. In the mainland China, with the use of social media, the large volume of testimonial accounts revealed by women is unprecedented, making these long suppressed experiences visible and pressure from the movement has resulted in a series of changes in sexual harassment-related policies and legislation (Huang, 2019). The second learning point is that when sharing their accounts and understandings of their lived experiences both women and mental health service users could face gaslighting with accusations of unreliable memory, emotionality and irrationality. Thus epistemic injustice as one of the existential inequalities that invalidate our experience because of our ascribed identities is a common challenge for both feminism, recovery and mad studies movements.

Conclusion

From its inception, the recovery movement has attempted to challenge power inequalities within the mental health system and, in so doing, to assert the validity and significance of experiential knowledge. Yet, the mainstreaming of recovery in mental health policies and services in Anglophone countries, where neoliberalism prevails, has been criticised for being co-opted and becoming a disciplinary discourse that can turn against service users. In this chapter, I have argued that while it is crucial to preserve a space for the production of experiential knowledge outside the psy-professions, dialogue and engagement with the recovery movement is still important – we should reclaim its meaning rather than leaving it to the professionals to define recovery for us. Upcycling recovery into a project of communities could provide a way of reclaiming its progressiveness, placing the focus on changing communities and challenging inequalities, rather than on changing and blaming individuals. Such a project requires cross-sectional movements to challenge systemic and multi-level inequalities with joint efforts.

For potential alliances among recovery, inequality and mad studies, the conceptualisation of vital, existential and resource inequality may offer insights when envisioning synergies for future research and activism. Mad studies challenges the failures of recovery and attempts to create and protect a space of 'in/discipline' for the production of experiential knowledge and protest narratives that celebrate madness and diverse forms of human existence (Ingram, 2016). When recovery is viewed as a community project to tackle inequalities, epistemic injustice offers a possible entry point for understanding the different kinds of invalidations and oppressions experienced by individuals within that community. This is where upcycled recovery as a project of communities could have shared interests with mad studies. Moreover, charting a new territory of mad studies outside the system to prevent co-option may inadvertently reproduce its marginalised position in knowledge production but maintaining dialogue with upcycled recovery may extend the reach of mad studies. Finally, for people who may not identify with 'mad' identity and politics, upcycled recovery may broaden the space for reflecting on their lived experience and producing experiential knowledge; knowledge which may work towards the same goal of challenging power inequality in the mental health system and beyond.

References

Anthony W A (1993). Recovery from mental illness: The guiding vision of the mental health service system in the 1990s. *Psychosocial Rehabilitation Journal*, 16(4): 11–23.

BBC (2018). Taiwanese novelist has left us for one year: Have *Fang Si-Qi*s changed the world?. *BBC Chinese* 25 April. https://www.bbc.com/zhongwen/trad/chinese-news-43891468. Accessed: 6 January 2019. (In Chinese.)

Brown S (1997). Excess mortality of schizophrenia: A meta-analysis. *British Journal of Psychiatry*, 171(6): 502–508.

Brunner R. (2017). Why do people with mental distress have poor social outcomes? Four lessons from the capabilities approach. *Social Science and Medicine*, 191: 160–167.

Deegan PE (1996). Recovery as a journey of the heart. *Psychiatric Rehabilitation Journal*, 19(3): 91–97.

Ferguson I (2017). *Politics of the Mind: Marxism and Mental Distress*. London: Bookmarks Publications.

Foucault M (1980). *Power/Knowledge: Selected Interviews and Other Writings, 1972-1977*. New York: Pantheon.

Fricker M (2007). *Epistemic Injustice: Power and the Ethics of Knowing*. Oxford: Oxford University Press.

Hopper K (2007). Rethinking social recovery in schizophrenia: What a capabilities approach might offer. *Social Science and Medicine*, 65(5): 868–879.

Huang SX (2019). The anniversary of China '#Me Too': journey, achievement and limitations. *The Financial Times Chinese*. 2 Jan. http://www.ftchinese.com/story/001080907. Accessed: 6 January 2019.

Ingram R (2016). Doing mad studies: Making (non)sense together. *Intersectionalities. A Global Journal of Social Work Analysis, Research, Polity, and Practice*, 5(2): 11–17.

Laursen T M (2011). Life expectancy among persons with schizophrenia or bipolar affective disorder. *Schizophrenia Research*, 131(1–3): 101–104.

Leamy M, Bird V, Le Boutillier C, Williams J and Slade M (2011). Conceptual framework for personal recovery in mental health: Systematic review and narrative synthesis. *British Journal of Psychiatry*, 199(6): 445–452.

LeFrançois B A, Beresford P and Russo J (2016). Editorial: Destination Mad Studies. *Intersectionalities: A Global Journal of Social Work Analysis, Research, Polity, and Practice*, 5(3): 1–10.

LeFrancois B A, Menzies R J and Reaume G (eds) (2013). *Mad Matters: A Critical Reader in Canadian Mad Studies*. Toronto: Canadian Scholar's Press.

McWade B (2016). Recovery-as-Policy as a form of neoliberal state making. *Intersectionalities: A Global Journal of Social Work Analysis, Research, Polity, and Practice*, 5(3): 62–81.

Morrow M (2013). Recovery: Progressive paradigm or neoliberal smokescreen? In RJ Menzies, G Raeume and NA LeFrancois (eds) *Mad Matters: A Critical Reader in Canadian Mad Studies*. Toronto, ON: Canadian Scholars' Press, 323–333.

Moth R and McKeown M (2016). Realising Sedgwick's vision: Theorising strategies of resistance to neoliberal mental health and welfare policy. *Critical and Radical Social Work*, 4(3): 375–390.

Newbigging K and Ridley J (2018). Epistemic struggles: The role of advocacy in promoting epistemic justice and rights in mental health. *Social Science & Medicine*, 219: 36–44.

Nussbaum MC (2000). *Women and Human Development: The Capabilities Approach*. Cambridge: Cambridge University Press.

Penney D and Prescott L (2016). The co-optation of survivor knowledge: The danger of substituted values and voice. In J Russo and A Sweeney (eds) *Searching for a Rose Garden: Challenging Psychiatry, Fostering Mad Studies*. Monmouth: PCCS Books, 35–45.

Pilgrim D (2008). "Recovery" and current mental health policy. *Chronic Illness*, 4(4): 295–304.

Recovery in the Bin (2016). The unrecovery star. *Asylum Magazine*, 23(3): 18.

Rose D (2014). The mainstreaming of recovery. *Journal of Mental Health*, 23(5): 217–218.

Russo J and Sweeney A (2016). *Searching for a Rose Garden: Challenging Psychiatry, Fostering Mad Studies*. Monmouth: PCCS Books.

Sen A (1999). *Development as Freedom*. Oxford: Oxford University Press.

Slade M (2009). *Personal Recovery and Mental Illness: A Guide for Mental Health Professionals*. Cambridge: Cambridge University Press.

Slade M, Amering M, Farkas M, Hamilton B, O'Hagan M, Panther G, Perkins R, Shepherd G, Tse S, Whitley R (2014). Uses and abuses of recovery: Implementing recovery-oriented practices in mental health systems. *World Psychiatry*, 13(1):12–20.

Spandler H and Calton T (2009). Psychosis and human rights: Conflicts in mental health policy and practice. *Social Policy & Society*, 8(2): 245–256.

Tang L (2017). *Recovery, Mental Health and Inequality: Chinese Ethnic Minorities as Mental Health Service Users*. London/New York: Routledge.

Tang L (2018a). Barriers to recovery for Chinese mental health service-users in the UK: A case for community development. *Community Development Journal*, 53(2): 358–374.

Tang L (2018b). Recovery, Hope and Agency: The Meaning of Hope Amongst Chinese Users of Mental Health Services in the UK. doi: 10.1093/bjsw/bcy033.

Tang L (2018c). Community development with Chinese mental health service users in the UK. In G Craig (ed.) *Community Organising Against Racism: 'Race', Ethnicity and Community Development*. Bristol: Policy Press, 109–122.

Tang L and Pilgrim D (2017). Intersectionality, mental health and Chinese people in the UK: A qualitative exploration. *Mental Health Review Journal*, 22(4): 289–299.

Therborn G (2013). *The Killing Fields of Inequality*. Cambridge: Polity Press.

Tse S, Ran M S, Huang Y and Zhu S (2013a). Mental Health Care Reforms in Asia: The urgency of now: Building a recovery-oriented, community mental health service in China. *Psychiatric Services*, 64(7): 613–616.

Tse S, Siu B W M and Kan A (2013b). Can recovery-oriented mental health services be created in Hong Kong? Struggles and strategies. *Administration and Policy in Mental Health and Mental Health Services Research*, 40(3):155–158.

TUC (2014). *TUC Equality Audit 2014*. https://www.tuc.org.uk/sites/default/files/Black%20workers%20 and%20unions%20-%20TUC%20Equality%20Audit%202014.pdf. Accessed: 6 January 2019.

Wallcraft J (2011). Service users' perceptions of quality of life measurement in psychiatry. *Advances in Psychiatric Treatment* 17(4): 266–274.

Ware N C, Hopper K, Tugenberg T, Dickey B, and Fisher D (2007). Connectedness and Citizenship: Redefining Social Integration. *Psychiatric Services*, 58(4): 469–474.

Wilkinson R and Pickett K (2018). *The Inner Level: How More Equal Societies Reduce Stress, Restore Sanity and Improve Everyone's Well-being*. London: Penguin.

28

BODIES, BOUNDARIES, B/ORDERS: A RECENT CRITICAL HISTORY OF DIFFERENTIALISM AND STRUCTURAL ADJUSTMENT

Essya M. Nabbali

Introduction

Looking out to the Burrard Inlet and Port of Vancouver from the privilege and ostensible safety of my north-facing patio, I debate the title of this work. Three cruise ships are docked at Canada Place, among the many tensions on display for a city striving to be the "greenest" by 2020. Last year, Vancouver (Unceded Coast Salish Territory) would have "welcomed" nearly a million cruise passengers on 243 ship visits (Jang, 2019), most of which travelled along the Inside Passage of British Columbia (BC), navigating through designated critical habitat for the Northern and Southern Resident killer whales. To give some perspective, the population of the city-proper is said to balloon by 50–60% during "cruise season," and the total number of Southern Residents, specifically, is 73. On the brink of extinction, these orcas grabbed international headlines in 2018 when they mourned the death of a calf by carrying the carcass for, at least, seventeen days and over 1600 kilometers in what researchers have described as an unprecedented "tour de grief" (Cuthbert and Main, 2018).

It has well been identified that the main threats to the survival of Resident killer whales in Canadian Pacific waters are prey availability, acoustic and physical disturbances from marine vessels, and polluted water (Fisheries and Oceans Canada, 2019). The cruise industry has been notorious for environmental crimes (Klein, 2008); Carnival Cruise Lines, including Princess and Holland America ships, both "regulars" of Canada Place, admitted on June 3, 2019, to violating terms of probation from a previous conviction for discharging oily waste and covering it up. Meanwhile, the Vancouver Port Authority projects a record-setting 22% increase of cruise passengers through Canada Place in this year of 2019, part of the "evolution" of cruise tourism and the larger, and larger ships (Jang, 2019).

The same day that Carnival Cruise pleaded guilty to deliberate acts of pollution (read: acts of extinction), the Canadian National Inquiry into Missing and Murdered Indigenous Women and Girls (MMIWG) and 2SLGBTQQIA[1] people released its final report to end, as established, the race, identity, and gender-based genocide across the country. Homicide rates for Indigenous

DOI: 10.4324/9780429465444-33

womxn[2] range up to twelve times higher than for non-Indigenous womxn and represent, more broadly, a quarter of all homicide victims in Canada (Mahoney et al., 2017). A human rights and Indigenous rights crisis, Canadian Prime Minister Justin Trudeau would lament "colonialist structures" and commit government action on the 231 recommendations of the report during his opening remarks later that evening at the 2019 Women Deliver Conference, hosted next door to Canada Place in the Vancouver Convention Centre. Just ten blocks away, a coalition of local grassroots organizations and activists emerged in the Downtown Eastside (DTES) to commemorate MMIWG2SLGBTQQIA[3] and champion a transformative agenda for gender justice.

Expanding on the lessons from June 3, 2019, this chapter confronts the complex entanglement of speciesism, environmental racism, and gender inequity, to make commensurable the structural violence, even if only a fraction of ecologies underpinning and effectively perpetuating poor health, suffering, and catastrophic biospheric illness. I begin by outlining the case for storying this momentous day in Canadian history and for eco/feminist organizings in Vancouver. I turn briefly to the passage of the 2012 Mental Health Act of Ghana and related ethnographic fieldwork to position my reflection against the charged backdrop of (global) mental health development. While this is not a comparative study, the analytical move reveals the relationship between critical race, Indigenous, and Mad Studies, allowing us to bring personal, public, and planetary wellbeing along two conceptual and concentric tracks: differentialism and structural adjustment. It is my contention that the pursuit of "difference," a pretext of rights abuse, historically for structural adjustment (qua social control), can be flipped to lend itself to problem definition and agenda-setting for contemporary policy purposes. In this regard, I argue that we cannot find anti-oppression (read: legitimacy) outside of structural adjustment for politics of difference.

Ecologies of entanglement

In September 2016, the Government of Canada launched a National Inquiry into MMIWG2SLGBTQQIA in response to calls from the Truth and Reconciliation Commission that had been set up as part of the Indian Residential Schools Settlement Agreement, the largest class-action settlement in Canadian history. Long had the disproportionate rates of sexual and gender-based violence experienced by Indigenous womxn loomed in policy discussions both nationally and abroad (Kuokkanen, 2019). Notably, gender-discriminating provisions (read: social determinants) in the federal Indian Act have been condemned for producing and consequently naturalizing a patrilineal (patriarchal) social order. With its passage in 1876, "Status" (read: enfranchisement) as an "Indian" was legislated to "any male person of Indian blood reputed to belong to a particular band, and any child of such person and any woman who is lawfully married to such a person" (Gibbins and Ponting cited in Comack, 2012: 70). In other words, Indigenous womxn who unioned with non-Status men (so, their children) were legally disenfranchised from band membership and therefore stripped of what marginalized political rights and "reserve" lands were afforded under the Act.

The National Inquiry (2019a) details the usurp that the Indian Act has had over Indigenous self-determination and how it has mainstreamed gender-based differential treatment. An amendment in 1985 introduced a "second generation cut-off" whereby Indigenous womxn and their children, but not grandchildren, could apply to have their lost status reinstated. Effectively, "it did not address all the inequality and discrimination" (Palmater, 2011: 20) as reinstated status remained inferior to that of paternal counterparts whose children could carry it forward (Cotter, 2006: 154). Subsequent court decisions, including from the United Nations

Human Rights Committee (2019), have ruled in favour of Indigenous womxn, finding that the Government of Canada discriminates against them and their descendants.[4]

The devastating impact of over 150 years of structural injustices have culminated with 64% of Indigenous womxn living off-reserves, and in many ways, the gruesome 1992 murder of a Coast Salish mother in Vancouver's DTES (Martin and Walia, 2019). Every Valentine's Day since then, a Women's Memorial March has honoured the womxn who have disappeared from the inner-city neighbourhood (Culhane, 2003: 594). Their names and often photographs, screen-printed or sewn across shirts and banners, weigh heavy on the vulnerabilities (read: targeting) of womxn in the area (Hunt, 2014: 83). Customarily stopping at the former Vancouver Police headquarters, the annual gathering draws attention to the pattern of political failures and resultant predatory violence on the basis of race, class, genders, and sexualities, glaring but forsaken by society at large and law enforcement in particular (Oppal, 2012).

It was no coincidence that Feminists Deliver, a collective of BC-based feminists and rights groups, hung red dresses[5] inside the old police building before a livestream of the Closing Ceremony of the National Inquiry. With free admission, lunch, refreshments, and child-minding services (Cloma and Holliday, 2019), what would be a four-day event in the heart of DTES sought to carve out space for, and within, the margins. It was in juxtaposition to Women Deliver, promoted as "the world's largest conference on gender equality and the health, rights, and well-being of girls and women," from behind a paywall in the city's flagship convention centre. As stated on the official Feminists Deliver website (www.feministsdeliver.com):

> Feminists Deliver is a grassroots collaboration of BC-based Two-Spirit people, non-binary folks, Indigiqueer, trans women, lesbian women, and cis women and girls, and the organizations that support them, that have come together, on account of the 2019 Women Deliver Conference taking place in Vancouver, to:
>
> 1. shed a light on the urgent issues facing marginalized communities in BC and the grassroots struggles leading the way for transformative change;
> 2. build transnational connections between grassroots intersectional feminist movements;
> 3. re-envision the global women's agenda as one that centers a diversity of grassroots intersectional feminist voices; and
> 4. host a four-day conference and tradeshow.

Sylvia McAdam, one of the keynote speakers and co-founder of the Indigenous-led movement, Idle No More, emphasized the importance of 'delivering' on the diverse and inclusive (read: anti-oppression) mandate of the coalition. McAdam framed marginalization as a local issue as much as a transnational one, signaling that the existing power relations "would collapse if womxn refused to maintain them" (June 5, 2019). The argument rests on the strength of numbers and collective action. Interestingly, Kwakwaka'wakw Jody Wilson-Raybould, another keynote and the former Minister of Justice and Attorney General of Canada, took a more macro approach to social justice and denounced the current Canadian parliamentary system, which advances a mathematical majority at the expense of broadening our political process and decision-making machinations (June 6, 2019).

For Melina Laboucan-Massimo, Lubicon Cree environmentalist, gender equity is inextricably tied to the environment, so, climate justice (June 3, 2019). Her talk, "Violence against the Land Begets Violence against Women," opened Feminists Deliver with an earnest discussion of the unresolved death of her sister amid the thousands of MMIWG2SLGBTQQIA and the devastation of industrial extraction zones. Noting the Athabasca bitumen tar sands in northeastern Alberta, Laboucan–Massimo explained "the connections between violence against womxn and violence against the lands" and the overwhelming ruin that this has had (and is having) on Indigeneity:

> Womxn are not only the carriers of water, but they are the carriers of culture. Families are not only fighting for our womxn, but we are fighting to protect the very lands and the very existence of who we are as Indigenous peoples.

Through tears, she argued that the colonial technologies of (racial) hierarchy, patriarchy, and capitalism co-organize the exploitation of womxn like lands, and in turn, the "pillaging and rape […] of the fabric of Indigenous societies." Such ongoing (social and economic) impositions, enforced by the Indian Act and para/military armament, clear a way for the Canadian government to blur, complicate, and secure the acceptance and normalization of extractive practices (Preston, 2017) – once the residential schools system and eugenic sterilization, and therefore, inseparable from the "logics of elimination" (Wolfe, 2006).

In the context of this "Canadianness" (Preston, 2017), premised on "non-consensual inclusion" (Jurgutis, 2018) toward the erasure of Indigeneity (Belcourt, 2015; Tuck and Yang, 2012), Laboucan-Massimo questioned official narratives of reconciliation, and by proxy, whatever efforts may derive from the National Inquiry. On a global scale, she rejected that Canada could nor would heed the 1997 Kyoto Protocol and 2015 Paris Agreement to reduce anthropogenic greenhouse gas emissions and slow climate change for our collective futurity, let alone Indigenous lifeways. Extreme weather events, such as earthquakes, tsunamis, and hurricanes, as well as the increased rates of mosquitos, desertification, soil salinization, glacial retreat and sea-level rise, are exacerbating unsafe living and working conditions (Wedeman and Petruney, 2018). Often gendered, the task of collecting water, as one example identified by Laboucan-Massimo, is becoming more difficult if possible. Displacements due to environmental threats are increasing consequentially and the associated experiences of loss adversely impact structurally marginalized populations, not least, womxn and girls (Freedman, 2016).

B/ordering difference

Critical race, Indigenous, and Mad Studies have been instrumental in centring the biopolitical violence in the creation of "ideal types," so, the processes of differentiation to mark, justify, and culminate in a taxonomy of beings. Power, accordingly, hinges on the intelligibility of "populations" in concert with statistics and the gross standardization of experience through which social control can be essentialized and masked by normative boundaries (Foucault, 1997). It is precisely this separating logic, the emergence of 'b/orders'[6] that I scope as the frontier to our most pressing public issues.

In other words, I share the focus on "difference" as a category of analysis or social construction (Johnson, 2010; Perry, 2011). Deeply relational and responsive to context, difference forces us to rethink division. For Brighenti (2007), difference is grafted to "visibility," a more strategic framework for the social sciences. Leveraging Foucauldian models of surveillance, including the medical gaze, alongside Goffmanian performance, and literatures on moral panic and identitarian movements, Brighenti construes that the more visible a demarcation the more inherent (and invisible) the differential treatment (and indifference) may be perceived.

Of course, in/visibility as the byproduct of discourse is subjection (Foucault, 2006). But it also brings to surface "common" (ableist/sanist) sense-making through the valuation or role of "seeing" as differentiating evidence. Here, there is a noteworthy double-entendre: Empiricists have devoted considerable efforts to experiential knowledge, complicit in the colonial project to "rationalize" for taking (control), on the one hand, of the "uninhabited" lands of what is now North America, home at the time of "discovery" to 18 million Indigenous peoples (Monchalin, 2016: 61), and yet, on the other hand, of the pathologizable "delusions" or other symptoms for any given nonconforming narrative. "Same institutions, different stories?" to draw wryly from Gorman (2013: 217) and to question, per foundational concerns in Mad Studies, the paradox in visibility and "disqualification" of lived experience where it breaks from fields of view.

The constructedness and shifty (fault)lines of difference have been vexed time and again. For instance, genealogical approaches to "race" have done much to illuminate the multiple contradictory dimensions used to visibilize and group humans based on appearance, family history, or symbolic and interactional inferences (Roth, 2016). The issue of policing methodology has served as a central axis for differentialism, an umbrella term being used similar to other 'isms' to describe the effect of b/ordering or confluence of boundary- and hierarchy-making at once. As Comack (2012: 70) unpacks, Canadian nation-building (read: settler–colonial imperialism) has involved a number of strategies, one of which is the mythology aforementioned of *terra nullius* ("empty land") that pivots on the politics (ergo, visibility) of racial formation directed under the Indian Act. With it, a list of civil, criminal, and moral "offenses" became applicable only to "Indians." What Comack (2012: 23) demonstrates is that (settler) colonialism produces "deviance" in its production of difference, and by extension, enacts racialized policing (qualitatively distinct from racial profiling) together with "correctional" interventions.

Taken up by Joseph (2019: 169), the social regulatory function of "punishing difference" can be traced to ideals of Whiteness, much in the way that Fanon (2008: 111) derived the pathologization of Blackness upon "the slightest contact with the white world." Smith (2004) also evaluates Whiteness akin to normativity. Menzies and Palys (2006: 158) remind us that the constellation of eugenic institutions, at least with respect to Canada, were assembled historically by the "white male professionals who were often indifferent." But it is just not enough to make visible differentialism as the blueprint and all-pervasive ethos for understanding the b/orders of Canada, and further, the world. Living differently has foreground "problem populations" relative to power, fraught in law and policy, which generate a continual movement to "contain" the disparities (read: antagonisms) in ways that materialize on/in the body (politic) and fuel differentialist distortions as if unproblematic. The phenomenon of "over-representation" (Menzies and Palys, 2006) or "hypervisibility" (Reddy, 1998) prevails in well-researched Indigenous morbidity and mortality rates, decidedly genocidal in the National Inquiry. Jurgutis (2018) employs the notion of "colonial carcerality" to underscore the overlay of spatial and social exclusion within colonial violence, "literally mapped onto geographic locations" (Owusu-Bempah, 2017: 26) such as Indian reserves and residential schools, but also, urban "ghettos" like DTES, mental health institutions, prisons, and the immigration system. Fabris (2011: 3) adds that emergent technologies incarcerate even in the public domain by "routinely imposing drugs as restraints."

Structural mal/adjustment

The concept of differentialism is invaluable in exposing the "problem" of difference. It has helped us to understand the victimization, criminalization, and pathologization continuum (Chan and Chunn, 2014), leaving little agency *for* difference. This has been a crucial point of the disability movement as well. Many working within the movement have challenged rationalist (empirical) modes of the norm as having permeated the ideal and centre-outward hegemonically oriented systems (Garland-Thomson, 1997). Above all, the rise of industrialization conflated human worth with the "able"-body in terms of "productivity" and "efficiency" (Barnes et al., 1999). The focus turned to correcting, however possible, those who were "underdeveloped" or "deficit" and "economically problematic" (Chappell et al., 2001: 46) – or else, removing them from society "to the point of death" (Foucault, 1990: 138). Using a rights-based approach, the disability movement has interrogated "non"-able-bodiedness and catalyzed critical legal protections and practice reforms, namely linked to barrier removal and poverty reduction (Davidson, 2006).

My previous research brings into stark relief the shortcomings of the disability movement to build solidarities (Nabbali, 2009) and manifest anti-oppression work beyond "a series of discrete factors that can be isolated, added, or removed" (Cosgrove et al., 2019: 2). This is not to overlook the saliency of socioeconomic exclusion in disabling conditions (Nepveux, 2009). But much like "healthy public policy," which has gained traction for embedding the prioritization of "health" in civic decisions and programs (Orsini, 2007: 348), the disability movement fails to scale up and account for environmental "trigger" events (Fabris, 2011: 19)—those "push factors" (Fein, 2007: 44) that lead to the proliferation of risks (read: "at risk" or "high risk" categorizations) and thereby exalt the carcerality of b/orders.

Another way of advancing the same point is to consider how policy responses continue the violence of boundary- and hierarchy-making that, frankly put, "often ends with lifelong impairment and sometimes with horrifying 'accidental' death" (Fabris, 2011: 18). Gorman (2013: 271) argues that the under-theorization of disability has eclipsed wider considerations and "disallowed a focus on disablement caused by war, imperialism, and environmental destruction." As contribution, Kazami Hill (2019) "re-narrates" the living conditions of survivors, including veterans, of the Iran–Iraq War. By having to quantify or "prove" what happened to them (in the very service of b/orders), survivors go without access to care and their lived experiences of (post)conflict violence are unrecognized, if not silenced in death (given the prevalence of suicide). Kazami Hill analyzes "global-southern-ness," similarly to the work of Razack (2011: 352) on the medicalization of Indigenous bodies, as "beyond help" so "already dead" when deaths occur. What is being highlighted is the ongoing displacement of responsibility sustained through the health field and "context stripping" (Raphael and Bryant, 2002) such to privilege certain ways of knowing over Others.

In February 2013, I travelled to the Greater Accra Region to study the implementation of the Mental Health Act (Act 846) of Ghana, which had passed less than a year earlier and came into law by the end of 2012, replacing legislation from 1972 never realized. Act 846 followed six years of advocacy on the heels of the Disabled Persons Act (Act 715) which sought to elevate the social participation of disabled people in accordance with the disability movement and in tandem with activities of the African Decade of Persons with Disability (1999–2009). Heralded as another major milestone and "'new dawn' for mental health" (Doku et al., 2012), Act 846 came with the technical (read: rational) support of the World Health Organization (WHO) and set as the "example of WHO best practice" (Walker, 2015: 267).

Act 846 specifies 100 clauses to decentralize custodial "care" from the three psychiatric institutions in urban areas along the southern coast of the country (per colonialist investment patterns), engage the informal sector of traditional and faith healers, and integrate the oversight of all forms of (psy) subjects and related service delivery to a governing body for whom the Chief Executive came to be the Chief Psychiatrist. It was the constitution of this Mental Health Authority that raised the most controversy during my research. As reads clause 4(1):

The governing body of the Authority is a Board consisting of

(a) a chairperson,
(b) the Chief Executive of the Mental Health Authority who shall be the secretary of the Board,
(c) one representative from the Ministry responsible for Social Welfare not below the rank of a director,
(d) one representative of the Attorney-General not below the level of Principal State Attorney,
(e) one representative from the Ministry of Health not below the rank of a director,
(f) one representative from the Ministry of Interior not below the rank of a director,
(g) one representative from the Ghana Health Service not below the rank of a director,
(h) one person from a tertiary medical institution nominated by tertiary medical training institutions, and
(i) three non-governmental persons nominated by the Minister, at least one of whom is a woman.

Notwithstanding the dominance of medical bureaucratization and the more insidious implications of security in the Board's makeup, there were calls to formalize and guarantee the inclusion (read: voting rights) of "persons with experience as service users" in lieu of their consultative function per clause 3(a). The Board was inaugurated a few weeks after I left Ghana with no known amendment.[7] Members were appointed for a period of four years and up to two terms, save the indefinite authority of the Chief Executive as posited in clause 5(2).

The ethnographic fieldwork related to this project had a profound impact on me to which I have only been able to discuss cursorily (Nabbali, 2016). I have struggled to reconcile my presence in Ghana and the range of experiences, relationships, and stories that intimately and intricately shaped my (research) landscape and lens. On the front line was a network of womxn that I met through the Mental Health Society of Ghana, and who had formed, in 1996, the Mothers' Club of Nima-Maamobi before branding under the Red Cross Society (Buerger, 2016). Their work, entirely voluntary, is grounded in resilience building. In addition to weekly meetings and house-to-house education, such as sanitation and hygiene campaigns, as well as a breastfeeding support program, the Mothers' Club has launched petitions to draw attention to their underserved community, including the lack of streetlights and garbage removal (Perelman and Young, 2011). The womxn mobilize an annual Nima Clean-Up to rake a large open drain, forthrightly known as "Gutter," that snakes through, and separates, Nima (specifically Nima-East) as a formally designated "third class residential area" within the capital city of Accra (Aggrey-Korsah and Oppong, 2013). The womxn also facilitate fellows in First Aid because the ambulances, they stressed in conversation with me, are not able to navigate the narrow corridors of the neighbourhood. In cases of emergencies, the nearest capable persons would be needed as human lift to an arterial road for pick-up.

Gutter incarnates the spatial asymmetries and immediate environmental disturbances that serve the "discourses in distress," as framed by Orsini (2007: 355) to convey the creeping (neo-liberal) "responsibilization" of health/care in a climate where we are increasingly aware of countervailing forces. *This is madness*—the mollification of agitations through the language of risk that readies vectors of power, expressed modestly as harm reduction, at best, and structural adjustment, at worst. I must admit, it feels particularly 'risky' to critique public health infra-structure given my own everyday praxes to 'reduce harm' within the harmful spaces, systems, and institutions through which I move on stolen occupied land under the omnipresence of

BC's Opioid Overdose Public Health Emergency. Certainly, I wish neither to dismiss the activities of the Mothers' Club. To be as clear as ever willing, I am raising instead an aspiration beyond public health and healthy public policy, which easily tokenize empowerment through the diffusion of information (read: knowledge translation). As Orsini (2007: 355) puts it, oversimplified cause-and-effect now make "you [...] responsible for your own health" and "communities are urged to get busy building the necessary 'social capital' that will enable them to take charge of issues that affect them."

Reminiscent of the structural adjustment programs that swept across sub-Saharan Africa, including Ghana, to reverse "global" marginalization in the absence of a paradigm shift (Fergusson, 2007: 11), there is a growing effort to expose WHO literature and global mental health initiatives (Mills, 2014; Titchkosky and Aubrecht, 2015). I would be remiss not to spotlight the interjection that such works pose to non-profit, medical, and pharma industrial complexes. They have also had a major influence on my own thinkings. But it is unclear to me how a "politically informed societal determinants of health framework" (Cosgrove et al., 2019: 6) will do away with "eco-anxiety" (Clayton et al., 2017) however historicized. I ask only rhetorically, thought-provokingly; I have no interest in a deep dive into the brand of "chronic fear" (Doherty and Clayton, 2011) that is being debated in connection with detrimental ecological and deteriorating life-sustaining climate conditions. I do worry, though, about obstructing far-reaching forms of social/epistemic justice (Liegghio, 2013). Let us never forget the now preposterous label of "drapetomania" (Melzl, 2010), recorded when African slaves ran away or disrespected their "masters" and the larger conversation that it offers for "cure."

Fatal Toxicity and Anticolonial "Deviance"

The Athabasca tar sands, to circle back to Feminists Deliver and specifically the keynote of Laboucan-Massimo, are visible from space. More than twenty-six First Nations and Métis peoples have reported being immediately affected by the pace and scale of extractive bitumen megaprojects (Preston, 2017). Over 480 million gallons of toxic wastewater byproduct are dumped daily into unlined reservoirs, which leach into the surrounding ecosystems and poison subsistence-related activities (Huseman and Short cited in Preston, 2017: 4). In Fort McKay First Nation, a community in closest proximity to the tar sands and along the Athabasca River, members complain of skin rashes, asthma, rare cancers, and premature births (McCarthy, 2017). Approximately 350 kilometres south in Beaver Lake Cree Nation, 200 animals and amphibians died and over 300,000 kilograms of oily vegetation had to be removed following a series of oil spills in 2013 (Lamenan cited in Preston, 2017: 6). By May 2016, a state of emergency would be declared when a "wild" fire ravaged the region, burning more than 5000 square kilometres and resulting in the "largest prolonged evacuation in Canadian history" (Stacey, 2018: 857). While the fire halted tar sands operations, infrastructure linked to extraction development carried on.

Months before the fire was declared under control, the National Energy Board (NEB) of Canada would recommend the approval of the Trans Mountain pipeline expansion (TMX) to triple the capacity to transport bitumen products from the tar sands in Alberta to export terminals, here, along the Burrard Inlet where I sit and write today. The number of oil tankers required to route these waters for shipping would sevenfold (from 30–50 to 400 per year), intensifying the plight of marine wildlife, especially the critically endangered Southern Resident killer whales. Amid legal efforts to suspend construction, including a federal court ruling[8] that criticized the NEB for neither meaningfully consulting First Nations nor considering the increased project-related marine traffic in the environmental assessment, the Trudeau government purchased TMX in summer 2018, seemingly proclaiming political surety and outright indifference.

Southern Resident killer whales have become a visible icon—a rallying cry—of the gross injustices or "intergenerational curse" (Yong, 2018) of this moment in time. They tell a horrible tale of urgency and entangled ecologies, which do not stop at our shores, but of course, come from them and filter back to them. The carcass of Scarlet (J50), the orca calf on display for the world to grieve, was never recovered for a biopsy, but overall chemical exposure (in part due to reproductive transfer) is presumed to have played a central factor in her failed health. Persistent, bioaccumulative, and toxic substances (PBTs) are a class of compounds that highly resist degradation and have found their way through rainwater runoff and industrial dumping into oceans (Fisheries and Oceans Canada, 2019), surely not unlike byproduct of the tar sands. Ingested by plankton and successively up the food chain, the average adult Resident male carries six times the toxicity threshold (so, a compromised immune system) whereas their female counterparts transfer PBTs to offspring during gestation and lactation (Gaydos et al., 2004).

If, as Laboucan-Massimo suggests, violence against the land begets violence against womxn, then the (mis)management of issues related to the orca highlight not the moral outrage that they are, but existential abyss. The message is also coming from caribou that range on the east side of the Athabasca River and are fighting extinction by 2040 (Smitten and Lameman, 2010). It is coming from the Anishinaabe community of Grassy Narrows and over 100 other official drinking water advisories in Indigenous communities across Canada (Preston, 2017). It is coming from the people of Iceland that gathered during my writing process to hold a funeral for Okjokull, a 700-year-old glacier, which at the turn of the twentieth century, spanned nearly 40 square kilometres (Teirstein, 2019). It is coming from my mother who, only weeks prior, was diagnosed with Stage 4 kidney cancer. It is coming from the Mothers' Club and other stakeholders of the Mental Health Act of Ghana, as well as survivors of the Iran–Iraq War, demanding the persuasive recasting of deserving, and so, its resounding structural adjustment.

Analytically, it is untenable that such mounting, totalizing (personal, public, planetary) violence is not obvious to everyone. In effect, Canada would declare a "Climate Emergency" exactly two weeks after the final reporting of the National Inquiry. Among the recommendations to which Trudeau pledged was:

> 13.4 We call upon the federal, provincial, and territorial governments to fund further inquiries and studies in order to better understand the relationship between resource extraction and other development projects and violence against Indigenous women, girls, and 2SLGBTQQIA people.
>
> *(National Inquiry, 2019b: 196)*

Imagine the emotional confusion when his government 'delivered' a re-re-approval of TMX on the day after affirming the climate emergency. Rage would soon follow with the jail sentencing (read: delegitimization) of Rita Wong for peacefully blocking the entrance of a TMX work site.

Conclusion: Rightfully Mad (Studies)

Speaking on a panel on "Taking up the Calls for Justice in the Final Report of the National Inquiry," Kwagu'ł Sarah Hunt queried the value of making MMIWG2SLGBTQQIA visible if there is no justice (September 30, 2019). My purpose in this chapter has been to wrestle with such concern by organizing a critical history that sheds co-productive light on recent in/actions for ending violence. At core of the reflection is the date of June 3, 2019, when the National Inquiry tendered its final report and legal imperatives to end the genocide in Canada to which the federal government committed, Feminists Deliver emerged, and the cruise industry was exposed for flagrant crimes that further the connivance of policy in climate destabilization qua deathways.

Weary of prescriptions (to say the least), I have found great strength in the defiance offered by the "chaos" or "anti-narrative" of Frank (1995: 98), what has been gleaned as "telling without mediation, and speaking about oneself without being fully able to reflect on oneself." This recalls the expressed aims of Liegghio (2013) who journeyed with her mother through liver cancer and "mad talk" to "bring back into existence" nonconforming ways of knowing and being. Specifically, Liegghio (2013: 127) charged:

> It is not enough to give voice but one must think of voice in different ways—in ways that recognize difference as legitimate rather than measuring differences against a standard of *normal*.

I make no mistake that there is a simple path to a politics of difference (Young, 1990). However, I have tried to approach the coalition ethic of McAdam and spirit of Feminists Deliver by portraying the ways in which critical race, Indigenous, and Mad Studies are working against b/orders toward legitimacy.

Dedication

To Elizabeth.

Notes

1 Two-Spirit, lesbian, gay, bisexual, transgender, queer, questioning, intersex, asexual.
2 Gender justice organizing, propelled by intersectional feminism, has tended to replace the 'e' with 'x' as a more inclusive term to operationalize the diversity of, and thus, binary opposition to "womanness." I have chosen to follow this convention, removed of proper nouns and titles, not only for myself but for oral quotations as well. I wish to note that data, if disaggregated and gendered, rarely captures the wide(r) context of gender oppression.
3 An interim report of the National Inquiry into MMIWG expanded its mandate to include 2SLGBTQQIA people in Canada. While MMIWG2SLGBTQQIA is a mouthful, I would not want to further invisibilize the many marginalized bodies for whom the National Inquiry explicitly seeks to support.
4 On August 15, 2019, indeed while writing this chapter, provisions were announced by the Trudeau government to eliminate "all forms of inequity in Indian registration."
5 The REDress Project (www.redressproject.org) began in 2011 as an outdoor installation by Métis artist Jaime Black to highlight the national issue of missing and murdered Indigenous womxn.
6 While the forward slash is often used to mark a fraction or division in formal writing, or a line break in the case of poetry and songs, it is being mobilized throughout this chapter to collapse presented ideas. Notably, 'b/orders' seeks to evoke the separated yet inseparable – indeed, to conflate shared history and convey a shared predicament in lieu of the Latin preposition of *cum* (e.g., borders-cum-orders). It allows me to continue to think through the "order of things" (Foucault, 1994) where the organizing principle has been discussed as a "color-line" (Dubois, 1994) to a "border-line," accounting for "the effort to restrict territorial access" (Andreas, 2003: 78).
7 It bears acknowledging that one of the non-governmental persons appointed under 4(1)(i) was a founding member of MindFreedom Ghana and community organizer with the World Network of

Users & Survivors of Psychiatry. To my knowledge, there are 10 (not 11) Board members. Only two (of three) non-governmental persons were named; the second being a former director with the Ministry of Health.

8 *Tsleil-Waututh Nation v. Canada* (2018).

References

Aggrey-Korsah E and Oppong J (2013). Researching urban slum health in Nima, a slum in Accra. In J Weeks, A Hill and J Stoler (eds.) *Spatial Inequalities, Health, Poverty, and Place in Accra, Ghana*. New York: Springer, 109–124.

Andreas P (2003) Redrawing the line: Borders and security in the twenty-first century. *International Security* 28(2): 78–111.

Barnes C, Mercer G and Shakespeare T (1999) *Exploring Disability: A Sociological Introduction*. Cambridge: Polity.

Belcourt B-R (2015) Animal bodies, colonial subjects: (Re)locating animality in decolonial thought. *Societies* 5: 1–11.

Brighenti A (2007) Visibility: A category for the social sciences. *Current Sociology* 55(3): 323–342.

Buerger C (2016) Contested advocacy: Negotiating between rights and reciprocity in Nima and Maamobi, Ghana. In B Oomen, M Davis and M Grigolo (eds.) *Global Urban Justice: The Rise of Human Rights Cities*. Cambridge: Cambridge University, 1–21.

Chan W and Chunn D (2014) Intersectionality, crime, and criminal justice. In *Racialization, Crime, and Criminal Justice in Canada*. North York: University of Toronto, 27–38.

Chappell A, Goodley D and Lawthom R (2001) Making connections: The relevance of the social model of disability for people with learning difficulties. *British Journal of Learning Disabilities* 29(2): 45–50.

Clayton S et al. (2017) Mental health and our changing climate: Impacts, implications, and guidance. Technical paper presented to the American Psychological Association and ecoAmerica. https://www.apa.org/news/press/releases/2017/03/mental-health-climate.pdf Accessed: 12 November 2020.

Cloma E and Holliday E (2019) Women Deliver/Feminists Deliver: Reflections on activism and space. *Sad Magazine* 20 June. https://www.sadmag.ca/blog/2019/6/16/women-deliverfeminist-deliver-notes-and-reflections Accessed: 12 November 2020.

Comack E (2012) *Racialized Policing: Aboriginal People's Encounters with the Police*. Halifax: Fernwood.

Cosgrove L et al. (2019) A critical review of the Lancet Commission on global mental health and sustainable development: Time for a paradigm change. *Critical Public Health* 394: 1–7.

Cotter A (2006) *Race Matters: An International Legal Analysis of Race Discrimination*. London & New York: Routledge.

Culhane D (2003) Their spirits live within us: Aboriginal women in Downtown Eastside Vancouver emerging into visibility. *American Indian Quarterly* 27(3–4): 593–606.

Cuthbert L and Main D (2018) Orca mother drops calf, after unprecedented 17 days of mourning. *National Geographic* 13 August. https://www.nationalgeographic.com/animals/2018/08/orca-mourning-calf-killer-whale-northwest-news/ Accessed: 12 November 2020.

Davidson M (2006) Universal design: The work of disability in an age of globalization. In LJ Davis (ed.) *The Disability Studies Reader (Second Edition)*. New York & London: Routledge, 117–130.

Doherty T and Clayton S (2011) The psychological impacts of global climate change. *American Psychologist* 66(4): 265–276.

Du Bois WEB (1994) *The Souls of Black Folk*. Mineola: Dover.

Doku V, Wusu-Takyi A and Awakame J (2012) Implementing the Mental Health Act in Ghana: Any challenges ahead? *Ghana Medical Journal* 46(4): 241–250.

Fabris E (2011) *Tranquil Prisons: Chemical Incarcerations Under Community Treatment Orders*. Toronto: University of Toronto.

Fanon F (2008) *Black Skin, White Masks*, trans. R. Philcox. New York: Grove.

Fein H (2007) *Human Rights and Wrongs: Slavery, Terror, Genocide*. New York: Routledge.

Fergusson J (2007) *Global Shadows: Africa in the Neoliberal World Order*. Durham: Duke University.

Fisheries and Oceans Canada (2019) Cumulative effects assessment for Northern and Southern Resident killer whale (Orcinus orca) populations in the Northeast Pacific. *Canadian Science Advisory Secretariat* 056. https://www.dfo-mpo.gc.ca/csas-sccs/Publications/SAR-AS/2019/2019_030-eng.pdf

Foucault M (1990) *The History of Sexuality, Volume I: An Introduction*, trans. R. Hurley. New York: Pantheon.

Foucault M (1994) *The Order of Things: An Archaeology of Human Sciences*. New York: Vintage.

Foucault M (1997) *Society Must be Defended: Lectures at the Collège de France 1975-1976*, trans. D. Macey . New York: Picador.

Foucault M (2006) *History of Madness*, trans. J. Murphy and J. Khalfa. New York: Routledge.

Frank A (1995) *The Wounded Storyteller: Body, Illness, and Ethics*. Chicago and London: University of Chicago.

Freedman J (2016) Sexual and gender-based violence against refugee women: A hidden aspect of the refugee 'crisis.' *Reproductive Health Matters* 24(47): 18–26.

Garland-Thomson R (1997) *Extraordinary Bodies: Figuring Physical Disability in American Culture and Literature*. New York: Columbia University.

Gaydos et al. (2004) Evaluating potential infectious disease threats for Southern Resident killer whales, *Orcinus orca*: A model for endangered species. *Biological Conservation* 117: 253–262.

Gorman R (2013) Mad nation? Thinking through race, class, and mad identity politics. In B LeFrançois, R Menzies and G Reaume (eds.) *Mad Matters: A Critical Reader in Canadian Mad Studies*. Toronto: Canadian Scholars, 269–280.

Hunt S (2014) *Witnessing the Colonialscape: Lighting the Intimate Fires of Indigenous Legal Pluralism*. Unpublished Ph.D. dissertation. Simon Fraser University.

Jang D (2019) Last cruise ship of the 2019 season departs Canada Place tomorrow. Press release by the Port of Vancouver (October 31). https://www.portvancouver.com/news-and-media/news/last-cruise-ship-of-the-2019-season-departs-canada-place-tomorrow/ Accessed: 12 November 2020.

Johnson A (2010) The social construction of difference. In M Adams, WJ Blumenfeld, R Castañeda, HW Hackman, ML Peters and X Zúñiga (eds) *Readings for Diversity and Social Justice (2nd Edition)*. New York: Routledge, 15–20.

Joseph A (2019) Contemporary forms of legislative imprisonment and colonial violence in forensic mental health. In A Daley, L Costa and P Beresford (eds.) *Madness, Violence, and Power: A Critical Collection*. Toronto, Buffalo, and London: University of Toronto, 169–183.

Jurgutis J (2018) *Colonial Carcerality and International Relations: Imprisonment, Carceral Space, and Settler Colonial Governance in Canada*. Unpublished Ph.D. dissertation. McMaster University.

Kazami Hill S (2019) Whose disability (studies)? Defetishizing disablement of the Iranian survivors of the Iran-Iraq War by (re)telling their resilient narratives of survival. *Canadian Journal of Disability Studies* 8(2): 196–226.

Klein R (2008) *Paradise Lost at Sea: Rethinking Cruise Vacations*. Halifax: Fernwood.

Kuokkanen R (2019) *Restructuring Relations: Indigenous Self-Determination, Governance, and Gender*. New York: Oxford University.

Liegghio M (2013) A denial of being: Psychiatrization as epistemic violence. In B LeFrançois, R Menzies and G Reaume (eds.) *Mad Matters: A Critical Reader in Canadian Mad Studies*. Toronto: Canadian Scholars, 122–129.

Mahoney T, Jacod J and Hobson H (2017) Women and the criminal justice system. *Statistics Canada*. https://www150.statcan.gc.ca/n1/en/pub/89-503-x/2015001/article/14785-eng.pdf?st=J4R8qle0 Accessed: 1 July 2021.

Martin C and Walia H (2019) *Red Women Rising: Indigenous Women Survivors in Vancouver's Downtown Eastside*. Vancouver: Downtown Eastside Women's Centre. http://dewc.ca/wp-content/uploads/2019/03/MMIW-Report-Final-March-10-WEB.pdf Accessed:12 November 2020.

McCarthy S (2017) Where oil and water mix. *The Globe and Mail* 12 November. https://www.theglobeandmail.com/news/alberta/where-oil-and-water-mix-oil-sands-development-leaves-fort-mckays-indigenous-communitytorn/article27151333/ Accessed: 12 November 2020.

Menzies R and Palys T (2006) Turbulent spirits: Aboriginal patients in the British Columbia psychiatric system, 1879-1950. In J Moran and D Wright (eds) *Mental Health and Canadian Society: Historical Perspectives*. Montreal and Kingston: McGill-Queen's University, 149–175.

Metzl J (2010) *The Protest Psychosis: How Schizophrenia Became a Black Disease*. Boston: Beacon.

Mills C (2014) *Decolonizing Global Mental Health: The Psychiatrization of the Majority World*. New York: Routledge.

Monchalin L (2016) *The Colonial Problem: An Indigenous Perspective on Crime and Injustice in Canada*. Toronto and Tonawanda: University of Toronto.

Nabbali E (2009) A 'mad' critique of the social model of disability. *International Journal of Diversity in Organisations, Communities and Nations*, 9(4): 1–12.

Nabbali E (2016) On becoming 'White' through ethnographic fieldwork in Ghana: Are ideas imperial by course? *Language, Discourse, & Society* 4(1): 83–110.

National Inquiry into Missing and Murdered Indigenous Women and Girls (2019a) *Reclaiming Power and Place: The Final Report of the National Inquiry into Missing and Murdered Indigenous Women and Girls* (Volume 1a). https://www.mmiwg-ffada.ca/wp-content/uploads/2019/06/Final_Report_Vol_1a-1.pdf Accessed: 12 November 2020.

National Inquiry into Missing and Murdered Indigenous Women and Girls (2019b) *Reclaiming Power and Place: The Final Report of the National Inquiry into Missing and Murdered Indigenous Women and Girls* (Volume 1b). https://www.mmiwg-ffada.ca/wp-content/uploads/2019/06/Final_Report_Vol_1b.pdf Accessed: 12 November 2020.

Nepveux D (2009) *"In the Same Soup": Marginality, Vulnerability, and Belonging in Life Stories of Disabled Ghanaian Women.* Unpublished Ph.D. dissertation, University of Illinois at Chicago.

Oppal W (2012) *Forsaken: The Report of the Missing Women Commission of Inquiry.* https://missingwomen.library.uvic.ca/wp-content/uploads/2010/10/Forsaken-Vol-3-web-RGB.pdf Accessed: 12 November 2020.

Orsini M (2007) Discourses in distress: From 'health promotion' to 'population health' to 'you are responsible for your own health. In M Orisini and M Smith (eds) *Critical Policy Studies.* Vancouver and Toronto: University of British Columbia, 347–363.

Owusu-Bempah A (2017) Race and policing in historical context: Dehumanization and the policing of Black people in the 21st century. *Theoretical Criminology* 21(1): 23–34.

Palmater P (2011) *Beyond Blood: Rethinking Indigenous Identity.* Saskatoon: Purich.

Perelman J and Young K (2011) Freeing Mohammed Zakari: Rights as footprints. In L White and J Perelman (eds) *Stones of Hope: How African Activists Reclaim Human Rights to Challenge Global Poverty.* Stanford: Stanford University, 122–145.

Perry B (2011) Framing difference. In *Diversity, Crime, and Justice in Canada.* Don Mills: Oxford University, 16–38.

Preston J (2017) *Racial extractivism: Neoliberal White Settler Colonialism and Tar Sands Extraction.* Unpublished Ph.D. dissertation. York University.

Raphael D and Bryant T (2002) The limitations of population health as a model for a new public health. *Health Promotion International* 17(2): 189–199.

Razack S (2011) Timely deaths: Medicalizing the deaths of Aboriginal people in police custody. *Law, Culture, and the Humanities* 9(2): 352–374.

Reddy M (1998) Invisibility/hypervisibility: The paradox of normative whiteness. *Transformations: The Journal of Inclusive Scholarship and Pedagogy* 9(2): 55–64.

Roth W (2016) The multiple dimensions of race. *Ethnic and Racial Studies* 39(8): 1310–1338.

Smith P (2004) Whiteness, normal theory, and disability studies. *Disability Studies Quarterly* 24(2), n.pg.

Smitten S and Lameman R (2010) First Nations call for federal emergency order protecting caribou. https://raventrust.com/first-nations-call-for-federal-emergency-order-protecting-caribou-press-release/ Accessed: 12 November 2020.

Stacey J (2018) Vulnerability, Canadian disaster law, and the Beast. *Alberta Law Review* 55(4): 853–887.

Teirstein Z (2019) Here's why Iceland is mourning a dead glacier. *Grist*, August 19. https://grist.org/article/heres-why-iceland-is-mourning-a-dead-glacier/ Accessed: 12 November 2020.

Titchkosky T and Aubrecht K (2015) WHO's MIND, whose future? Mental health projects as colonial logics. *Social Identities* 21(1): 69–84.

Tuck E and Yang KW (2012) Decolonization is not a metaphor. *Decolonization: Indigeneity, Education, & Society* 1(1): 1–40.

United Nations Human Rights Committee (2019) Views adopted by the Committee under article 5(4) of the Optional Protocol, concerning communication no. 2020/2010. *International Convenant on Civil and Political Rights, January 11.* https://webcache.googleusercontent.com/search?q=cache:63c7xZdqjhQJ:https://tbinternet.ohchr.org/Treaties/CCPR/Shared%2520Documents/CAN/CCPR_C_124_D_2020_2010_28073_E.pdf+&cd=1&hl=en&ct=clnk&gl=ca Accessed: 12 November 2020.

Walker G (2015) Ghana Mental Health Act 2012: A qualitative study of challenges and priorities for implementation. *Ghana Medical Journal* 49(4): 266–274.

Wedeman N and Petruney T (2018) Invest in girls and women to tackle climate change and conserve the environment: Facts, solutions, case studies, and calls to action. *Women Deliver* (Policy Brief).

https://womendeliver.org/wp-content/uploads/2017/09/2019-10-D4G_Brief_ClimateChange.pdf Accessed: 12 November 2020.

Wolfe P (2006) Settler colonialism and the elimination of the Native. *Journal of Genocide Research* 8(4): 387–409.

Yong E (2018) The lingering curse that's killing killer whales: Long-banned pollutants called PCBs could wipe out many orca groups within the next century. *The Atlantic* September 27. https://www.theatlantic.com/science/archive/2018/09/pcbs-are-killing-killer-whales/571474/ Accessed: 12 November 2020.

Young I (1990) *Justice and the Politics of Difference*. Princeton: Princeton University.

29

SPIRITUALITY, PSYCHIATRY, AND MAD STUDIES

Lauren J. Tenney

Introduction

Some people uncomfortably chuckle when to their question of my academic field of practice I respond I am a Mad Social Scientist/Environmental Psychologist who conducts Survivor Research. Mad, in my thinking here is used to describe a righteous rage type of mad that does in fact exist and is not in the realm of psychiatrization. Psychiatrization, using this just as an example from an unlimited range of examples that people in the field of psychiatry have created, is the labeling of any person's actions as rooted in an inappropriate biologically instigated emotional response. This supposed inappropriate display of emotion is said by people in the fields of psychiatry and psychology, which are at odds with many people who have had spiritual experiences that include voices and visions, to be spurred by some kind of yet-to-be-proven-to-exist-biological damage.

People having their emotional responses or experiences of emotions psychiatrized is nothing new. Rae Unzicker, a grandmother of the modern human rights movement of people with psychiatric histories, who is sorely missed for her passions and organizing skills detailed what it was "To Be A Mental Patient":

> To be a mental patient is to never say what you mean, but to sound like you mean what you say. To be a mental patient is to act glad when you're sad and calm when you're mad, and to always be 'appropriate.' ... To be a mental patient is not to die, even if you want to – and not cry, and not hurt, and not be scared, and not be angry, and not be vulnerable, and not to laugh too loud – because, if you do, you only prove that you are a mental patient even if you are not. And so you become a no-thing, in a no-world, and you are not.
>
> *(Unzicker, 1984)*

People in the field of psychiatry, and some people in the field of psychology, support the notion that what are called symptoms of a 'mental illness' can be controlled with the (purchase and) use of biological or behavioral products, procedures, or practices that people in the field have labeled as medicine. However, these drugs, procedures, and practices often are not understood

DOI: 10.4324/9780429465444-34

in their form or function and are known to cause injuries and a multitude of damages and harm, including death.

Being psychiatrically assigned and confined to a psychiatric institution at fifteen years of age is what prompted what I see as my early righteous rage and determination to expose this system for the truth about it and its institutional design. The design of the system exploits real experiences of human suffering to help perpetuate itself; its purpose is clearly to maintain social control at a profit. This I have learned from stories people who have experienced severe forms of oppression and torture via the psychiatric system have shared with me over more than twenty-five years. My involvement with the Psychiatric Survivor and Human Rights Movements began around 1991. I was locked up in 1988. These factors remain my fuel for the work I do to try to expose the historical and contemporary realities of the institutional and structural design of psychiatry and its often non-cooperation with, but rather benefit from, tax-payer resources.

Guiding values and framework

In 1982, in Toronto, Canada, at the Tenth Annual International Conference on Human Rights and Against Psychiatric Oppression, a Declaration of Principles was written and adopted, and the human rights movement agreed to work toward implementing those principles. The principles speak for themselves and I will be relying on several of them throughout this chapter.

> Principle Three: We oppose involuntary psychiatric intervention because it is a violation of the individual's right to control his or her [their] own soul, mind, and body.
>
> *(Declaration of Principles, 1982)*

When someone has a spiritual experience, too often the psychiatric response is to fail to obtain the person's full informed consent, fail to explain their possible choices, and force them into compliance with clinical practices, procedures, and products. When constituting torture, murder, and slavery, these are all violations of human rights. A person's spiritual experience, which some people may identify as occurring within the realm of their souls, was considered as in need of mention to protect the rights of those involved with psychiatry by those who wrote the Declaration of Principles in 1982. This inclusion of the idea of a soul may be because the issues of the soul, or what others may describe as human experiences which one has the opportunity to seriously and deeply contemplate, has been a concern of the Human Rights Movement for those who experience psychiatric oppression.

Yvonne Z. Smith is a person for whom I have immense respect for and love. Throughout this piece, there are sections where I share Yvonne's direct review of an early draft of this work with you. She has some ideas about the way the world is that are quite different from mine. As I am someone who also rejects organized religion, although perhaps for differing reasons than Smith does, it is Smith's guidance that I go by when writing this piece:

> *I personally do not find religion comforting or faith at all but an assault on sensible things. If your condition is uncomfortable fight it, do not submit. As a rabid atheist, part of my recovery has been to throw off such beliefs.*
>
> *In fact, Lauren they serve as an irritant. Much more than an irritant I only think of God when I wish harm on someone. I never say I will pray for a person because that means I will pray for you to die. It conjures up uncomfortable feelings of helplessness. All manner of religious*

practices actually make me super angry. I don't like gospel music. I hate it when there is prayer in a group setting and usually will just leave its very unbearable. There is no grand design for us by somebody greater than me.

That is my opinion and I respect others beliefs if it gives them comfort. Psychiatry is doing the same as the slave breakers.

Also, I did not come to my conclusions on spirituality by any psychiatrist but on my own for what was making me uncomfortable in thought. Now for others it might be the opposite.

Everyone should find his or her own path.

For some people their religion or spirituality I think might serve the same as a rape victim who blacks out to avoid the horrible memories. For others it is a horrible memory the spirituality of helplessness. And pain.

I am sorry I cannot contribute more than this since I don't believe in religion.

It is my belief (lol) that Mad Studies can create opportunities for people to explore aspects of experiences concerning the soul, about which they are passionate and curious, and that Mad Studies can make this possible in ways that no other way of thinking might do.

Demons and deities: Possession states and rude awakenings

Over time, there have been fierce pendulum swings between making the heart of the problem either religious or biological. Ossa-Richardson points to a medical doctor, Richard Mead, who rejected the spiritual explanations of supposed insanity and in "1749, denied the existence of possession, and prescribed medical treatment for the insane: blood-letting, emetics, purgatives and other drugs, diet, and exercise" (2013: 553).

Possession, of course is still included as a concept in the newest diagnostic manual (*DSM-5*) published by the American Psychiatric Association, which is officially a lobby group. The diagnosis of Dissociative Identity Disorder includes possession-form presentations which are culturally determined for their level of acceptability versus diagnosability per the culture in which the said possession is experienced, and different than experiences of possession which are deemed a problem, which are now thought to be a part of Dissociative Identity Disorder:

> Possession-form identities in Dissociative Identity Disorder typically manifest as behaviors that appear as if a 'spirit,' supernatural being, or outside person has taken control, such that the individual begins speaking or acting in a distinctly different manner. For example, an individual's behavior may give the appearance that her identity has been replaced by the 'ghost' of a girl who committed suicide in the same community years before, speaking and acting as though she were still alive. Or an individual may be 'taken over' by a demon or deity, resulting in profound impairment, and demanding that the individual or a relative be punished for a past act, followed by more subtle periods of identity alteration. However, the majority of possession states around the world are normal, usually part of spiritual practice, and do not meet criteria for Dissociative Identity Disorder. The identities that arise during possession-form dissociative identity disorder present recurrently, are unwanted and involuntary, cause clinically significant distress or impairment (Criterion C), and are not a normal part of a broadly accepted cultural or religious practice (Criterion D).
>
> *(American Psychiatric Association, 2013: 293–294)*

Psychiatrized for spirituality: Emerging topics in survivor research

I present different ideas I have around these issues of spirituality, psychiatry, and Mad Studies that all have multiple dimensions gone fractal. But to be clear, for me, what it means to be a Survivor Researcher has forced me into spiritual crises I never even imagined possible.

The environmental community-based participatory action research project, (de)VOICED (Tenney, 2014) that was the basis of my dissertation research in the field of Environmental Psychology, explored the multiple ways in which people are silenced and retaliated against by organized psychiatry. For those who work in the peer industry, the retaliation is in response to what it is they say or do when publicly challenging the role of psychiatry, especially when trying to hold their employer accountable to the truth of the situation, including pointing out the lack of any actual science people in the field have for what they do and plenty of biological evidence of the injuries and death caused by psychiatric 'treatments.' Sometimes the retaliation people who work in the peer industry face takes place at an individual level, through psychiatric (re)assignment – where one is (re)diagnosed with some fraudulent psychiatric diagnosis instead of acting on the complaints.

Through the (de)VOICED research processes, patterns of the retaliation and silencing of people who challenged psychiatric authorities were uncovered as being committed at a systemic level. People who participated in (de)VOICED had worked in roles where they were 'out' as someone with a psychiatric history. Role titles such as: 'director of consumer affairs,' 'psychiatric survivor and activist,' 'ex-patient and advocate,' 'recipient affairs specialist,' 'person with lived experience,' 'survivor researcher,' 'ex-patient researcher,' 'consumer researcher,' 'psychiatrist with schizophrenia,' 'consumer liaison,' and/or 'peer counselor, peer specialist, peer leader,' and so on.

The types of retaliation people who challenge the status quo of organized psychiatry when they are employed in roles within the organization described included experiencing: being fired; being demoted; and being removed from a public platform, where opportunities of having an amplified voice as a conference speaker or spokesperson for an agency were removed, taken away, or canceled.

Part of my initial interest for looking at issues of spirituality and religion was directly related to issues that were sometimes brought up in (de)VOICED and discussed later in this chapter. Other Survivor Research such as the work of David Webb is also discussed later in this chapter, in the section, "What Are We Yet To Know?".

Critical feminist psychology and anti-psychiatry

Psychiatrization, or the act of psychiatrizing, is the act of medicalizing someone's experience because another person is dissatisfied with the first person's actions or speech or using the first person's behavior or speech … and that other person labels them with a psychiatric diagnosis. Thinkers and visionary leaders in the field of psychology, psychologists such as Paula J. Caplan, PhD (2020, 2015, 1995), in the United States and Bonnie Burstow, PhD in Canada, who is sorely missed, have each been researching and publishing about these realities of psychiatric diagnosis as a root of damage for decades.

Caplan calling the diagnosis itself the "first cause" of all other harm that follows under a psychiatric regime. Over the course of decades of research and involvement in professional activities at the highest levels of organization of the fields of psychiatry and psychology, Caplan has shown in a variety of ways, through research and exposing actual activities of the American Psychiatric Association, how people in the field of psychiatry have perpetrated fraud against those they claim to 'help.' Caplan does not only have vision but backs her work with actions.

Burstow, also for decades in a multitude of publications, research efforts, organizing, and activism, demonstrated the illegitimacy of the supposed science that people in the field of psychiatry puts forth and the breaks in conscience and ethics that proponents of the field have to take to implement the psychiatric agenda. For example, in *Psychiatry and the Business of Madness*, Burstow traced part of the development of psychiatry back to the fifteenth century classification systems that "distinguish witchcraft from insanity" (2015: 30) and directly linked these actions to the oppression of women and told how a "rather disturbing story involving power evolves" (2015: 30).

Burstow identifies The Church and women healers as "two of the medical doctors' major competition" (2015: 30) and that their competition wrongly, "positioned mad-doctoring itself as inherently humane and liberatory" (2015: 30). The development of psychiatry rested not only on the "business of psychiatry" but also the large variety of people, places, systems, laws, and regulations that act to sustain the structural design of psychiatry within societies.

Even though it can feel lonely, we must remember we are not alone in these efforts. Other people who publicly identify as having a psychiatric history also have focused on issues of spirituality both inside and outside of academic systems. Additionally, there are psychiatrists, psychologists, academic researchers, lawyers, and medical doctors who have spent lifetimes shining light on the ways in which psychiatric assignment harms people.

Prison psychiatry: Spirituality psychiatrized within the walls of a legalized system of slavery

A participant in (de)VOICED urged us to remember both the conditions created by prison psychiatry as they relate to spiritual experiences and to the development of policy and regulation. When discussing his experiences of forced psychiatry while in the prison system he offered:

> It'll make you cry. It'll make you bow down. You can't do nothing about it, man. You try and they will beat you down. Dope you up more. Give you more meds. Straightjacket you.
>
> *(Tenney, 2014)*

These were physical repercussions that came from expressing his spiritual experiences. He explained that it was when he was in prison that he was assigned a psychiatric diagnosis and that in part that psychiatric decision was based on his religious beliefs and spiritual experiences, he said:

> Your best bet, I guess with them, is to go ahead and go along with the program. Don't try to buck the system. They will make you move. But I do, I kind of buck the system, because I bring up God … Doctor asked me, you still hearing voices? No doc, I hear, I feel the voice now, and I feel it. Is it violent? No. It's like love, Doc, it's like, and it's like love. But I have to be careful, when I talk about G-O-D, because they think that's delusional. I'm delusional thinking or talking, so ante up his medication.
>
> *(Tenney, 2014)*

Later in my conversation with him, this person discussed a meeting he attended hosted by the Substance Abuse and Mental Health Services Administration (SAMHSA) of the United States as part of his work. He explained to me how at this meeting he discussed the importance of religious experiences – his own religious experiences. He explained how even among those who worked in the same capacity as himself, a 'peer' or someone who relies on personal experiences with psychiatry to do their work, many other People of Color understood what he meant, but white people did not express support for what he stated. He explained to me his spiritual perspective is part of the African American culture. And psychiatrists, and, he underscored, even white people who have been involved with psychiatry, often dismiss it. He offered:

> It's in the community. It goes deep, like I told you. It goes deep to slavery, all the way to slavery about that higher power. They were singing songs about Christ and God, coming over here. Being whipped and worked. Abused. Lynched. Burnt up. They were raising God at every aspect of their life. That's in me … I'm like, this is real.
>
> *(Tenney, 2014)*

For as many people as there are, there will be as many perspectives. What can we be sure of? It is our moral and ethical imperative to respond to the entirety of a situation, not just the way we experience it or want it to be. When reviewing an early version of this chapter, Yvonne Smith offered this response:

> *Spirituality in the sense as it is used in Psychiatry is a double-edged sword. Health care professionals compartmentalize religion, which commonly means that you say you are a person of faith but, you don't really believe that a deity can speak to you.*
>
> *Culture is discounted.*
>
> *For many people who have been raised in a particular faith religion is the fall back to things that they cannot answer. You will hear people say when someone, or a situation, or contact is unbearable that they will leave it all up to God. For some this is steeped in their cultural tradition. It also has allowed some to bear very uncomfortable situations without action. In fact, it is what White America, early on, has trained Black people to do. In the early days of slavery, Whites justified slavery because Africans were not converted to Christianity. Initially conversion was a pathway to freedom. That did not last long.*
>
> *Soon, one's skin color became a convenient reason to keep people enslaved a lifetime and to pass that condition to any children produced. It was convenient. In the Americas not only was skin color a way of identification, but it came with economic conveniences. For example, in many of the colonies importing slaves meant more land for the white settler. Labor was needed to produce crops for the British companies to send back to England.*
>
> *Not just in British colonies in North America but South America also.*
>
> *Africans who were kidnapped to America had their own religions but part of the breaking of the slave was to do away with their culture. People were forced to speak English.*
>
> *People were strongly penalized for worshipping their gods. People were indoctrinated into White man's religion with a promise of a freedom upon death.*
>
> *Bible stories provided relief. The bible is full of people being talked to and even having conversations with God and or other bodies.*
>
> *Much is made of the explanation of evil in the world.*
>
> *There was a war in heaven. Between god and the Devil. The devil lost and was kicked out, so the story goes. So why cannot humans have a battle like this going on, also?*
>
> *Psychiatry discounts the acculturation of people, black and white. For some people religion explains and gives comfort. For others it's a call to arms. Just as in some who have taken on a militarized form of Islam, Jihad, so to speak? Why do people fly into a building or become a*

suicide bomber? It is because they believe they will be rewarded in the afterlife. This is the concept that religions have of reward and comfort. Also, that they have a personal relationship with God. But this is or has been a conditioning technique used by others.

So why does a person have to be of deep belief in compartments? By compartment, I mean, the belief only is on the religious days and not all during their life, because religion is convenient for at first the government and now for psychiatry.

This is a good time to return to the Declaration of Principles (1982), Principle Eight reads: "We oppose the psychiatric system because it is an extra-legal parallel police force which suppresses cultural and political dissent." Fundamental to the conversation is how the modern U.S. police force and prison system, as well as criminal court system, are part of the maintenance of the modern system of slavery in the U.S., that was made legal through the Thirteenth Amendment, as a punishment for a crime duly convicted in 1865.

Many people are offended by this. It is offensive. However, we are so conditioned into accepting this system, that to challenge it causes uproar. To be clear, this argument in total considers the way someone's spiritual experiences or religious practices can and is used by psychiatry to involuntarily detain people, as an extra-legal police force.

As the asylum model in the US grew in the nineteenth century, the model was portrayed as a Quaker model. A model of "moral treatment" where there were beautiful fields for inmates to work and shops for them to build things. Labor was the treatment. As Phebe Davis (1855) explained, concerning her "two years and three months" stay at the Utica State Lunatic Asylum, it was equal to that of slavery, being forced to labor, in her situation, being forced to being a seamstress. From the establishing reports of the Utica State Lunatic Asylum, the Managers reported profits to the New York State Legislature from the products and wares the inmates created in the shops and cultivated on the farms. In the late nineteenth century, the managers used taxpayer resources to buy buildings and farmlands just for those purposes.

Certainly to the point of discussing how psychiatry maintains itself as a system through all of the other various actors and entities that hold it up, Burstow's (2015) *Psychiatry and the Business of Madness* explains in very plain terms how inter-related this all is and how it all relies on these fundamental frauds sold to the American people, and as Burstow points out, people around the world.

Religion and spirituality are essential parts of culture. Some people, however, consider religion as a center point of social control. Spiritual and religious practices that are out of the bounds of contextual norms are used as reasons that people can be apprehended and confined in psychiatric institutions, under the auspices of an extra-legal parallel police force to be institutionalized via psychiatry.

Psychiatrists, in terms of legal consequences, in 2020 still have a tremendous amount of power. Sadly, in a U.S. courtroom, and I suspect elsewhere, the testimony of a psychiatrist often has more power than the truth has power. Psychiatrists routinely also have more power than police, judges, and nearly anyone involved in jurisprudence, including the defendant. This was established as the focus of a committee on the first day of the American Psychiatric Association's existence, in 1844, when it was called the Association of Medical Superintendents of American Insane Institutions, ultimately creating the fields of forensic psychiatry and forensic psychology.

This matters to the issue of spirituality because since before the beginning of psychiatry's formal existence in the United States, people in its field have supported locking up people as inmates. The stripping of someone's identity kit (Goffman, 1959) and the mortification of self (Goffman, 1961), combined with deprivation of personal liberty and civil rights is sometimes enacted as punishment for a supposed crime but it is also sometimes enacted for 'religious excitement' and other subjective cultural ways of being, like possession-form presentations described in the modern psychiatric codes, the *DSM-5* (American Psychiatric Association, 2013).

What are we yet to know?

People's psychiatrization because of their spiritual or religious or other cultural beliefs and practices, or lack thereof, has been of concern as long as our modern human rights movement has existed. If you asked Elizabeth Packard (1868) in the nineteenth century if she thought psychiatrization based on religious ideas was a concern for human rights, she would probably say the concern was real then too. She names human rights as a concern in her expose of being institutionalized for her differing beliefs from her husband's. Her husband was a religious leader who mounted a petition campaign against Packard to have her locked away. She upon her release, became involved with the nineteenth-century Lunatics Liberation Movement and fought for the rights of freedom and for free communication while institutionalized.

It is the position of this work that in part, Mad Studies must take on issues of oppression and human rights violations caused by psychiatry with spirituality or religious issues as entrance points to the exploration. This work utilizes an anti-psychiatry framework, which does leave one to question what the point of creating any kind of research design concerning the field of psychiatry is, and the work that those in this field do.

A frustration that comes with using an antipsychiatry framework is that by focusing on psychiatry we just add to and build the system of psychiatry, even if the goal of the research is to deconstruct the phenomena or search for evidence for legitimacy for calls for abolishing certain practices, procedures, and products.

No matter how prepared we think we are for what we will learn when we take on the goal of trying to create research with emancipatory and liberatory underpinnings, our true aim of research is to find out information we did not even think to ask about in our initial inquiry. The goal of research is not to find information that confirms what one thinks they already know. We ought never stop there, particularly when asking questions about something as multifaceted as spirituality.

'What we are yet to know' realms exist and it is in those realms, when we reach them, if we reach them, that we can begin to explore places we never imagined, trying to see and understand larger patterns that may emerge over varying spans of time or snapshots of its moments.

Sometimes, prior to our understanding of its relevance, a 'what we are yet to know' place we find in data looks to us like utter nonsense.

When unsure of which way to go, consider returning to the individual, back to the original questioning point, or back to the idea that what we are trying to do is rip away the fraudulent notions that there is something medical underlying any psychiatric or psychological category.

David Webb is specific about this issue, and one of the recommendations he makes is to "demedicalise suicide" (2016: 94). When fraudulent psychiatric categories are called on to describe a spiritual experience by the people around that person who may not understand or agree with the expression of spirituality, an assault on the integrity of the person's spiritual experience is being made. The public has been conditioned to call in a psychiatric 'authority' to 'stop' it from occurring, resulting in the potential need for the person whose lived experience perhaps having a worse experience due to the psychiatric response to the spiritual experience rather than the spiritual experience itself.

Separating how you will examine what was direct to the spiritual experience and what was direct to responding to the assault of psychiatrization may be something you consider taking into your research design. In other words, when conducting research on spirituality and psychiatric response, try to separate what part of the result for the individual was from the spiritual experience, and what of the result, if any, was from the psychiatrization due to discussion or response to that spiritual experience. A negative response to a spiritual experience may actually be a negative response to the ways the spiritual experience was responded to by those surrounding the person. Through Mad Studies on spirituality and psychiatry, we have opportunities to create generalizable knowledge about both spirituality and the responses of psychiatry to spirituality.

User-led research conducted by Davidson et al. specified that:

> some participants talked about the valuable role their own spirituality or connection to something greater than themselves had played in their survival.
>
> *(2010: 111)*

Webb underscores this sentiment, "The suicidal urge to die only passed for me when I finally attended to the spiritual crisis that lay at its heart" (2010: 87). Kathryn Cascio, a survivor and human rights activist, responds to this work in the following way:

> *I agree with David Webb that someone contemplating suicide is in a spiritual crisis. I say this even if someone is an atheist. I am someone who has thought seriously about ending my life several times. My experience has taught me that when I am contemplating death, I am actually evaluating my life.*
>
> *It is so important for people to be able to talk about suicidal feelings safely, meaning without judgment, without someone trying to fix them or forcing them into the psychiatric industry.*
>
> *Although I am not a fan of labels, for the purpose of this response I will identify as a Buddhist, or more accurately, a student of Buddhist dharma. What I like about Buddhism is that it is not a religion. Buddhism is a philosophy. You work on yourself. It is about stripping away the ego and getting back to your primordial soul.*
>
> *I do not believe in an afterlife. This may change, but right now my belief is that we are energy and energy does not die.*
>
> *While I am here some days, I want it to end. Other days, days are a gift. I am trying my best to love people. After all, we are all stardust.*

The myriad ways spiritual experiences are denied, belittled, and diagnosed by organized psychiatry remains a staggering problem for protecting the human rights of people who are psychiatrically assigned. So, furthering Peter Beresford's suggestion that we take charge of our own research (2016: 30), I ask you, future Mad Studies people – in relation to spirituality, how do we create emancipatory lines of questioning that will aim to free people from the trappings of organized psychiatry? It is entirely necessary and centuries overdue.

I am not a religious person. I have some kind of agreement with some kind of entity greater than myself that excuses me from having to know the difference between left and right, east and west, or which phase of the calendar the moon may be in at any moment. I am someone, particularly as I entered my teens and early adulthood, who was psychiatrized (in part) for my beliefs about the etherworlds. Throughout my life I have sometimes been surprised by how some people have reacted to my ideas.

Each person on Earth has had these experiences of spirituality to some degree or another. Humans, whether accepting or rejecting the concepts, in all cultures across time, in all places in the world, have been thought to somehow contemplate how we are connected to the universe, what our purpose is, and if there is something greater than us, within us, or that we can join.

David Webb's work is an alternate analysis for how as a society we can think about one of the most difficult subjects for humans to discuss. Webb gives a concrete map to how the designs of organized psychiatry could immediately be changed by eliminating certain debasing practices that seem unnatural to have to even mention to trained professionals, such as his first suggestion, "Prohibit psychiatric violence – stop beating us up" (Webb, n.d.).

He brings forward terrific insights about what will happen if people begin to listen to those who have been suicidal and include our voices in descriptions of what it means to be suicidal. This is yet another prime example one would think we would not have to instruct researchers studying suicide to explore, and yet, here we are having to make these explanations. The perceived right of organized psychiatry to commit violence against people who are contemplating suicide is poignantly acknowledged by Webb:

> But the main reason, I believe, why suicidology pays so little attention to the suicidal person is that suicide is considered irrational madness, so, almost by definition, such people are seen to have nothing useful to contribute to the rational, scientific study of suicide. This is just one of numerous examples of how suicidology uses its scientific pretensions to exclude not only the spiritual and the subjective but also anything that it deems to be irrational. I think this also suits many suicidologists very nicely because many of them really do not want to have any real contact with actual suicidal people.
>
> *(2016: 87)*

Designing Mad Studies about spiritual or religious experiences

I do not define spirituality or religiosity or define the line (if any exists) that separates the two, with the exception that it seems to be as subjective and individual as any other aspect of what is to be discussed when it comes to any individual. Perhaps, as Sen and Sexton discuss, there is no direct guidance on how to get around the issue of where our inquiry begins – at the level of the individual, or at the collective. While the issue at hand is entirely different than the issues resulting from a participatory archive, Sen and Sexton pose a question that is entirely relevant to the design of spirituality-focused survivor research within mad studies:

> This raises questions around whether it is legitimate to take a life history approach that is individualistic, rather than collective, in its starting point … all starting points have strengths and weaknesses: in a collective there is a danger that the individual is lost; with an individual approach there is a danger that the collective (and its power) is dissolved. It seems that perhaps both are necessary and legitimate approaches that answer different needs.
>
> *(2016: 170–171)*

I do not at any point claim to have answers as to how to go forward, but perhaps, offer some questions to think about as you are plotting if and how you incorporate or reject ideas of spirituality within the dimensions of work that might be done using a lens of Mad Studies. I do see 'mad' as righteous rage.

You decide whether there is a battle among the etherworlds taking place or not over this, for I cannot be sure.

Perhaps it all comes simply to planetary motion, fate, and destiny. The work of David Lawrence Palmer (2020), a celebrity astrologer and intuitive known as the The Leo King, informs me. As Palmer instructs, there is a clear mathematical science of Astrology. Whatever one thinks about fate and destiny, the solar system inside of which we live, which undeniably exists, and can be mathematically charted backward and forward for centuries, as Palmer points out, even accommodating for differing calendars over millennia. Astrology possesses much more science than psychiatry has ever offered.

One of the ways that Psychiatry props itself up is by diminishing the role of spirituality in people's lives. It's been my experience that Introduction to Psychology courses actually use the study of Astrology to define pseudoscience. A basic (sacrilege) Wikipedia (2020) search will show, Astrology was ousted as "pseudoscience" as the "scientific revolution" began in the nineteenth century. To me, the degradation of the system of Astrology by people in the emerging field of Psychiatry was to divert attention from the fact that the alienists had no science of their own. It is my perspective that the only science psychiatry has today to show any evidence of what it does, is to show the immense damage and death that it causes. No other biological tests are available to confirm any supposed diagnosis they have created and believe one day they will find the scientific proof to match.

Whatever it is you or I believe, there is an unspoken weight about trying to construct a framework for something that can be so mysterious, so grand, so complex, and yet seen in the smallest fractions of time, in specs, glances, moments that sometimes can take a lifetime to process or understand. Often the type of spiritual experiences I am talking about are routinely denied as not even existing, and quickly pointed to as evidence for largely undefined, completely non-biologically based and socially determined psychiatric assignments.

Sometimes terrifying, sometimes exhilarating, often some mixture of unnamed moments adding to an incredible version of understanding that often when one tries to explain to someone who has not had their own, moment, shall we say, leads to the beginning of one's then being questioned, belittled, dismissed as insane. That cutting of what can seem to be the most genuinely clear moment an individual might have had, to something that is at the root of the problem, as opposed to, perhaps, the root of the solution, can be as much an issue of what it means to address spirituality within Mad Studies as any other thing can.

But a spiritual or religious experience is not always a message, or an insight, or the idea that you have some purpose to communicate to others. Sometimes it is something that happens when all other means of escape from the realities of one's life no longer serve one's needs and one has to come face to face with their own soul. The darkest moments can provoke the most beautiful light. What happens when one realizes that no one else, no one else at all being there will matter? We must be able to sit with ourselves without distractions, without our edges softened, without outright obliteration. We come to the point of where we accept ourselves for all our faults, misdoings, shortcomings, and outright failures, and come to believe that we have worth and are part of something larger. Or we don't. One outcome can lead us to a sense of euphoria and the other to a sense of torment, just being numb, or a range of possibility as wide as there are individual experiences, and within each experience, never-ending capacities for range.

Perhaps rejecting spirituality entirely seems attractive when one contemplates what it means to explore the darkness within us, around us, perhaps there is a fear that comes with it, what if we cannot find the light, what if the idea of the light is a fraud? Perhaps rejecting spirituality is the correct thing to do.

Some people do have positive, peaceful, and loving experiences of spirituality. Perhaps I have yet to reach that place of spirituality in earnest. Perhaps that is why I still even question at all or attempt to be able to express ideas that for those who are firmly rooted in a spiritual path may have trouble to understand. Perhaps a true sense of spirituality is still yet to come for me, perhaps questioning is part of the truth of it, for me.

My not knowing how others describe their senses of spirituality does not make their experiences any less necessary to contemplate than mine, or mine less than theirs, there is enough contemplation for everyone. The fact that in one reality it does not exist, does not make it not exist in other realities. Firmly, my own thoughts, my own intentions in this reality, do in reality influence the physical world and physical body in which I live and therefore, there is a consequence of actions that exist and are interchangeable, it becomes easy to understand, we really all are, one.

Oh, I know, for some we are still truly at the rejection or contemplation stages of multiple realities. This all makes it so difficult. My intention of having an honest contemplation of the subject as I experience these issues of spirituality is to encourage by practice others to consider their own stance, forthrightly with themselves. My goal is not for you agree with me. The goal is that you agree with you and one of the first and best ways of being sure of that is to really map out, or further detail, how you feel about these domains. This is important to do, so we will know how our own thoughts may be contributing to our research as our values and worldview seep into and inform every aspect of our work, at unconscious and conscious levels. It is important that we bring these motivations to the front of our thinking.

How do we choose or dismiss topics for research? What are the questions we ask, of whom, in what fashion? How do we track and analyze the information we collect? How and by whom will we have our work reviewed? In what ways will we present and disseminate our findings and analyses? How will the research enterprise be constructed? How will issues of informed consent be addressed? Who shall fund the execution of the design and under what terms? How will the research processes be evaluated and by whom? Who do we want to publish our conclusions and under what circumstances? What kinds of conflicts of interest might exist?

We would take all safeguards on such an endeavor as we would with any other type of study, including the possibility of results that dispute our own theories.

How can spirituality be taken on and explored by Mad Studies? How can it not be? How ought we talk and think about spirituality? In all ways except to ignore those aspects that are in direct competition with our own ideas, are things we disagree with, are seemingly impossible to us, or make us uncomfortable, or are things that we want to avoid. We were asked, are there other ways, other than organized psychiatry/psychology's horrendous or diminished attempts to ask questions as they relate to spirituality, within Mad Studies, to respect a person's ideas, to take seriously their experiences, to approach what they bring forward from the position of that individual or the collective, as the situation warrants.

The aspiration is that simply by including this chapter with all its limitations, that it will inspire future research designs focusing on spirituality via Mad Studies.

Are we inspired to produce future research designs grounded in values that lead us to think about spirituality away from psychiatry? Are we willing to pull apart the complexities of the topic of spirituality through our firsthand experiences? Are we ready and able to not be guided entirely by our rational brain, but that our knowledge comes in together with our hearts, and our talents, and our goals? Our souls? Can we write together from our thinking and feeling experiences? Can we try to give a sense of what is possible within Mad Studies that is not possible elsewhere? What kinds of approaches in our design can we take? What kinds of analyses can we potentially make through the data we collect? What kinds of knowledge do we urgently need to create?

I do not pretend to have these answers. Mad Studies, however, may offer us some avenues for conversations that will get us closer to understanding the variety of ways the topic of spirituality and Mad Studies intersect.

Foremost, this is a call to you, if you have not already done so, and if you are so inclined, to begin to develop your own research design about spirituality through the lens of Mad Studies.

References

American Psychiatric Association (2013) *Diagnostic and Statistical Manual of Mental Disorders*. 5th edn. Arlington, VA: American Psychiatric Association.

Beresford P (2016) The role of survivor knowledge in creating alternatives to psychiatry. In J Russo and A. Sweeney (eds) *Searching for a Rose Garden: Challenging Psychiatry, Fostering Mad Studies*. Monmouth: PCCS Books, 25–34.

Burstow B (2015) *Psychiatry and the business of madness: An ethical and epistemological accounting*. Palgrave Macmillan. https://doi.org/10.1057/9781137503855.

Burstow B (2020) The works of Doctor Bonnie Burstow, PhD. Retrieved on August 8, 2020 http://bizomadness.blogspot.com/.

Caplan P J (1995) *They say you're crazy: How the world's most powerful psychiatrists decide who's normal*. Reading, MA, US: Addison-Wesley/Addison Wesley Longman.

Caplan P J (2015) Diagnosisgate: Conflict of interest at the top of the psychiatric apparatus. *Aporia*, 7(1): 30–41.

Caplan P J (2020) The works of Doctor Paula Joan Caplan, PhD. Retrieved on August 8, 2020 http://www.paulajcaplan.net/.

Cascio K (2019) Personal communication. Review of this material.

Davidson, L., Shaw, J., Welborn, S., Mahon, B., Sirota, M., Gilbo, P., McDermid, M., Fazio, J., Gilbert, C., Breetz, S., Pelletier, J.F. (2010) "I don't know how to find my way in the world": Contributions of user-led research to transforming mental health practice. *Psychiatry: Interpersonal & Biological Processes*, 73(2), 101–113.

Davis, P B (1855) Two years and three months in the New York Lunatic Asylum and outlines of twenty years' peregrinations in Syracuse. Phebe B. Davis. http://resource.nlm.nih.gov/101173345

Goffman E (1959) *The Presentation of Self in Everyday Life*. New York: Anchor.

Goffman E (1961) *Asylums: Essays on the Social Situations of Mental Patients and Other Inmates*. New York: Anchor.

Ossa-Richardson A (2013) Possession or insanity? Two views from the Victorian lunatic asylum. *Journal of the History of Ideas*, 74(4), 553–575. Retrieved on June 30, 2021 http://www.jstor.org/stable/43290161.

Packard E P W (1868) *The Prisoners' Hidden Life: Insane asylums unveiled: As demonstrated by the report of the investigating committee of the Legislature of Illinois together with Mrs. Packard's coadjutors' testimony*. Chicago: A. B. Case Printer.

Palmer L D (2020) The works of David L. Palmer. The Leo King. (website). Retrieved on September 3, 2020 www.TheLeoKing.org.

Sen D and Sexton A (2016) More voice, less ventriloquism: Building a mental health recovery archive. In J. Russo and A. Sweeney (eds) *Searching for a Rose Garden: Challenging Psychiatry, Fostering Mad Studies*. Monmouth: PCCS Books, 163–171.

Smith Y (2019) Personal communication. Review of this material.

Tenney L J (2014) *(de)VOICED: Human rights now. (An environmental community-based participatory action research project)*. CUNY Academic Works. Retrieved on November 10, 2020 https://academicworks.cuny.edu/gc_etds/296.

Unzicker R (1984) To be a mental patient. Retrieved on November 10, 2020 http://www.narpa.org/reference/to_be_a_mental_patient.

Webb D (2010) *Thinking about Suicide: Contemplating and Comprehending the Urge to Die*. Ross-on-Wye, Herefordshire, UK: PCCS Books.

Webb D (2016) Thinking (differently) about suicide. In J Russo and A Sweeney (eds) *Searching for a Rose Garden: Challenging Psychiatry, Fostering Mad Studies*. Monmouth: PCCS Books, 86–96.

Webb D (no date) *Thinking about suicide.* Retrieved on September 23, 2018 https://thinkingaboutsuicide.org/.

Wikipedia (2020) *Astrology.* Retrieved on November 10, 2020 https://en.wikipedia.org/wiki/Astrology.

Acknowledgments

Special thanks to David Webb for his work and Yvonne Z. Smith, Kathryn Cascio for their reviews and comments on this piece. I am grateful to Jasna Russo, Kathy Boxall, and Peter Beresford for the opportunity to explore the topics of spirituality and psychiatry using a lens of Mad Studies. For their endless support, I am appreciative of Tracy Puglisi, Celia Brown, and Jennifer M. Padron. It is with much gratitude that I thank Richard J. Hall, and Paula J. Caplan for their thoughtful reviews and countless edits of this work. All errors are my own.

PART 5

Inquiring into the future for Mad Studies

30

TAKING MAD STUDIES BACK OUT INTO THE COMMUNITY

David Reville

Introduction

This chapter takes as its starting point an earlier chapter I wrote for *Mad Matters – A Critical Reader in Canadian Mad Studies* (LeFrançois et al, 2013), which was about the Mad Studies courses taught at Ryerson University in Canada. The Ryerson Mad Studies courses began in 2002, when Mad People's History was taught for the first time by Geoffrey Reaume, though the term 'Mad Studies' was not in use at that point. An outline for a second course, A History of Madness, was also written by Geoffrey Reaume but this wasn't offered until 2004, when I was hired to teach both courses – Mad People's History, and A History of Madness. The chapter I wrote for *Mad Matters* (Reville, 2013) talked about my experience of developing and delivering these courses at Ryerson and concluded with 'a recipe' for developing Mad Studies in the academy:

1. Find a way into the academy.
2. Once you're in, you have to find your way around.
3. That includes making alliances with like-minded people and making nice with the bureaucrats who make things happen.
4. You have to bring Mad students and teachers in, too.
5. Then you have to find your way back out into the community again (2013: 179).

The last stage of the recipe included a section headed *Taking Madness Back Out into the Community*, which argued that Mad people's history shouldn't be cloistered in the university. It also listed the Mad people's history talks I'd given, some of which were to the Mad community – organisations of mental health service users, or people who have survived psychiatry. Other talks were to mental health organisations or community groups. I also suggested using the internet as a way of getting Mad Studies out of the university. For example, Ryerson's School of Continuing Education uploaded three videos to YouTube in 2010 and 2011; these discuss Mad people's history, the consumer/survivor/ex-patient movement and self-labelling and identity. By 2018, these videos have had more than 45,000 views between them.[1]

In 2018, Kathy Boxall (who's based in Australia) got in touch asking if we could talk about what I'd written in *Mad Matters*. In November 2018, Kathy and I met via Skype for a

DOI: 10.4324/9780429465444-36

conversation about taking Madness back out into the community; the remaining pages of this chapter document that conversation.

Kathy   I wanted to ask you about what you say in your *Mad Matters* chapter (Reville, 2013: 178) about taking Madness back out into the community.

David   What I meant was to take Mad Studies back. I see Mad Studies as, not just an academic activity, but an activist activity. Given that Mad Studies is founded in the stories of Mad people, it's wrong to sequester those stories. Those stories need to be shared broadly – but primarily with Mad people. It worries me that Mad people don't know their own history of resistance and struggle and I think it's important that they do know that. I also think that dialogue between the community and the university is critical because a good part of that knowledge is going to come from the Mad community.

Kathy   But I was interested that you talked about taking *Madness* back out to the community. So, is there a difference between taking Mad Studies back out and taking Madness back out? I suppose what I'm asking is do we need Mad Studies, or could we do the Madness stuff, the Mad people's history stuff, without the academy?

David   I don't know. I don't know. Certainly, some of that work has indeed been done by the Mad community, without reference to the academy and I'm thinking of the work that Louise Pembroke (1996) did on self-harm, for instance. That wasn't an academic project, that was a grassroots knowledge creation exercise. And I'm thinking that some of Judi Chamberlin's historical stuff was the movement recording its history, although she did get connected with the Center for Psychiatric Rehabilitation at Boston University at some point.

Did you ever read a book called *Women look at psychiatry*? One of the editors was Dorothy Smith, the sociologist – Judi wrote a couple of chapters in that book (Chamberlin, 1975a, 1975b). It was in 1975 and Judi takes after feminists for speaking on behalf of Mad women. After reading that, I remember thinking, Wow was she ever astute – a very clever woman. She wrote her own book too – *On Our Own* (Chamberlin, 1988).

Kathy   A book I remember reading was Mary O'Hagan's (1993), *Stopovers On My Way Home from Mars*, where she compares extracts from her psychiatric records with what was going on for her at that time.

David   Yeah, I met Mary O'Hagan, she did some work in Canada.

Kathy   For me it was amazing when I read Louise Pembroke and Mary O'Hagan's books. I found out about them when I joined Survivors Speak Out. Before that, I had no idea that anything like that had been written. I was trying to make sense of my own experiences of psychiatry, with nothing from anyone else who'd had similar experiences, and it was an absolute revelation to read those books. But they didn't come from Mad studies, or from the academy – so the question I was asking before was: Do we need the academy, or can we do those things without the academy?

David   I think we can.

Kathy   So, what can the academy add to that fantastic work that was being done before? And you will know (because you will have been involved far earlier than me) all about the early Mad movement and what was done then. What does the academy add to that?

David It creates a location from which all sorts of things can happen. For instance, I used to teach Mad People's history informally with survivor groups. One of the things I benefited from was the presence of survivor groups to which I could go – they had their own structure and membership, which created an opportunity. If you don't have those groups, then the university can be the place that creates that opportunity. And maybe they can complement one another – the survivor groups and the university.

I think the other thing is the ability to run research projects. We've been able to bring in members of the Mad community as part of the research team, which is another way in which the academy can be beneficial for the Mad community. In 2009, we put together a group of Mad people and academics (some Mad, some not) to ask users what they thought about "recovery" (Mental Health "Recovery" Study Working Group, 2009). And in 2012, we put on an event called "Recovering our stories: a small act of resistance" (Costa et al, 2012).

One of the difficulties I spent time trying to figure out how to overcome was that many people in the Mad community don't go to university. They can't go to university, so how do you get them into the university, so I developed this workshop idea, but then I had to spend time finding sponsors for each of the students because they didn't have any money, and the academy doesn't do stuff for free. But I keep thinking that if you had tenured professors, they'd be in a position to do some of that stuff in way that contract staff can't.

Kathy But even if you've got tenured professors, you've still got the problem of students needing to pay fees to do the course.

David Yes, that's right.

We're taking one small step to solve the fee problem. Working for Change is an organisation which provides employment and education opportunities for people disadvantaged by systemic barriers.[2] The David Reville/Working for Change bursary in Mad People's History pays the fees for a member of the Working for Change community to take Mad People's History. We did the work earlier this year to make this an endowed award which means that it can go on in perpetuity (Ryerson Today, 2018).

Kathy I'm playing devil's advocate here, but it sounds like what you're saying is: bring the Mad people into the academy, so we can take Madness or Mad Studies back out to the community, and I'm wondering about that. Why do we need to bring everyone in, so we can take everything out again?

David Alright, because the other way to do that is for the academy to go to the community, as I used to do often. There's a wonderful survivor run organisation in Toronto called Sound Times[3] so I spent an afternoon at Sound Times, and spoke about Mad People's History. It was like a workshop and it was their space and I took a colleague with me, a Mad-identified student so that she could get a bit of practice in doing this kind of stuff, and I think that's a great thing for the academy to be doing. I think I said in my *Mad Matters* chapter that I did 20 or more speaking engagements in a year. I would always be talking about something to do with the Mad movement and, of course, that was to a wide range of audiences.

And I want to tell you about this new thing that I'm going to do. I discovered that there's something called The Life Institute,[4] it's an organisation that provides educational opportunities for people over the age of 50. There's a partnership between Life Institute and Ryerson University and I'm taking a course there right now. The course is called The Rock and Roll Era! I got to thinking that maybe I should teach a course at the Life Institute, so in January, I'm going to teach a version of A History of Madness to these students aged 50 plus – that will be a new venture for me. We will see if that takes Madness out to the community, or not!

Kathy   Another thing I wanted to ask was, when I read your *Mad Matters* chapter again yesterday, you talked about the numbers of students doing Mad People's History and mostly they weren't Mad-identified students. In a way, isn't that taking Madness back out into the community? Aren't those students who are not Mad-identified going to take their learning out with them when they finish university, to whatever they're going to do in life.

David   Many of them say that they will do that, particularly the ones in the helping professions, who say that the course was transformational, and that they will be approaching their clients or patients differently because they took that course.
I think one of the things that's amazing is that Ryerson has two courses – one is A History of Madness and the other is Mad People's History. The people who take the History of Madness are from all five faculties – so we have Engineers taking A History of Madness, as well as Social Workers, and people from Performing Arts – and it really has turned out to be an interesting opportunity to present an alternative to the medical model.

Kathy   I think there's no doubt that that kind of work has an impact on students, but I wonder about what happens when they get back out there into the mental health organisations, or even the ordinary social work or social welfare organisations where the medical model is so dominant. Can we teach enough students to be able to make a difference in those kinds of organisations, where the power's held by the people at the top, who've been around for the longest and haven't done Mad People's History at Ryerson University?

David   And they should be made to do it *[Laughs]*. I agree with you that we send these young people out with a new way of looking at things and they step into a space where that new way of looking at things is not welcomed, and what do they do about that? I think some of them manage to do their best with that. And some, not so much.

Kathy   That's no criticism of them really, given how powerful all these ideas are in those sorts of organisations, how powerful dominant medical model and individual deficit views are.

David   Yes, and I wonder the same thing often. I go to the Convocation and see the students from Disability Studies graduating, with a whole new way of looking at disability, and then they go back to work. And I think, 'Oh my God, we have made things so hard for these people?' And particularly in disability studies the students are primarily women, many of them are what we call 'visible minorities', many of them are mothers, some of them are single mothers. And they are all amazing, really amazing.

Kathy   And they have to earn an income when they finish their studies, and sometimes in order to do that they have to work in organisations where those medical model views dominate. I think it can be really hard for people to resist that, to work in those organisations and resist the medical model.

David   We have some managers now, the School has been around long enough now that some of our graduates are now managers, so they would be able to resist some of that pressure, I would think. One of our graduates, who comes to the summer awards that we have each year, runs an agency for people with developmental challenges, and she's the boss, so I think that would be a very different organisation.

Kathy   That's the work I did when I got out of the psychiatric hospital, working with people with developmental disabilities. I think it's easier in that arena than in the so called 'mental illness' arena, because people think we're mad and bad; but people with developmental disabilities are seen as deserving in a way that we're not.

David   Yes, yes.

Kathy   David, I like what you did in your Mad Matters chapter, at the end where you talk about a 'recipe' for Mad Studies, for getting Mad Studies *into* the academy. And I'm wondering if we could have a recipe for taking Madness, or Mad Studies *back out* to the community?

David   *[Laughs]* What do you think?

Kathy   Well I'm thinking, bring them in – bring Mad people into the academy – to start with, at the beginning of the recipe.

David   Certainly, bringing the Mad people in is part of the recipe. What I talked about in my *Mad Matters* chapter was how do you make sure that Mad knowledge is coming into the academy? And you do that by bringing in Mad teachers as well as Mad learners. But I think the really critical thing is to keep Mad Studies from becoming elitist, and one way you can do that is to make sure that you're in strong communication with the Mad community. The way I've seen that working is when those of us who are in the university have really strong connections with the Mad community and with people that aren't in the university. That's the trick I think, if the connections are strong between the university and the Mad community. Of course, it's easier if the Mad community is well organised and that certainly won't be everywhere.

I came into the university after a lifetime of community activism. That isn't the case for the high-knowledge crazies coming up. However, scholars like Jijian Voronka, Lucy Costa, Jenna Reid and Danielle Landry are active in the Mad community. What a resource these four women are! Jenna and Danielle are teaching A History of Madness and Mad People's History at Ryerson these days. Lucky Ryerson. Me, I continue to be on the board of Working for Change.

This brings me to another important topic: mentoring. I've been glad to be a mentor to others; and Danielle Landry and Kathryn Church write about mentoring in *Searching for a Rose Garden: Challenging Psychiatry* (Landry and Church, 2016).

Kathy   You talked about the Mad community being well organised, or not so well organised, can I ask about the inclusion of Indigenous people and other minorities in the Mad movement in Canada? In Australia, where I am now, there are university preparation courses, scholarships and support schemes for Aboriginal or Indigenous students – not for Mad Studies courses, but for courses generally – and it looks like you have similar schemes in Canada; for example, Indigenous Services Canada's programs to support First Nations and Inuit students.

David   Yeah, that's a place where maybe the academy can be especially helpful. Ryerson University is committed to supporting Indigenous students[5] – but outside the academy, my experience of the Mad movement is that it's mostly white. There are better connections with LGBTIQ people than there have been; but for visible minorities, not so much; Indigenous people, not so much. And part of that, I believe, is that being out as a Mad person is more dangerous, way more dangerous than it is for me – it's not dangerous at all for me, anymore. And the university, at least Ryerson University, is wonderfully multicultural, but there's still the issue around inclusion of Indigenous people in Mad scholarship. We just started to see some scholarship from visible minorities who are Mad-identified who are looking at those kinds of issues, but I'm not aware of anything like that from the Indigenous community in Canada.

Someone who's written about Indigenising the Mad movement is Louise Tam, one of the first South East Asians I knew in the Mad community – she has a chapter in *Mad Matters* (Tam, 2016).

Kathy   OK, so going back to this recipe – the recipe looks like you bring the Mad people into the academy or the university, and the university has a role to play here in bringing in students from diverse groups, and staff from diverse groups. So, what's the next stage of the recipe.

David   Well I think the academy has to go out into the community and to be very purposeful about that as well.

Kathy   So, do we want to offer a list of ways that they could do that?

David   Well, I think it's really a question of developing relationships with community leaders and then ways for the academy to assist will come to mind – I know they will – once those relationships have been built.

Kathy   When you say community leaders, do you mean community leaders in general? You don't just mean the mental health organisations, you mean the local politicians, the people that organise events in the Town Hall – do you mean all of those people?

David   Well that's becoming a very tall order to try and have that many relationships. I mean, clearly, you need to start with building relationships with leaders of the Mad community and sometimes that will include service providers, and sometimes not. There's an organisation in Canada called the Schizophrenia Society,[6] which is not a friend to the Mad movement at all. It's a carer organisation, they want the Mental Health Act amended so it's really easy to lock people up and force treatment on them! We've been at loggerheads with them forever. But that's certainly not the case with all individual family members and sometimes you can find an organisation which is very progressive.

One organisation is called the Canadian Mental Health Association,[7] which is organised provincially and locally and the local branch provides services. Parts of that organisation are very progressive, but they change from time to time too, so you have to sort of be alert, so for instance the local Canadian Mental Health Organisation sponsored students to come to my workshops and I think they sent a couple of staff as well as participants, so that's great when that can happen.

Kathy   I think we're getting there with the recipe. We've got that you bring the Mad people in, as learners, teachers and researchers, and the academy can help because universities have requirements around diversity and lots of diverse students are coming into the university, including Indigenous students. And then you start to take Mad Studies back out again, but we need to do that in a purposeful way, by building relationships and making connections with the community out there. That needs to start with Mad people's organisations, but can also be a range of other organisations. And we've also got the students from diverse backgrounds who come into the university to do the courses and take what they've learnt out to the community as well.

Is there anything else you want to add?

David   I can't think of anything else right now! Maybe it will come to me in the middle of the night!

Notes

1 See https://www.youtube.com/watch?v=AKBFYi6A6pA
2 See http://workingforchange.ca
3 http://soundtimes.com
4 https://www.thelifeinstitute.ca
5 https://www.ryerson.ca/content/dam/aboriginal-news/aboriginal-report-web.pdf
6 http://www.schizophrenia.ca
7 https://cmha.ca

References

Chamberlin J (1975a). Women's oppression and psychiatric oppression. In D E Smith and S David (eds) *Women Look at Psychiatry: We're Not Mad, we're Angry*. Vancouver: Press Gang Publishers, 39–46.

Chamberlin J (1975b). Struggling to be born. In D E Smith and S David (eds) (1975) *Women Look at Psychiatry: We're not Mad, We're Angry*. Vancouver: Press Gang Publishers, 53–57.

Chamberlin J (1988). *On Our Own: Patient Controlled Alternatives to the Mental Health System*. London: Mind.

Costa L, Voronka J, Landry D, Reid J, McFarlane B, Reville D and Church K (2012). "Recovering our stories": A small act of resistance. *Studies in Social Justice* 6(1): 85–101.

Landry D and Church K (2016). Teaching (like) crazy in a mad-positive school: Exploring the charms of recursion. In J Russo and A Sweeney (eds) *Searching for a Rose Garden: Challenging Psychiatry, Fostering Mad Studies*. Monmouth: PCCS Books, 172–182.

LeFrançois B, Menzies R and Reaume G (eds). (2013). *Mad Matters: A Critical Reader in Canadian Mad Studies*. Toronto: Canadian Scholars Press Inc.

Mental Health "Recovery" Study Working Group (2009). *Mental Health "Recovery": Users and Refusers. What do Psychiatric Survivors in Toronto Think about Mental Health "Recovery"?* Toronto: Wellesley Institute, Ryerson-RBC Institute for Disability Studies Research and Education.

O'Hagan M (1993). *Stopovers On My Way Home from Mars: A Journey into the Psychiatric Survivor Movement in the USA, Britain and the Netherlands* . London: Survivors Speak Out.

Pembroke L (ed). (1996). *Self-harm: Perspectives from Personal Experience*. London: Survivors Speak Out.

Reville D (2013). Is mad studies emerging as a new field of inquiry. In B LeFrançois, R Menzies and G Reaume (eds). *Mad Matters: A Critical Reader in Canadian Mad Studies*. Toronto: Canadian Scholars Press Inc., 170–180.

Ryerson Today (2018). *Disability Studies Award Carries David Reville's Legacy*. https://www.ryerson.ca/news-events/news/2018/07/disability-studies-award-carries-david-revilles-legacy/. Accessed: 20 December 2020.

Tam L (2016). Whither indigenising the mad movement? Theorizing the social relations of race and madness through conviviality. In B LeFrançois, R Menzies and G Reaume (eds) *Mad Matters: A Critical Reader in Canadian Mad Studies*. Toronto: Canadian Scholars Press Inc., 281–297.

31

INTERROGATING MAD STUDIES IN THE ACADEMY

Bridging the community/academy divide

Victoria Armstrong and Brenda A. LeFrançois

Introduction

We come together for the writing of this chapter as mad[1] activists from two different countries who have both advocated for, struggled with and actively engaged in the 'doings' of mad studies within the academy through the teaching and learning process. One of us (Victoria) hails from the north of England and was first inspired to 'do' mad studies in the community with the North East Mad Studies Forum after reading *Mad Matters* (LeFrançois et al., 2013). Victoria was then invited to co-teach a mad studies course at Northumbria University. The other one of us (Brenda) lives and works in the East Coast of Canada and, in addition to being one of the three co-editors of *Mad Matters* (LeFrançois et al., 2013), has been teaching mad studies courses at the undergraduate and graduate levels for several years at Memorial University of Newfoundland.

We first met each other in person in 2014 at the Mad Studies conference that was organised by the North East Mad Studies Forum (NEMS) and hosted at Durham University (LeFrançois, 2015; NEMS, 2015), although we had been meeting with each other virtually for several weeks leading up to the conference. Our communications with each other at the time and since have been mostly intense, with the sharing of our varied experiences of 'doing' mad studies and with critical debates about how it is done inside and outside the academy, including our visions for its democratic potentials and our concerns over neoliberal and power-infused co-optings. This chapter represents our bringing together on paper some of these experiences and theorisings that we have engaged in both separately and within our conversations with each other.

What follows, then, is a discussion of our experiences of bringing mad studies into the university, and our analyses of what mad studies courses might be, distinguishing them – however messily – from 'critical mental health' courses. In addition, we interrogate issues relating to power and mad knowledge dissemination in the classroom, including service user tokenism. In the spirit of engaging in mad democratic (Beckman and Davies, 2013; Davies and MPA Documentary Collective, 2013) pedagogical practices, we offer insights into the construction of a mad studies that bridges the academy/community divide.

DOI: 10.4324/9780429465444-37

Mad studies in the university: our experiences

Victoria

The publication of Mad Matters (LeFrançois et al., 2013) sparked my interest and involvement in 'Mad Studies'. I use inverted commas because I feel somewhat detached from it, unsure of what it means to me, and have reservations about the power at play in its doing. This chapter considers some of those challenges, along with the possibilities, in the telling of that journey which began for me in 2013 whilst I was part way through my PhD studies at Durham University, UK. My PhD (Armstrong, 2016) involved exploring concepts of stigma and discrimination in voluntary sector organisations designed to support people experiencing, or having experienced, mental distress. Whilst I was engaged in fieldwork in 2013 to 2014, I read Mad Matters and found it contemporary, critical, and innovative. The experiences of Mad people and their accounts were the focus of each and every contribution, chiming with some of the themes I was exploring and trying to understand via my fieldwork. For example – and I highlighted this in my review of Mad Matters (Armstrong, 2017) – the co-optation of Mad peoples' knowledge; the political appropriation of notions of peer support, anti-stigma campaigns and recovery models; and the collaborative exploration of new ways to resist oppressive practices and languages of a largely un-democratised psychiatry. I also surmised that whilst Mad Matters does not provide a blueprint to challenge oppression or necessarily do Mad studies, I felt that it provided us with a number of critical starting points and a foundation to move forward as activists, academics, and practitioners. Along with being critically cognisant that we occupy and negotiate many roles at any one time, and how that negotiation takes shape depends on a range of complex power relations.

Just before Mad Matters was published, me and Roz Austin, a postgraduate colleague from geography also studying at Durham University, were keen to set up a reading group of sorts to discuss 'mental health'. Due to our own lived experiences we both felt strongly that the group should foreground personal experience and knowledge in our engagement with texts and social theories. We both had good networks inside and outside of the university and so e-mails were sent, a small group of us got together, and we agreed to meet bi-monthly. When I became acquainted with Mad Matters, I enthusiastically introduced it to the group. I think that the group embraced the doing of Mad Studies because it provided us with a vehicle to do things our way, to organise ourselves, and think and speak collaboratively and critically of medical and psychiatric orthodoxy, the psy-disciplines, the impact of other experience(s) on madness such as family, abuse, work, welfare systems, along with failing public and health services, and the dominance of below par services which had shaped many of our lives. We agreed that we would call ourselves the North East Mad Studies Forum (NEMS) or some variation of that title. Due to our interest in Mad Studies, we also applied (with support from Durham University) to the Wellcome Trust for funding to hold the first international mad studies conference. An overarching aim of the conference was to create space to spark meaningful discussion.

Many people were invited and attended the bimonthly meetings, but a core group of us had crystallised by the time we found out that we had been successful in our Wellcome Trust bid and we made plans to hold the conference in Autumn 2015. Despite some criticism, it felt like a very special and engaging event, and what made it such an unforgettable and invaluable experience for me, was the way in which we organised ourselves and, in my opinion, did Mad Studies. It wasn't about someone taking the lead or dictating how it should be. Around five of us at any one time would sit down and discuss what the conference needed to be, what should be included, how it should be included. There were emotive discussions, hard discussions, each of us had our own experiences which we brought to the table impacting upon what we thought Mad Studies should be. But we sat together, listened to one another, cried and shouted a little too. It wasn't easy and it wasn't conventional. It was exhausting at times, but there was a democratic sense of equality about those working meetings that I have never before experienced. Although I had one foot in the academic camp, I understood that to do Mad Studies with the democracy it demanded, we had to work as a collective. This collaborative way of working was the only way through and it had something to do with equality. What I mean by equality isn't necessarily about coming from the same place or point of view, but there was a desire by all contributors to make it equal, along with a commitment to respect, and giving space to differing opinions. Often an easier way of doing things may be to give up, not give time or space, because it was too hard. However, to do this would be to emulate the institutions that had so often let us down, and we wanted no part in that sort of practise. We were very proud of what we achieved with that conference.

The group had been galvanised by the doing of the conference, the way we worked together, and facilitated the event. We had been particularly inspired by the folk at Queen Margaret University in Edinburgh (Bain et al., 2015), and began considering developing and delivering our own community course at Waddington Street in Durham.[2] Waddington Street is a small independent mental health resource centre with over 35 years of experience offering a wide range of informal educational activities and support services. The staff, trustees, and volunteers at the centre had been extremely supportive to our group and kindly provided a meeting space. As a result, we set to work on designing our 'community course' to be delivered in the Summer of 2016.

In terms of bringing mad studies into the university, in addition to the conference, I had also been involved in two other modules in 2014, which were instrumental in shaping my thoughts over this time. The first involved working with Toby Brandon who is a Reader in Disability and Mental Health at Northumbria University UK. Toby had a particular interest in research as co-production and wanted to develop and deliver a Mad Studies module, along with Alisdair Cameron who is Director of ReCoCo (The Recovery College Collective – a peer led mental health charity[3]) and team leader at Launchpad (a charity that offers the chance for anyone who uses mental health services in Newcastle upon Tyne to have their voice heard by the people who run these services[4]). Both Toby and Alisdair had attended a number of the North East Mad Studies Forum meetings and in 2014 I helped co-deliver an optional module for students on the joint honours BA degree programme linked to Disability Studies at Northumbria University. The module aimed to equip students with a cutting-edge critical appreciation of the meaning of madness within contemporary society, how it is constructed from different perspectives, and in doing so how both power and stigma are created and exercised. It was delivered via a combination of 'traditional' higher education methods (i.e. lectures and seminars) and assessed by a 3000-word written essay. The lecture topics were largely influenced by sociology and disability studies, and Toby and I often discussed whether we were teaching critical mental health studies as opposed to Mad Studies. For me, it didn't compare to what I had experienced when I was part of the collective and 'doing' Mad Studies to prepare for and deliver the conference, and how we were working to develop a community course. I think that the root of this was because there wasn't a particularly democratic division or sharing of power. It was the lecturers with the 'power'. That said, I explored other models for mad studies in the UK, specifically the Mad Studies course at Queen Margaret University in Edinburgh, and I was invited to deliver a guest lecture on my work on stigma. Influenced by the work at Ryerson University (Reaume, 2019; Reville, 2013) the course at Queen Margaret was developed in partnership with mad identified and mad positive academics and activists. It made me consider how mad studies could have a place in the academy, working more collaboratively, with a different distribution of power. Privately I wondered whether Mad Studies actually could ever belong in the academy. I felt that a rethink was in order and I was inspired by a relatively unrelated endeavour – the Inside-Out programme.

In 2014 I had become involved with the development and delivery of a criminology module exploring contemporary issues in criminal justice as part of the Inside-Out prison exchange programme at Durham University.[5] From 2014 until 2016, I was a teaching assistant on the programme and it strongly influenced how I began to think about how we might better do Mad Studies in the academy. I don't want to conflate criminality with madness, and I think that point ought to be made. Although there are parallels with incarceration and institutionalisation. Namely stereotypes, labels, and how experience is shaped by institution, as well as by exploring wider social structures which shape social inequalities and inequities such as those based on family composition, racism, classism, etc. Essentially, Inside-Out involves a class made up of 'Outside' students enrolled at Durham University and 'Inside' students incarcerated in the local prisons who were partners in the programme. The module provides the opportunity for 'Outside' students to connect with real world criminal justice issues, including imprisonment, and for 'Inside' students to place their own experiences of the criminal justice system in a wider academic context. The module is led by Professor Fiona Measham, facilitated by Durham University criminology staff, and places emphasis on the experience learning about crime and justice in the prison context and on learning with and from each other. 'Inside' and 'Outside' students work collaboratively as peers towards creating a critical and reflective dialogue around issues in criminal justice. The programme was first introduced and developed by Lori Pompa in the United States in 1997[6] with the aim of breaking down barriers and challenging stereotypes and prejudices by providing 'Inside' students and 'Outside' students with a unique opportunity to study together as peers behind the prison walls (Pompa, 2013). Most importantly, the context and method of delivery placed 'Inside' and 'Outside' students on an equal footing, as co-learners working together. It was also important that both inside and outside students received the same credits and the inside students could put these credits towards their degree studies. Taking all of my experiences together at that time, and upon reflection, I began to think that a similar approach could be developed for Mad Studies to work in the academy.

The Mad Studies module at Northumbria University is running again in 2018–19 as an option for the integrated health and social care degree programme. I am no longer part of its delivery, but it now involves 'service users' as students. However, as I understand it, they are not enrolled as students of the university because this would be too costly. Even when academics or institutions have the most honourable of intentions, we have seen how chasms open up and divisions are perpetuated. For example, the co-option of mad people in health services and in research, when mad people aren't paid the same rate or are rolled out to tell their stories as material for study (LeFrançois and Voronka, forthcoming). The power dynamics are inequitable, and it feels tokenistic. There is a violence to this tokenism, a sort of 'jolly violence' where we are told we are all the same ("let's all smile and use the language of inclusion"), whilst they capitalise on experiences of oppression for which the oppressed should be made to feel grateful.

The NEMS collective delivered their community course at Waddington Street in the summer of 2016 and we approached its development and delivery in a similar way to the conference. We opted for three-hour sessions for six weeks and included topics such as resistance, mad people's history, big pharma, and the history of confinement. The sessions involved creative exercises, much discussion, and reflective journals which were private to the participants unless they chose to share their thoughts. Members of the collective involved in each of the sessions were referred to pilots and co-pilots, we weren't lecturing or teaching, we were on a journey together.

During this time, many members of the core group also secured full-time employment and it was becoming difficult to find time to meet for any significant length of time. There was a realisation about how much time it took to really do mad studies. In addition, there was the emotional labour i.e., being prepared to spend more of yourself in a way that regular teaching or lecturing didn't demand. That said, I think every member of the group at that time would have been happy to be paid a proper salary to work on and deliver mad studies and do mad work, but the reality was that no institutions or funding bodies were queuing up to pay us. It was clear that we needed time and space to develop ideas and that couldn't happen when we were working 37-hour weeks (and the rest) in other roles. And so, for mad studies to work in the academy it requires time and space; components which are not natural bedfellows with the growing commercialisation of higher education, winning research funding, and writing publications. This is just my own account and journey. For me, at the moment, the battle for social justice, equality and equity IS mad studies rather than the content of what is being delivered.

Brenda

My context of bringing mad studies into the academy starts a bit earlier in time, when I was a student on the M.A. in Mental Health course between 1995-1997, a degree convened by psychiatric survivor Prof. David Brandon (1991), at Anglia Ruskin University in the UK. 'Mad studies' as a term had not yet been used at that point in time, but I understand myself to have been a student of mad studies through this course, nonetheless. Although very little is written about this programme of study (Khoo et al., 2004) and indeed as I understand it, the programme dissolved into a mainstream mental health nursing course shortly after David's death in 2001. It stands out to me, nonetheless, as an example of an early point in the evolution of what ultimately is now known as mad studies.

At its inception, the modules were co-developed between David and mad community members (or local service user groups, as they were termed at the time). The modules in this programme were mostly taught by academics who were also service users or psychiatric survivors, although the politics of the time did not demand being 'out' about these experiences. This is at a time when 'service user involvement' in education initiatives were only starting to be discussed, and in my view[7] this programme fell outside of those efforts, as the tokenism, sanist othering, stereotypical understandings/biomedical readings and disability tourism (Costa et al., 2012) that eventually came to characterise these 'inclusion' efforts did not appear to be present. The lecturers who taught us sometimes discussed their personal experiences but mostly did not. Their job was to teach us about mental health from a critical perspective, and given the hierarchical nature of the academy, they were in the position to make choices of concepts to cover, required readings and assignments, which were all undoubtedly influenced heavily by their personal experiences of psychiatrisation and (forced) treatment as well as by the mad communities who co-developed the modules. Indeed, the mental health module started with the study of what we now term mad people's history (Reaume, 2019; Reville, 2013; Bain et al., 2015), starting with Marjorie Kemp and following mostly the historical analyses of Roy Porter (1989, 1990). It then discussed psychiatric oppression followed by psychiatric survivor activism and current day mad cultural production. Being in this position of power as mad lecturers, allowed for a reversal of the typical imposition on students of professional knowledge as superior. However, as Victoria and I discuss below, this nonetheless remained a non-democratic process where mad students were not involved in the shaping of the courses nor were they overtly accepted into the programme as students,[8] which still leads us to question how we might truly madden the academy.

In addition to this course being taught mostly by mad lecturers, David also organised the bringing of mad communities into the classroom, in order to attempt to bridge the academic/community divide. There were members from politicised psychiatric survivor organisations and user-led services who came into the classroom throughout the two-year programme to discuss what activism and alternative interventions were taking place at a grassroots level. One such invited guest sticks out to me now as he did then. Peter Campbell (2006) of Survivors Speak Out (SSO) came in to discuss the activism taking place organised by SSO as well as to discuss the violence and oppression experienced by people within the mental health system. I particularly remember his discussion of adverse effects of psychiatric drugs such as tardive dyskinesia, demonstrating the effects to us in an embodied way. This was at a time when very few professionals in the UK ventured to suggest that psychiatric oppression was anything other than a delusion of patients. Peter Campbell's talk and presence in the classroom had a profound impact on me and marked the beginning of the (formal) politicisation of my own lived experiences of psychiatrisation. This was a life-changing moment; a moment of radicalisation from which I would not return. I continue to think that mad studies courses in the academy can offer such experiences to students today, however, the context in which we teach and the world we live in has changed dramatically since the mid-90s, and so too then must the way in which we think about mad studies in the academy.

Filled with fire in my belly, empowered by the mad teachings from this programme, I applied to do my PhD at the Tizard Centre at the University of Kent at Canterbury, making overt in my application form my status as someone who had been deemed 'mad'. I was surprised to see the question on the application form: Are you or have you ever been a mental health service user? This seemed progressive at the time and led me to assume that I was entering a space that was as politicised as the one I was leaving.

However, my experiences there were on the whole painful, distressing, isolating and oppressive. My 'service user' status being made known administratively, I was very quickly targeted by others in this space as problematic, as somehow wrong, as an unacceptable outsider. By many of the academics in the centre, my contributions were actively dismissed and expectations of me were low, in addition to other forms of sanist aggressions such as those that have been well detailed in Poole et al. (2012) as well as experiencing the type of epistemic injustice detailed by LeBlanc and Kinsella (2016) and the aspects of ethical loneliness detailed by de Bie (2019). I, however, was most caught unawares and was especially harmed by the viciousness I endured at the hands of other PhD students – students who were, unsurprisingly, intent on doing research 'on' instead of 'with' mad and disabled people, or who engaged academically in other forms of epistemological and methodological sanism and/or dis/ableism (LeFrançois and Voronka, forthcoming). It seems my presence in the academy most offended them, and in hindsight, perhaps intimidated them. I was harassed daily, my personal life was invaded and interrogated, and I was overtly made to feel unwelcomed and detested through an ever-changing violent barrage of being shouted at, ridiculed or ignored and excluded. I never asked for or expected support from those around me at the centre, but I also didn't expect to be actively attacked. That is, I just didn't expect them to put and keep their feet on my neck (Kadi, 1996). That being said, I did eventually share close friendships with some other PhD students, including some who were also deemed mad. Clearly, however, mad bodies were neither welcomed nor valued in this particular space at this particular time, which contrasts with the experiences detailed by Wolframe (2013) in a different space and time and leaves me with some hope for the maddening of the academy. Regardless, I left this space knowing it was not safe to be 'out' in the academy as mad. All of this provides us with important context to explain how it is that I did eventually come to bring mad studies into my own teachings, however hesitantly.

So how then do we bring mad bodies into the academy, when the potential for experiences of sanist violence is ever present? How do we even bring mad studies into the academy, if the experiences of mad people can be so violent and oppressive? My answers to those questions are exemplified in how I went about establishing myself in academia in Canada. Before completing my PhD, I was made to leave England (after almost a decade of living there) and return to Canada as I ran out of funding and was not able to demonstrate to the Home Office that I had sufficient funds to warrant an extension to my student visa (despite working three jobs whilst being a full-time student). Upon arrival in Canada, I found myself homeless in Hamilton for close to a year. While in provisional accommodation, I applied for many academic jobs, with little success given my status as ABD.[9] Eventually, I was offered an interview and later an academic position. Given my experiences of sanist violence and then homelessness, I re-invented myself as an ally to psychiatric survivors and service users and remained hidden inside this identity up until I was given tenure, and hence security and permanency in my work.

Over the past several years, I have been teaching what I consider mad studies courses at both the undergraduate and graduate levels at Memorial University in Newfoundland. I cannot stress enough that although there is the existence of some politicised mad people as well as mad cultural production in the East Coast of Canada (see for example, 'Our Voice/Notre Voix',[10] 'Mad Pride on the Rock' and 'Cracked on the Rock'[11]), in general mental health services remain mostly unaware of these critiques and continue to foster mainstream oppressive practices unchecked. Unlike in Canadian cities like Toronto, Vancouver and Montréal, both urban and rural spaces alike in the East Coast do not contain a critical mass of dissent towards psychiatric oppression. Mad communities, in their varied forms, remain tiny to non-existent within most of these spaces. This has created room for services to continue to openly oppress patients without any accountability, and with little to no criticism or public/community scrutiny. To exemplify this, when some community members got together in 2014 at the grassroots level to create a Hearing Voices Network (HVN) for Atlantic Canada – an alternative service that has been long established in the UK and other places and, indeed, has now been criticised by mad communities as being co-opted into the mainstream and reproducing psychiatric oppression[12] – it failed to take off effectively. Its failure was largely due to the psychiatric system fighting back hard against its establishment, including with threats to patients that their medication dosages would be increased if they dare attend any HVN meetings, as such attendance would demonstrate that they were becoming more 'unwell' (i.e.: not adhering to the psychiatric script of ignoring their voices and understanding them wholly as symptoms of psychopathology that need to be medicated away). There is no need for mental health services to attempt to co-opt grassroots alternatives in the East Coast, if they can merely squash with an iron fist such efforts from the beginning through threats and reprisals to those mad people who they are forcibly treating, either as involuntary patients in hospital and in the community, or as voluntary patients who need to toe the line in order to maintain their public housing arrangements, or keep custody of their children, etc.

It is in this context of uncompromisingly repressive power relations wielded by the psychiatric regime in the East Coast that I have begun to develop and teach mad studies courses geared to social work students. The first course I developed is an on-campus course, held for three hours once per week over twelve weeks. We cover topics starting with mad people's history, mad pride and mad cultural production to issues relating to psychiatric oppression and sanism. Social work students are asked to deconstruct the impact of social work's allegiance with oppressive practices within mental health services and to discuss their accountability to service users, based on anti-racist and anti-sanist values. Mid-term assignments involve getting students out into mad communities (usually virtually) and learning about survivor led services and other mad grassroots resources. The final assignment involves writing a paper outlining how they might work differently given the mad knowledges learned about in the course. I developed the reading list with the focus of both de-centring whiteness and de-centring sane-identified contributions. That is, at least two-thirds of the readings are authored by mad scholars. To de-centre whiteness, like Reaume (2019), I avoided putting Foucault and other dead white men as required reading, although there are many such academics and allies whose scholarship is useful for any discussion of mad studies. Given the need not to overload students with too many readings, I prioritise publications written by mad people of colour and by mad people who actively combine critical race, transnational feminist and anti-colonial theories with their mad theorisings. This is not a difficult de-centring task, given that I would say at the moment the most cutting-edge scholarship tends to be coming from mad people of colour and other authors who understand the deep connections between sanism, racism and colonialism (see for example Aho et al., 2017; Bruce, 2017; Chapman et al., 2014; Cohen, 2014; Davar, 2016; Joseph, 2014, 2015; Gorman, 2017; Gorman et al., 2013; Kalathil and Jones, 2016; Kanani, 2011; King, 2016; Meerei et al., 2016; Mills and Fernando, 2014; Nabbali, 2013; Patel, 2014). In one of the last iterations of this course, I consulted with an online mad studies community, regarding readings, and I had some guest speakers from the local community come in to lecture. The graduate level course I developed follows from this course although it is online only.

Not surprisingly, since the inception of my first undergraduate mad studies course, complaints rolled in from students, parents and colleagues. Indeed, mad studies was even mentioned disparagingly in an unrelated course in the university's medical school, presumably so as to make medical students aware of its subversive and supposedly dangerous doings. I am encouraged to think that they felt the need to take time to complain; the courses must be having an impact to elicit such strong reactions. I remain empowered by my tenured rank to continue this work knowing that formal reprisals against me are now prohibited. That being said, the informal reprisals – which are many – continue to take their toll on me, both physically and emotionally. Nonetheless, I remain uplifted by overwhelmingly strong anonymous student evaluations of both the mad studies courses that I am now teaching regularly. I am now developing a PhD-level mad studies course.

Regardless of these barometers of success, there remain problems with the delivery of these courses, that leads me, like Victoria, to question the extent to which mad studies has a place within the academy. I remain committed to the notion that one of the important characteristics of mad studies courses is that they bring students into the mad community and the mad community into the academy. However, the courses I teach do the former without the latter. Although some social work students in the courses identify as mad, this occurs by chance, and there is no way of purposefully opening up the courses to the wider mad community as enrolled students. In addition, unlike Reaume (2019), I am unable to allow mad people to audit the course, due to strict policies around students needing to meet the requirements of the programme in order to take the course. Regardless, I continue to look for ways to disrupt these requirements. Mad studies cannot exist without mad community (LeFrançois, 2016), and one mad body in the classroom does not a community make.

Mad Studies or critical mental health?

This leads us to a conversation we have both been having individually and with each other. How does mad studies in the academy differ from critical mental health courses? We remain inspired by the Oor Mad History course offered in Scotland (Bain et al., 2015), and greatly value the important pedagogical innovations engaged in by so many who have taken on the teaching of mad studies (Castrodale, 2017; Poole and Grant, 2018; Reaume, 2019; Reville, 2013; Snyder et al., 2019). We suggest that the difference must lay in the creation of courses that take up mad democratic principles (Beckman and Davies, 2013; Davies and MPA Documentary Collective, 2013) and are co-developed by mad community members and academics, whether those academics are mad-identified or not. The power relations endemic to the academy which bestows much status and power to individual academics must be rethought and re-managed so as to level the playing field for such collaborations to take place in an equitable manner. In addition to the co-development of courses, we also suggest that mad studies courses in the academy must be open to mad people as students, and in a way that neither requires the paying of expensive tuition nor denies mad people academic transcripts that indicate a mark and credits earned for having taken the course. How do we really bring mad studies into the university in this way, given the hierarchical, competitive and increasingly market-driven nature of the academy (Sweeney, 2016)? At the same time as we introduce mad studies to the academy, we witness the academy becoming more and more entrenched within white neoliberal ideals that exclude, bar, reject and pathologise mad people, some of whom may not have the finances to cover tuition, the academic credentials to be admitted into a course nor the confidence to take a seat next to those privileged students for whom the elitist academy ultimately exists. We remain concerned that the academic industrial complex is more likely to co-opt mad studies, turning it into something that is marketable and sanitised, rather than to open a wider space for mad communities and mad people to stake rightful claims to a place within the university as knowledge producers (Mills and LeFrançois, 2018) and as students.

Mad knowledge dissemination or service user tokenism?

We also question the extent to which mad knowledge may be disseminated within mad studies courses in the university. Even if the lecturer/instructor is mad, as was stated earlier by one of us: 'one mad body does not a community make'. In addition to mad people being students in the courses and mad scholarship being required reading, epistemic justice (LeBlanc and Kinsella, 2016) demands that mad people be valued as providing important contributions as co-instructors and/or as guest lecturers. We acknowledge vast differences here in relation to how this issue plays out both in Canada and in England. In the British context, service user involvement in higher education has meant the steady co-option and de-radicalisation of psychiatric survivor and mad politics, the tokenistic and stigmatised othering of service users' voices and the proliferation of disability tourism (Costa et al., 2012), without a hint of redressing the social inequalities and epistemic injustice (LeBlanc and Kinsella, 2016) that typically characterises mad–sane relations in the academy. In the Canadian context where service user involvement never really took off in higher education, we find in most universities, limited to no funding available to invite mad people into the classroom as guest lectures, and a complete devaluing by university administrators (and by academic colleagues) of the merits of such contributions. There remains little to no political impetus to force a change in this regard, which leaves mad studies courses in the hands of assigned (albeit usually mad) academic lecturers with little to no mad community involvement, unless mad people are willing to volunteer their time to guest lecture without being paid. The power relations and inequities inherent to this situation reproduce and magnify every sanist injustice found in the academy.

Conclusion: Bridging the community/academy divide

We hope that we might all begin to find ways to madden the academy sufficiently in order to create mad studies courses that are truly collaborative, epistemically just, and that bridge the academy/community divide in innovative ways. Based on a more democratic collaboration between mad people, mad communities and the academy, we suggest that perhaps a mad elaboration of the Inside-Out model might generate challenging solutions to some of the problems we have discussed above. That being said, it takes time to do things democratically, it takes emotional labour, but we owe it to Mad Studies to avoid easy wins in the academy by developing and delivering something that fits a more socially just and collaborative model. We need to avoid the soundbites that are the hallmarks of contemporary western life, from anti-stigma campaigns to recovery stories we should all aspire to. A way to do this may be to follow the Inside-Out model by ensuring all (mad) students are enrolled onto the module as students with credits to contribute towards degrees, that we reconsider the academy as the place to do Mad Studies and that we look instead to institutional and/or community settings to deliver modules. However, this will be hard with cutbacks and in times of 'austerity' but if universities want to trailblaze they will have to want us to be there, put in the graft, not see us as a nuisance, and provide the practical and financial support.

Notes

1 We use the term 'mad' as it is the language that is most often used by people who ascribe to mad studies, especially in Canada. We acknowledge, however, following Gorman et al. (2013) that not all people who have been deemed mad choose to use the term 'mad'. Using this type of political language is not always safe, especially for more marginalised mad community members, whose experiences of psychiatrisation may be further complicated by the violences of racism, sexism, classism, cisgenderism and heterosexism. We, nonetheless, choose to use the term 'mad' here as a reclaimed term in order to unsettle and contest notions of psychiatric and biogenetic reductionism in understanding experiences of altered states of mind, extreme emotions as well as unusual thoughts and behaviour. As such, we refer to 'mad people', 'mad community members', 'mad lecturers', 'mad bodies', 'mad students', 'mad theorisings', 'mad history', 'mad activists', 'mad scholars', 'mad democratic practices', mad knowledge', 'mad communities', 'mad politics', 'mad teachings', 'mad pride', etc., in the spirit of contestation and reclamation.

2 https://www.waddingtoncentre.co.uk/

3 https://www.recoverycoco.com/

4 https://launchpadncl.org.uk/

5 https://www.dur.ac.uk/sociology/crim/insideout/

6 See http://www.insideoutcenter.org/

7 My view here is in contrast to the ways in which the course has been framed within Khoo et al. (2004). However, I do not believe that we would be in disagreement today (the article having been written in 2004) about the ways in which this course differed dramatically from the ways in which service user involvement in education has ultimately become established.

8 See Snyder et al. (2019) for innovating pedagogical approaches to student collaboration, including rhizomatic learning.

9 *All But Dissertation:* A designation for PhD students in Canada that denotes that all requirements for the doctorate have been completed other than the written dissertation.

10 https://www.ourvoice-notrevoix.com/

11 https://www.facebook.com/Madontherock/

12 The point I am trying to make here is that even alternative services that are no longer seen as radical in most places in the Western world – and are no longer even seen as critical or potentially empowering by mad communities as their grassroots origins and visions become distorted through psychiatric co-option – are still fought off by the monolithic psy system in places where mad dissenting voices are less organised and influential.

References

Aho T, Ben-Moshe L and Hilton L (2017) Mad Futures: Affect/theory/violence. *American Quarterly*, *69*(2), 291–302.

Armstrong V E (2016) *Mental Distress and Stigma: Exploring the Significance of Interactions in the Context of Support Provision*. Doctoral thesis, Durham University. http://etheses.dur.ac.uk/11435/ Accessed: 14 July 2020.

Armstrong V E (2017) Mad matters: A critical reader in Canadian mad studies. *Qualitative Social Work*, *16*(1), 152–155.

Bain M, Ballantyne E, Bell C, Collie S-A and Fullerton L (2015) *Doing Mad Studies: Experiences, Influences and Impacts. How Was It for Us?* Paper presented at the conference Making Sense of Mad Studies, Durham University, Durham, UK.

Beckman L and Davies M J (2013) Democracy is a very radical idea. In B A LeFrançois, R Menzies and G Reaume (Eds.). *Mad Matters: A Critical Reader in Canadian Mad Studies*. Toronto, ON: Canadian Scholars' Press, 46–63.

Brandon D (1991) *Innovation Without Change? Consumer Power in Psychiatric Services*. London: Palgrave Macmillan.

Bruce L J (2017). Mad is a place: Or, the slave ship tows the ship of fools. *American Quarterly*, *69*(2), 303–308.

Campbell P (2006). Changing the mental health system – A survivor's view. *Journal of Psychiatric and Mental Health Nursing*, *13*(5), 578–580.

Castrodale M A (2017). Critical disability studies and mad studies: Enabling new pedagogies in practice. *The Canadian Journal for the Study of Adult Education, 29(1)*, 49–66.

Chapman C, Carey A C and Ben-Moshe L (2014). Reconsidering confinement: Interlocking locations and logics of incarceration. In L Ben-Moshe, C Chapman and A Carey (Eds.). *Disability Incarcerated: Imprisonment and Disability in the United States and Canada*. New York: Palgrave Macmillan, 3–24.

Cohen B M Z (2014) Passive-aggressive: Maori resistance and the continuance of colonial psychiatry in Aotearoa New Zealand. *Disability and the Global South, 1*(2), 319–339.

Costa L, Voronka J, Landry D, Reid J, McFarlane B, Reville D and Church K (2012). "Recovering our stories": A small act of resistance. *Studies in Social Justice, 6*(1), 85–101.

Davar B (2016) Alternatives or a way of life? In J Russo and A Sweeney (Eds.). *Searching for a Rose Garden: Challenging Psychiatry, Fostering Mad Studies*. Wyastone Leys, UK: PCCS Books, 14-19.

Davies M J and MPA Documentary Collective (2013). *The Inmates are Running the Asylum: Stories from MPA* [Documentary]. Canada: History of Madness Productions.

De Bie A (2019). *Living a Mad Politics*. (Doctoral dissertation). McMaster University, Hamilton, ON, Canada.

Gorman R (2017) Quagmires of affect: Labor, whiteness, and ideological disavowal. *American Quarterly*, *69*(2), 309–313.

Gorman R, saini a, Tam L, Udegbe O, and Usar O. (2013) Mad people of color—A manifesto, *Asylum*, *20*(4), 27.

Joseph A J (2014) A prescription for violence: The legacy of colonization in contemporary forensic mental health and the production of difference. *Critical Criminology, 22*, 273–292.

Joseph A J (2015) The necessity of an attention to Eurocentrism and colonial technologies: An addition to critical mental health literature. *Disability & Society, 30*(7), 1021–1041.

Kadi J (1996). *Thinking Class: Sketches from a Cultural Worker*. Boston, MA: South End Press.

Kalathil J and Jones N (2016) Unsettling disciplines: Madness, identity, research, knowledge. *Philosophy, Psychiatry, Psychology*, 23(3/4), 183–188.

Kanani N (2011) Race and madness: Locating the experiences of racialized people with psychiatric histories in Canada and the United States. *Critical Disability Discourse, 3*, 1–14.

Khoo R, McVicar A and Brandon D (2004) Service user involvement in postgraduate mental health education. Does it benefit practice? *Journal of Mental Health*, *13*(5), 481–492.

King C (2016) Whiteness in psychiatry: The madness of European misdiagnoses. In J Russo and A Sweeney (Eds.). *Searching for a Rose Garden: Challenging Psychiatry, Fostering Mad Studies*. Wyastone Leys, UK: PCCS Books, 69–76.

LeBlanc S and Kinsella E A (2016). Toward epistemic justice: A critically reflexive examination of 'sanism' and implications for knowledge generation. *Studies in Social Justice, 10*(1), 59–78.

LeFrançois B A (2015) *Acknowledging the Past and Challenging the Present, in Contemplation of the Future: Some (Un)doings of Mad Studies.* Paper presented at the conference Making Sense of Mad Studies, Durham University, Durham, UK.

LeFrançois B A (2016) Preface. In J Russo and A Sweeney (Eds.). *Searching for a Rose Garden: Challenging Psychiatry, Fostering Mad Studies.* Wyastone Leys, UK: PCCS Books, v–viii.

LeFrançois B A and Voronka J (forthcoming) Mad epistemologies and the ethics of knowledge production. In T Macias (Ed.). *Unravelling Research: The Ethics and Politics of Knowledge Production in the Social Sciences.* Toronto: Canadian Scholars' Press.

LeFrançois, B A, Menzies, R and Reaume G (2013) *Mad Matters: A Critical Anthology of Canadian Mad Studies.* Toronto: Canadian Scholars Press.

Meerei S, Abdillahi I and Poole J M (2016) An introduction to anti-black sanism. *Intersectionalities, 5*(3), 18–35.

Mills C and Fernando S (2014) Globalising mental health or pathologizing the global south? Mapping the ethics, theory and practice of global mental health. *Disability and the Global South, 1*(2), 188–202.

Mills C and LeFrançois B A (2018) Child as metaphor: Colonialism, psy-governance and epistemicide. *World Futures, 74,* 503–524.

Nabbali E M (2013) "Mad" activism and its (Ghanian?) future: A prolegomena to debate. *Trans-Scripts, 3,* 178–201.

North East Mad Studies (NEMS) (2015) Making Sense of Mad Studies conference. Durham University, Durham, UK.

Patel S (2014) Racing madness: The terrorizing madness of the post-9/11 terrorist body. In L Ben-Moshe, C Chapman and A C Carey (Eds.). *Disability incarcerated: Imprisonment and disability in the United States and Canada.* New York, NY: Palgrave Macmillan, 201–215.

Pompa L (2013) One brick at a Time: The Power and Possibility of Dialogue Across the Prison Wall. *The Prison Journal, 93*(2), 127–134.

Poole J M and Grant Z (2018) When youth get mad through a critical course on mental health. In S Pashang, N Khanlou and J Clarke (Eds.). *Today's Youth and Mental Health.* Cham, Switzerland: Springer International, 305–320.

Poole J M, Jivraj T, Arslanian A, Bellows K, Chiasson S, Hakimy H, Reid J (2012) Sanism, 'mental health', and social work/education: A review and call to action. *Intersectionalities: A Global Journal of Social Work Analysis, Research, Polity, and Practice, 1,* 20–36.

Porter R (1989) *A Social History of Madness: The World through the Eyes of the Insane.* London: Plume.

Porter R (1990) *Mind Forg'd Manacles: History of Madness in England from the Restoration to the Regency.* London: Penguin Books.

Reaume G (2019) Creating mad people's history as a university credit course since 2000. *New Horizons in Adult Education and Human Resource Development, 31*(1), 22–39.

Reville D (2013) Is Mad Studies emerging as a new field of inquiry? In B A LeFrançois, R Menzies and G Reaume (Eds.). *Mad matters: A critical reader in Canadian Mad Studies.* Toronto, ON: Canadian Scholars' Press, 170–180.

Snyder S et al. (2019) Unlearning through Mad Studies: Disruptive pedagogical praxis. *Curriculum Inquiry, 49*(4), 485–502.

Sweeney, A. (2016) Why mad studies needs survivor research and survivor research needs mad studies. *Intersectionalities, 5*(3), 36–61.

Wolframe P (2013) *Reading through Madness: Counter-psychiatric Epistemologies and the Biopolitics of (In)sanity in Post-World War II Anglo-Atlantic Women's Narratives (Doctoral dissertation).* McMaster University, Hamilton, ON, Canada.

32

MADNESS, DECOLONISATION AND MENTAL HEALTH ACTIVISM IN AFRICA

Femi Eromosele

Introduction

I recently concluded my doctoral research on madness in African literature, and, for several reasons, it has been a most interesting historical juncture to engage such research. In particular, not only is mental health advocacy gaining more visibility, renewed calls for decolonisation frame the expectations around what kind of knowledge is produced in and about the continent. Frantz Fanon has been an inevitable encounter at many turns as the arbiter of decolonisation and a pioneer in critical ethnopsychiatry. He is, however, but a voice – a very important one – amongst many. The strands that connect decolonisation and madness go in many directions. The resistance to definition that characterises both terms has meant that writers understand and evoke the decolonisation of madness or mental health in different ways. This chapter is a modest attempt to engage this body of work. Besides surveying the strands of decolonisation that appear in mad scholarship, I focus specifically on activism in Africa. What circumstances surround the demand for social justice? How is the call for decolonisation influencing local responses to the predominant discourse of human rights? How do these developments reverberate in the concerns of activist groups? These questions animate this chapter.

Decolonising madness

Mad experience and research as sites of (de)colonisation

The most prominent of the decolonisation narrative in mental health scholarship is that which aligns psychiatry with the position of coloniser. In the forward to *Mad Matters*, Peter Beresford talks about the "psychiatric empire [that] continues to grow, domestically and globally", and "its ever-widening diagnostic categories, its increasing pretense of providing solutions to structural and social problems, and its unholy alliance with global pharmaceutical corporations" (ix). Jacqui Dillon and Rufus May (2002), in their much cited "Reclaiming Experience", understand clinical categories as a "colonising discourse" imposed on those who experience the world in non-normative ways. The relationship of unequal power drawn between psy expertise and the mad is considered most manifest in the way subjective experiences are suppressed, dismissed, in favour of a seemingly more objective language and way of knowing. This is a thread that runs through several works, including Hornstein (2013), Geekie and Read (2009) and many others. John Read (2005:597) in particular considers this "a colonisation of the psychological and social by the biological", one which "has involved the ignoring or vilification of research showing the role of contextual factor such as neglect, trauma (inside and beyond the family), poverty, racism, sexism, etc in the etiology of madness". Resistance to this domination of psychic territories comes to be seen as efforts at decolonisation, a rhetorical move that gathers all psychiatrically oppressed individuals into a transnational, transcultural and transethnic (post) colonial community. What this does is that it effectively erases the ways that both madness and psychiatric oppression are experienced differently. I elaborate further below.

In a closely related vein, (de)colonisation is invoked with particular reference to research. In this case, what is colonised or in danger of being so is not the experience of madness itself, but the knowledge it generates. The relationship between these two is expressed by Jasna Russo and Peter Beresford:

> If the first problem was getting any kind of recognition for such narratives, then now this has begun to be achieved it appears we may have moved on to a further stage when an additional issue emerges. This is how to ensure that they are not just colonised or reduced to a new area for academic activity – taken from the control of their own authors.
>
> *(2015:155–156)*

Rather than the opposition between mad subjects and clinical experts, what is emphasised is the unequal relations between those who experience and the academic experts who mine their stories for research. The typical anthropological stance that is brought to bear during this process undermines the owners of the narratives as equals in knowledge production; their own analysis and understanding of their experience are taken over by those who consider them data for interpretation and commoditisation. But the problem is not just resident in misguided researchers. It persists in the very structures that sustain the valuation of what constitutes knowledge; proper "evidence" tends to be understood as that obtained through a certain distance from what is studied, an inherently objectifying process (Glasby and Beresford 2006; Landry 2017; Faulkner 2017; Beresford 2010). Unwittingly or otherwise, researchers who work with madness reproduce the power differential and epistemic injustice they seek to shed light on. The implications of this are manifest in very practical ways such as the kind of funding made available to user-/survivor-led researches (Rose 2017:777). These issues are taken up in much literature on service user/survivor contributions and sometimes in similar language of reclamation used in opposition to psychiatry (See e.g. "Recovering Our Stories" by Lucy Costa et al.).

Critiquing (de)colonisation as analogy

Louise Tam (2013) notes how the above conception of decolonisation, signalled in the use of maps and natural paths and the promotion of non-Western spiritual practices as alternative to psy, surfaces the "gap in mapping relations of race *to* and *in* madness" (283). This extends to the inability of such figuration to engage with the complicity of psy knowledge in the colonial endeavour as well as the enduring legacies of that violence in the majority world. Tam focuses on the works of two prominent user/survivor organisations, the Icarus Project and MindFreedom International. The language of decolonisation and "occupy" that permeates their literature exposes the problematic thinking that follows the metaphorisation of one form of struggle in the pursuit of another. Not only is the force of one category emptied into the other, identities are reified. Her critique echoes the warning by Eve Tuck and K. Wayne Yang that decolonisation must not be approximated with other expressions of oppression. It is neither metaphor nor "a swappable term for other things we want to do to improve our societies and schools" (2012:3). The authors are rightfully incensed about the way the term tends to be appropriated to occlude white settler guilt.

Decolonisation as analogy also does the two-fold work of stabilising what it means to colonise or decolonise and the identity of those involved in the struggle. If anything is apparent in the scholarship, it is that the project is a multifaceted endeavour that cannot be reduced to a single action or event. The violence of colonisation touches on every sphere of life of the colonised; it is material, epistemic, ontological, and so on. The path to decolonisation is thus neither straight forward nor predefined. It holds different meanings to different people, inaugurating different notions and strategies, some of them in contradiction with others. "A programme of complete disorder", Frantz Fanon calls it, a historical process that "cannot become intelligible nor clear to itself except in the exact measure that we can discern the movements which give it historical form and content" (2001 [1961]:27). Metaphor distils the meaning of this process, as if the ramifications and legacies of the colonial experience can already be grasped and summarised.

The rhetoric of decolonisation in certain strands of mad activism positions the mad movement as a homogenous collective. This is the critique Gavin Miller (2018) makes of Gail Hornstein's *Agnes's Jacket*. In this ethnography of Hearing Voices Network, Hornstein relies on the motif of a piece of clothing by Agnes Richter (1844–1916), a German seamstress incarcerated in several psychiatric institutions through the course of her life. Agnes's jacket is embroidered with text, which, in its indecipherability, represents for the author a coded message, a linguistic teaser into an unknown world, the world of madness. This world is that which has been colonised by psychiatry and from which its inhabitants like Agnes must smuggle their messages in hopes of being heard by those on the outside or who share similar experiences. Her jacket is the equivalent of modern-day patient blogs, websites and advocacy. Miller considers Hornstein's rhetorical manoeuvre contentious in the way it retrospectively ascribes political intention to Agnes's jacket, thereby creating the mad community as a diasporic and postcolonial nation. The heterogeneity of voices within the movement is compressed into one transnational citizenry. Miller's critique reiterates Rachel Gorman's (2013) contemplation about how the "appeal to an imaginary historical subject reproduces a particular ontology in the political present, and vice versa" (270). The normative subject of the imagined nation is unsurprisingly Western and white. Therefore, while relying on the notion of decolonisation, Hornstein's work and others like it occlude engagement with actual instances of historical and ongoing modes of colonial experience (Eromosele 2020). In fact such discourse may even be seen to constitute its own form of colonisation.

Non-western worlds as sites of (de)colonisation

The third application of decolonisation captures the intensified spread of Western psychiatry to the majority world. China Mills (2014), in a study that pulls together the senses of decolonisation already mentioned, examines this trend through the prism of Global Mental Health and WHO policy – the way psychiatrisation "creeps into domains of experience previously taken to be 'normal', and creeps across geographical borders" (146). With particular focus on India, Mills observes the way biomedical psychiatry invades new territories, fuelled by pharmaceutical capital and the political-economic power of industrialised nations. She points out the strange irony of the situation: that in a time when strident criticism has been levelled at Western psychiatry, there is also increasing clamour to spread such services across the globe, more and more into previously unsaturated regions. The body of knowledge that psychiatry constitutes not only creates a market for medication, but also works to silence the ways of being and knowing in non-Western climes – conceptions of self, of health and illness, and so on. Positioned as universal knowledge, psychiatry is exported across the world, where it relegates indigenous and home-grown modes of therapy. Systems of classification such as the Diagnostic and Statistical Manual (DSM) and the International Classification of Diseases (ICD) are effective instruments of dispersal. They enable the scientific legitimacy of such knowledge. Adebayo Akomolafe (2013) recounts how these tools are uncritically adopted by clinicians in Nigeria as the touchstone for deciphering mental ailments; complex stories are quickly sorted into symptoms and a diagnostic category, enabling the clinician to avoid the life-history of the patient. Ultimately, this move sometimes ends up creating even more harm. Akomolafe concludes that "[f]ar from being a promoter of mental health in Nigeria, Western clinical praxis effectively silences competing paradigms and colonises indigenous behaviour – successfully constructing only one way to experience life difficulties and, thus, only one way to 'treat' them" (2013:731).

Questions about the portability of psychiatry outside Western cultures have a longer history than their recent uptake. The impulse to make psychiatry amenable to Africans motivated the innovations of physicians like Thomas A. Lambo, Tigani El Mahi and Frantz Fanon (from Nigeria, Sudan and Martinique respectively). They understood the racism embedded in the practice of psychiatry and its complicity in the colonising mission of European powers (Britain and France, most notably). Their reworking of its categories was therefore seen as part of the efforts at political decolonisation. The most prominent – and subsequently most criticised – colonial psychiatrists such as J.C. Carothers, H.L. Gordon and Antoine Porot were hardly original when they theorised that the adult African is mentally inferior to the European. They were drawing on knowledge about the African that had become commonplace at this time, knowledge that structured the very foundations of their discipline. Psychiatry began to strive for scientific legitimacy in the eighteenth and nineteenth centuries, a time when barely-concealed racist thinking passed for "science". All scientific endeavours at this time were subtended by the crucial belief that the European was at the top of a process of evolutionary development (Fernando 2002, 2011). Through their "scientific" investigation in Kenya, Carothers and Gordon concluded that African culture stunted the social and intellectual development of the African and made them similar to a European child or leucotomised adult. Unlike psychiatric investigations in other parts of the world, the focus was on defining the "normal" African mind rather than the mad subject (Vaughan 1991). Constructing the African as always already "other", psychiatry justified the civilising mission of colonial powers. But it was also quick to caution the over-exposure of the African to European ways, for when met with actual cases of "mad" Africans, this was attributed to "deculturation" (Keller 2001:308; Vaughan 1991). Having trained into such a compromised body of knowledge, African psychiatrists considered it imperative not only to correct the racism of the profession but also to fashion therapy that responds to the particularity of their patients' lifeworld. Lambo started the Aro psychiatric village in Nigeria, where he combined indigenous healing methods with psychiatry. Patients were accompanied by at least a family member and assigned to local hosts (Akyeampong 2015; Asuni 1967). Fanon initiated a sociotherapy programme at Blida-Joinville Hospital in Algeria and a day hospital in Tunis (Fanon 2018).

While the work of early African psychiatrists constitute radical departure from the racist psychiatry of their times, in retrospect, it is easy to see how they remained constrained by the limitations of the discipline itself. They not only worked with psychiatric categories, but also continued to use therapeutic methods now considered cruel. Both Lambo and Fanon used methods such as ECT on patients, and as much as Lambo posed a departure from colonial psychiatry, he remained embedded, long after political independence, in the networks facilitated by the imperial sweep of Europe. He was from 1973 to 1988 the Deputy Director General of the World Health Organization. Heaton (2011) argues though, that it is exactly these scientific networks that facilitated his decolonisation project.

Mad activism as a site of (de)colonisation

Lastly, decolonisation enters the discourse of madness through the caution about generalised forms of advocacy. This, like the homogenised notion of psychiatry it seeks to combat, assumes a universal mode of relating to issues of mental health justice. Miller (2018) points this out. To export the sort of identarian advocacy espoused by Hornstein – and certain mad activism – he says, "could be simply to impose an extra layer of (literal) neo colonialism – a Western response to the West's own problems with biomedical psychiatry – one that overlooks the resources in LMICs for dealing with severe mental illness" (314). He echoes Fernando's comment about movements critical of psychiatry becoming just as racist as what they criticise. "[U]nless one customizes the alternatives we are trying to build up, unless we make active efforts to be anti-racist, racism is likely to pervade these too" (Fernando 2011:52). This mode of decolonisation is articulated as pre-emptive, as the need for a solution before the problem erupts. However, as we will see below, advocacy organisations in Africa are already querying the hegemony that attends connections/collaborations with international organisations that impose their own ideas of social justice.

Tracing (dis)continuities

The notion of decolonisation shifts as the referent of the process of colonisation, discursively and historically, changes. What is colonised, for some, is the realm of experience itself. In this regard, psy is not just a professional practice, but an apparatus of Reason which places itself in an oppositional relationship to what it is not. The work of the French philosopher and historian, Michel Foucault, is often a valuable resource for this kind of understanding. For others – and this is the second sense described above – it is the knowledge production that derives from this experience that is being colonised. To undo this would involve a reformulation of the relations between researchers and participants; survivor/user stories are not data to be commercialised or used as fodder for theory by experts. And yet others see colonisation in a slightly more literal sense of the spread of biomedical psychiatry to non-Western parts of the world, in a way that recalls and repeats the imperial spread of colonial powers. The referent of domination here are non-Western subjects and their ways of understanding self, illness and health. In close proximity, colonisation speaks historically to the subjection by European powers of populations they considered inferior. Psy is shown to be a veritable apparatus in this project. At stake at this historical juncture was not just independence in the political or economic sense, but a redefinition of subjectivity, an escape from the space that the white gaze had fixed the black person (Fanon 2008 [1952]). Because of the ramifications of madness for understanding human relations across many spheres, proposals for decolonisation remain necessarily expansive, embracing of different dimensions. What it means to decolonise mad experience is hardly what it means to decolonise its research; this is also not equivalent to decolonising psychiatry or modes of therapy. The meaning shifts according to the referent, and, sometimes, to centre a particular one reproduces the violence of colonisation itself.

If one would find a common denominator in these discourses of decolonisation, it would be in the call for a non-hierarchical multivocality; the need to fashion knowledge and praxis in a way that is both just and speaks to the particular situation it attends to. Distilling the ideas for change in her book, Mills argues that

> frameworks for understanding and responding to mental distress need to be 'home-grown' within the contexts from which distress emerges, privileging the knowledge of those with lived experience of distress and enabling interventions based on community collaboration, self help and peer support.
>
> *(2015:149)*

This of course resonates with Fernando's admonition to "customise the alternatives" and Akomolafe's proposal for the push for "new spaces of critical enquiry, the co-creation of indigenous research methods, the unravelling of knowledge production systems and the legitimisation of indigenous praxis" (737). Evidently, this is where Fanon continues to be a major voice in the advocacy for decolonisation. In his exemplary quest for understanding that is situated, despite the limitations of psy knowledge and the seductiveness of universalist thinking in his time, Fanon espouses an attitude to emancipatory work that takes nothing for granted, that questions constantly and weighs the relevance of received knowledge against the circumstance it is called to serve.

The above involves a good measure of reflexive criticism. Undoing or preventing colonial structures and thinking is a project that has no termination point, for every new formulation is always in danger of reconstituting previous violence. This is also the risk that identity-based advocacy faces in its dependence on the idea of a specific identity that is the locus of rights and recognition. Gorman (2013) expresses this well enough, reminiscent of Lennard Davis's argument that anti-discriminatory struggle based on such will always produce minorities, precisely because "an inherent limitation of permitted or favoured identities is built into the definition of the project" (1998:324). Essentialised notions of identity in the global sphere reproduce a white, Western Mad Subject (Gorman 2013:270). Even when localised, such a strategy fares no better, for the favoured identity (way of being Mad) and the rights that accrue to it can be "instrumentalised by state discourses of inclusion" not only to obscure those that do not fit into the model, but also to engender the conditions that produce them (Puar 2017:xvi). The alternative is to understand subjectivity or identity as perhaps a little less fixed than assumed, especially with categories like madness and disability. These positions are not eternal spaces that people occupy. Rather, depending on geographical, historical, and cultural placement, not to mention legal regimes, one may come to occupy them in very distinct ways. "'Madness' as a discourse changes based on the social', says Tam (2013), and by social she means "the convivial interaction of bodies in the dissemination of knowledge, the institutionalisation of policy, and the creation of cultural artifacts" (286).

I have so far been arguing in largely general terms, skirting somewhat the contextual specificity I consider essential to the discourse of decolonisation. From the foregoing, there are many geographic or discursive junctures to situate such a conversation. I will, however, focus on mental health activism in Africa in the rest of the chapter. While decolonisation in this regard is sometimes proffered as a pre-emptive measure, I examine how it is already a concern.

Decolonising activism

Since around the start of the century, peer-led advocacy organisations at national and regional levels have been on the rise in Africa. One of the very first of these, Mental Health Uganda, was established in 1999, and others have since cropped up in other parts of the continent. There is the Ubuntu Centre in South Africa, the USP in Kenya, MindFreedom International in Ghana, and many others. Some of these organisations are members of the continent-wide Pan African Network of People with Psychosocial Disabilities (PANUSP), affiliated to the World Network of Users and Survivors of Psychiatry. Not only are the organisations usually supported by or affiliated to international bodies, they base their appeal for legitimacy on the provisions in the United Nations Convention on the Rights of Persons with Disabilities (UNCRPD) and hence grapple with the implications of this alignment.

One of the major issues that have been raised is the appropriateness of the mode of advocacy in terms of priority. While international mental health organisations favour an anti/critical psychiatric emphasis, what those in Africa often have to contend with also involves issues of poverty and development. It is a situation where "Poverty, human rights violations and psychosocial disability go hand in hand" (PANUSP 2011). Disability benefits are hardly available in most countries, and the rampant poverty not only creates conditions of mental distress but limits the kind of care a person can afford. Psychiatry does not have the same level of presence it does in developed countries, and, as such, engenders a different kind of response. This is the motivation for PANUSP's change of name from Pan African Network of Users and Survivors of Psychiatry, which was considered inadequate in capturing the challenges of the mentally distressed in Africa (Kleintjes et al. 2013:193). As one member of an advocacy group puts it,

> In Africa, we have to have our own situation in perspective before we roll out our advocacy agenda, we cannot just go with what western advocacy are saying … people from the West are talking of people who have survived the services. In Africa … it's very few who can get to those services.
>
> *(Kleintjes et al. 2013)*

Though such remarks often seem homogenising, one must resist the impulse to assume the presence of psychiatry is the same across Africa. South Africa, for example, with its higher level of development relative to other African countries, also has a higher psychiatric presence. Advocacy organisations remain conscious of this and pay attention to how "[t]he history of psychiatry haunts our present. Our people remain chained and shackled in institutions and by ideas which our colonisers brought to our continent" (PANUSP 2014).

Critiquing rights-based discourse

The attempt to decolonise mental health advocacy in turn puts in relief the contradictions in the framework within which such organisations have to operate. While highlighting the relative absence of psychiatric service compared to indigenous healing systems, advocacy often has to be carried out in the register of biomedicine. Legibility through the lenses of the rights-based provisions of the CRPD compels people to understand themselves within a language that is perceived to be universal, even as they emphasise the specificity of their situation. PANUSP changes its name to convey distinction from the industrialised West, yet the "psychosocial disability" it adopts intimates the influence of the social model, itself an "import" of disability scholarship and activism outside Africa already subject to criticism of oversight (Mills 2015; Connell 2011; Meekosha 2011). Relying on the formulations of the social model, it has been observed, may assert the assumption of impairment and its position as the domain of medical expertise (Mills 2015; Spandler 2012). To what extent can the work of decolonisation be carried through within a framework that already presupposes a hierarchy in how conditions ought to be interpreted? How do people who do not see themselves through the prism of disability/impairment connect with such provisions? Where is the space for understandings that emphasise the spiritual dimensions of psychic experiences? While undoubtedly enabling a platform for articulating issues around mental distress and stigma on a national and more calculable scale, provisions like the CRPD constrain the sort of response that can be articulated.

The universality embedded in CRPD extends to the issue of human rights. Meekosha and Soldatic (2011) have examined the limitations and potentially harmful implications of disability rights as entrenched in the CRPD. The limitations accrue from certain paradoxes of human rights: the fact that nation-states are supposed to be the enforcers of rights but are sometimes the perpetrators of their violation, and the presumed universality of human rights, which simply entrenches the idea of the global North as the epicentre of modernity out of which civilisation flows to the rest of the world. In addition, human rights can be a diversionary instrument, a way of sidestepping the effects of invasion, colonisation, globalisation, and the power differential that persists between the global North and the majority world. Through the naturalisation of impairment in the CRPD and the construction of disability as social, claims for retributive justice for impairments wrought by imperialism and colonialism may be easily brushed aside. Meekosha and Soldatic draw on the critique of human rights that have emerged from thinkers in/from the South, particularly that of de Souza Santos and Makau Mutua. Their final observation, that "human rights for disabled people in the global South are extremely complex and the lived reality is often distant from the legal rhetoric" (2011:1394), remains crucial especially in mental health activism in Africa.

The crux of the criticism of human rights as has been promoted by organisations like the UN is that it needs to be modified to apply to non-Western contexts. Makau Mutua, in *Human Rights: A Political and Cultural Critique*, expounds some of the bases of this critique. The human rights corpus, if for nothing else, is suspect, for having been dominated so far by a region of the world that has been responsible for so much carnage and dehumanisation of the rest of humanity. "[A] historical understanding of the struggle for human dignity should locate the impetus of a universal conception of human rights in those societies *subjected* to European tyranny and imperialism" (2002:12; emphasis in original), Mutua argues. Rather than dismiss the human rights corpus outrightly, he calls for a "multi-culturalisation" (xi), a realisation on the part of its adherents that the corpus as it is does not have the final say on what is just and how the fight for that must be engaged. Instead of positioning the grammar of human rights as universal, one must realise that for it to be so, it has to interact convincingly with the local contexts it is brought into. The people have to own it. This cannot be done by ignoring indigenous forms of understanding. Human rights framework necessitates liberal democracy, a political model that has so far been largely inadequate for the postcolonial condition of many African nation-states. Not only this; a rights-based political and legal structure relies on a conception of personhood much different from what is commonly understood in Africa. This has been a major point of critical attention in recent times.

Seeking alternatives to human rights: Ubuntu

The individualised, self-contained and autonomous subject evoked in human rights has been unfavourably juxtaposed with the communitarian notion of personhood in Africa. Though it has been a concern in African philosophy for a while now, a concept that has recently resurfaced in capturing this aspect of African thought is ubuntu. The popular uptake of the term is evident in the existence of a computer operating system that bears the name. Regardless of its commercialisation and ubiquity, ubuntu remains an important concept activists and thinkers on social justice are eager to work with as an alternative to Western individualism. The first independent advocacy organisation run by and for people with psychosocial disability in South Africa goes by this name.[1] Ubuntu, short form of the Zulu saying *umuntu ngumuntu ngabantu*, is often translated as "a person is a person through other persons". With variants across Africa, especially the Nguni languages, it encompasses a particular philosophy of life, an ethical framework and the moral character of a person (Graness 2018). Ubuntu is predicated on the idea that personhood is attained through complex processes of interactive exchange between people and the totality of their environment – inclusive of the natural environment and other dimensions of living such as the living dead (ancestors) and the unborn. Because the community is always evolving, personhood is not a static and once-and-for-all state; it is acquired and may be lost. It is a process, a becoming, "one continuous wholeness rather than a finite whole" (Ramose 2001:n.p). Activism guided by this notion does not just marshal the political tools of human rights but appeals as well to the very ontological status of the society. Preserving human dignity is simultaneously political, ethical, and spiritual.

In addition to the criticism of collectivity, anachronism, and vagueness (Metz 2011), the processual conception of personhood in certain versions of ubuntu has been a subject of contention. If personhood is an acquired attribute, such criticism goes, then the exclusion of certain categories of people like women, children, and the disabled may be easily justified. The latter is of much importance because it is exactly the problem of discrimination that mental health activists work to address. Thaddeuz Metz (2011), in his reformulation, has responded to some of these criticisms. But one must bear in mind that ubuntu is an ethical stance, a way of judging relationship with oneself and others. Its values provide "grounds for a moral critique of social and other forms of exclusion, and it does not matter whether the basis of this form of exclusion or discrimination is gender, race or class" (Ogude 2018:4). Disability and madness can obviously be added to the list. Suspicion of the term tends to be influenced by the idea of community as a collective of individuals. As Augustine Shutte clarifies,

> the human self is not something that first exists on its own and then enters a relationship with its surroundings. It only exists in relationship to its surroundings; these relationships are what it is. And the most important of these are the relationships we have with other persons.
>
> *(2018:83)*

Providing the conditions of flourishing for everyone is the duty of the community; not just as a means of fostering the self-determination of one, but of keeping itself healthy, of affirming the basis for its own existence. The refusal to honour the humanness of another is what renders an individual a non-person, and what invalidates a community.

A number of scholars have proposed ubuntu as a veritable resource for the African disability movement. Maria Berghs in her 2017 article draws attention to how this can help in decolonising the disability thinking predicated on the narrow distinction between impairment and disability. According to this model, disability activism embraces and tackles all forms of injustice that threaten a common humanity. It connects physical, cognitive, and psychological impairments as well as concerns with environmental degradation and reclamation of indigenous lands. Ubuntu, interpreted as a concept that embraces otherness – "a human being is a human being through [*the otherness of*] other human beings" – recognises and even encourages the diverse experiences of humanness. Tsitsi Chataika et al. (2015) also challenge disability activists in Africa to adopt the notion as a basis for the struggle for rights. While mental health activists do not explicitly use the term, ideas associated with it are assumed to be the overarching motivation for groups like the Ubuntu Centre in South Africa. Concerns with disability and wellness appear in key texts on the concept. Augustine Shutte (2001), in his early intervention, devotes a good portion to health care in South Africa. Though it is difficult to tell to what extent it will keep shaping activist agenda, one can conjecture that versions of the notion will continue to surface, the more current human rights discourses show themselves incapable of effecting desired change.

Admittedly, ubuntu and its communitarian variants are easily practiced in much less complex social and political configurations than the nation-states that currently exist. Not only this; like other systems of knowledge the world over, it is hardly perfect. It has its blind spots, which tend to be more obvious with regards to certain categories of people than others. Discrimination against madness is not exactly a phenomenon of the postcolonial age. It was also a feature of some of the so called traditional or precolonial societies – albeit in a different shade, one that did not necessarily render an individual a non-person. The much better prognosis in rural locales attested to by early ethno-psychiatric research was not just a function of the therapeutic methods, but also about how the distressed person was perceived and related to by the community. However, mad activism and advocacy are emerging and attempting to gain ground at a time when the political structures are not only shifting but the questions of their suitability are even more strident. The challenge lies in articulating the demand for justice when the larger social configuration is yet unsure what grammar it can understand. The "distinctive style of political improvisation" (Mbembe 2015:102) that characterises African polity makes it doubly imperative for advocacy organisations to fashion tools that may not necessarily look like what obtains with organisations in Euro-America, or to deploy them in a complementary relationship.

Conclusion

This chapter begins by exploring some of the ways the discourse of decolonisation has tended to surface in the literature on mental health. I have been keen to reiterate that decolonisation means different things to different people, and sometimes, its rhetoric is used in ways that even obscure actual experiences of colonial domination. The chapter focuses on mental health advocacy in Africa, with the aim of elaborating the milieu under which it is striving not only to articulate itself, but to resist becoming a mere conduit for the agenda of organisations based outside the continent. In the wider search for an alternative to the language of human rights and its attendant political model of democracy, African communitarian ethic and notion of personhood have proven most seductive. Especially in Southern Africa, thinkers have turned to ubuntu and its variants.

In sum, what it might mean to decolonise mental health advocacy in Africa is scattered throughout the chapter. Significantly, it must go beyond a resort to mere indigenisation – the uncritical adoption of certain models or ways of knowing just because they emanate from the continent. As already mentioned, no system is perfect. One must be attuned to the contradictions that exist therein, in addition to recognising that societies are never static. The desire for indigenisation is sometimes projected as a return to some pristine "African" way of doing things. No such thing exists. Africa's encounter with the rest of the world, whether through trade or the experience of colonisation or globalisation, has contributed to the complex world which its people inhabit. Even when one talks of the communitarian ethic of ubuntu, its manifestation and capacity to be mobilised for emancipatory work cannot be understood outside the contemporary situation it has been called upon to serve. It is difficult, and perhaps most uncritical, to excise an idea from its histories of emergence, but decolonisation, whatever its referent, must focus not so much on the regional provenance of ideas but on their ideological import and usefulness for the immediate context. What I mean is akin to how Kwasi Wiredu describes what he calls "conceptual decolonisation":

> What it calls for is the reviewing of any such thought materials [of colonial provenance] in the light of indigenous categories, as a first step, and, as a second, evaluating them on independent grounds … If, upon such a review, some Africans should become confirmed exponents of some Western mode of thought, they would, of course, be within their rational rights. The considerations leading to the sought-after intellectual liberation merely enlarge our options, they do not decide them.
>
> *(Wiredu 2004:15)*

Note

1 See more information at https://ubuntucentre.wordpress.com/

References

Akomolafe A C (2013). Decolonising the Notion of Mental Illness and Healing in Nigeria, West Africa. *Annual Review of Critical Psychology*, 10, 726–740.

Akyeampong E (2015). A Historical Overview of Psychiatry in Africa. In E Ayeampong, A G Hill and A Klienman (eds.). *The Culture of Mental Illness and Psychiatric Practice in Africa*. Indiana: Indiana University Press, 24–49.

Asuni T (1967). Aro Hospital in Perspective. *American Journal of Psychiatry*, 124 (6), 763–777.

Beresford P (2013). Forward. In B A LeFrancois, R Menzies and G Reaume (Eds.). *Mad Matters: A Critical Reader in Canadian Mad Studies*. Toronto, Canada: Canadian Scholars' Press, ix–xii.

Beresford P (2010). Re-Examining Relationships between Experience, Knowledge, Ideas and Research: A Key Role for Recipients of State Welfare and Their Movements. *Social Work and Society International Online Journal*, 8 (1). www.socwork.net/sws/article/view/19/56. Accessed: 14 July 2020.

Berghs M (2017). Practices and Discourses of Ubuntu: Implications for an African Model of Disability? *African Journal of Disability*, 6, a292. https://doi.org/10.4102/ajod.v6.292. Accessed: 14 July 2020.

Chataika T, Berghs M, Mateta A and Shava K (2015). From Whose Perspective Anyway? The Quest for African Disability Rights Activism. In A de Waal (ed.). *Advocacy in Conflict: Critical Perspectives on Transnational Activism*. London: Zed Books, 187–211.

Connell R (2011). Southern Bodies and Disability: Re-thinking Concepts. *Third World Quarterly*, 32 (8), 1369–1381.

Costa L, Voronka J, Landry D, Reid J, Mcfarlane B, Reville D and Church K (2012). Recovering Our Stories: A Small Act of Resistance. *Studies in Social Justice*, 6 (1), 85–101.

Davis L (1998). Who Put the "the" in "the Novel"?: Identity Politics and Disability in Novel Studies. *NOVEL: A Forum on Fiction*, 31 (3), 317–334.

Dillon J and May R (2002). Reclaiming Experience. *Clinical Psychology*, 17, 25–77.

Eromosele F (2020). Fanon in the Time of Mad Studies. *World Futures*, 76 (3), 167–187.

Fanon F (2001) [1961]. *The Wretched of the Earth*. Trans. C. Farrington. London, UK: Penguin.

Fanon F (2008) [1952]. *Black Skin, White Masks*. Trans. R Philcox. New York, NY: Grove Press.

Fanon F (2018). *Alienation and Freedom*. Trans. Steven Corcoran. London: Bloomsbury.

Faulkner A (2017). Survivor research and Mad Studies: The Role and Value of Experiential Knowledge in Mental Health Research. *Disability & Society*, 32, 4, 500–520.

Fernando S (2002). *Mental Health, Race and Culture*, 2nd Edition. Basingstoke: Palgrave.

Fernando S (2011). Cultural Diversity and Racism: An Historical Perspective. In M Rapley, J Moncrieff and J Dillon (eds.). *De-Medicalizing Misery Psychiatry, Psychology and the Human Condition*. Basingstoke, Hampshire: Palgrave Macmillan, 44–52.

Geekie J and Read J (2009). *Making Sense of Madness: Contesting the Meaning of Schizophrenia.* New York: Routledge.

Glasby J and Beresford P (2006). Who Knows Best? Evidence-Based Practice and the Service User Contribution. *Critical Social Policy*, 26, (1), 268–284.

Gorman R (2013). Mad Nation? Thinking Through Race, Class, and Mad Identity Politics. In B A LeFrancois, R Menzies and G Reaume (Eds.). *Mad Matters: A Critical Reader in Canadian Mad Studies.* Toronto, Canada: Canadian Scholars' Press, 269–280.

Graness K (2018). Becoming a Person: Personhood and its Preconditions. In J Ogude (ed.). *Ubuntu and Personhood.* Trenton, New Jersey: Africa World Press, 39–59.

Heaton M M (2011). Thomas Adeoye Lambo and the Decolonization of Psychiatry in Nigeria. In B M Bennett and J M Hodge (eds). *Science and Empire. Britain and the World.* London: Palgrave Macmillan.

Hornstein G A (2013). Whose Account Matters? A Challenge to Feminist Psychologists. *Feminism & Psychology*, 23 (1), 29–40.

Keller R (2001). Madness and Colonisation: Psychiatry in the British and French Empires, 1800–1962. *Journal of Social History*, 35 (2), 295–326.

Kleintjes S, Lund C and Swartz L (2013). Organising for Self-Advocacy. Mental Health: Experiences from Seven African Countries. *African Journal of Psychiatry*, 16, 187–195.

Landry D (2017). Survivor research in Canada: 'Talking' Recovery, Resisting Psychiatry, and Reclaiming Madness. *Disability & Society*, 32 (9), 1437–1457.

Mbembe A (2015). *On the Postcolony.* South Africa: Wits University Press.

Meekosha H (2011). Decolonising Disability: Thinking and Acting Globally. *Disability and Society*, 26, 6, 667–682.

Meekosha H and Soldatic K (2011). Human Rights and the Global South: The Case of Disability. *Third World Quarterly*, 32 (8), 1383–1397.

Metz T (2011). Ubuntu as a Moral Theory and Human Rights in South Africa. *African Human Rights Journal*, 11, 532–559.

Mills C (2014). *Decolonizing Global Mental Health: The Psychiatrization of the Majority World.* London: Routledge.

Mills C (2015). The Global Politics of Disablement: Assuming Impairment and Erasing Complexity. In H Spandler, J Anderson and B Sapey (eds.). *Madness, Distress and the Politics of Disablement.* Bristol: Policy Press, 199–213.

Miller G (2018). Madness Decolonised? Madness as a Transnational Identity. In G Hornstein (ed.) *Agnes's Jacket. Journal of Medical Humanities*, 39 (3), 303–323.

Mutua M (2002). *Human Rights: A Political and Cultural Critique.* Philadelphia: University of Pennsylvania.

Ogude J (2018). Introduction: "Ubuntu and Personhood". In J Ogude (ed.). *Ubuntu and Personhood.* Trenton, New Jersey: Africa World Press, 1–9.

Pan African Network of People with Psychosocial Disabilities (PANUSP) (2014). The Cape Town Declaration (16th October 2011). *Disability and the Global South*, 1 (2), 385–386.

Puar K J (2017). *The Right to Maim: Debility, Capacity, Disability.* Durham: Duke University Press.

Ramose M (2001). An African perspective on justice and race. *Polylog.* http://them.polylog.org/3/frm-en.htm. Accessed 14 May 2020.

Read J (2005). The Bio- bio- bio Model of Madness. *The Psychologist*, 18, 10, 596–597.

Rose D (2017). Service User/survivor-led Research in Mental Health: Epistemological Possibilities. *Disability & Society*, 32(6), 773–789.

Russo J and Beresford P (2015). Between Exclusion and Colonisation: Seeking a Place for Mad People's Knowledge in Academia. *Disability & Society*, 30 (1), 153–157.

Shutte A (2001). *Ubuntu: An Ethic for a New South Africa.* Pietermaritzburg: Cluster Publications.

Shutte A (2018). The Primacy of the Personal. In J Ogude (ed). *Ubuntu and Personhood.* Trenton, New Jersey: Africa World Press, 79–113.

Spandler H (2012). Setting the scene. In J Anderson, B Sapey and H Spandler (eds.). *Distress or Disability? Proceedings of a Symposium Held at Lancaster University, 15–16 November 2011.* Lancaster: Centre for Disability Research, 14–17.

Tam L (2013). Wither Indigenizing the Mad Movement? Theorizing the Social Relations of Race and Madness through Conviviality. In B A LeFrancois, R A Menzies and G Reaume (eds.). *Mad Matters: A Critical Reader in Canadian Mad Studies.* Toronto: Canadian Scholars' Press, 281–297.

Tuck E and Yang K W (2012). Decolonization Is Not a Metaphor. *Decolonization: Indigeneity, Education & Society*, 1 (1), 1–40.

Vaughan M (1991). *Curing Their Ills: Colonial Power and African Illness*. Cambridge: Polity.

Wiredu K (2004). Introduction: African Philosophy in Our Time. *A Companion to African Philosophy*. Massachusetts: Blackwell Publishing, 1–27.

33

NAVIGATING VOICES, POLITICS, POSITIONS AMIDST PEERS

Resonances and dissonances in India

Prateeksha Sharma

A first, gut response when I heard the word 'Mad' was a shudder and a rejection. In sound you do not hear the case – lower or upper, the word is pure sound carrying culturally relevant symbols. It conjures images, ideas, faces, eyes, reactions. It is not neutral, for 'Mad' means something to everyone. I cannot jest about it, and for sure I cannot call anyone 'mad' – nor claim it for myself. Perhaps it comes from being *there*, having seen the other side, been called so. What may seem 'mad' to another made perfect sense to me when I was *there*: what others saw as my 'madness' then. I know there is a logic going on – regardless of whether it makes sense to another.

I write this piece with this attitude, as I walk amid peers, amid families, among contributors to my research, and also the ordinary citizens of my country, as one of them. We are a segment of humanity that suffers the sheer inhumanity and injustice of this unequal world – a world which wants to trim us all to one size. I walk in reflections, in reverie, tuned to sounds of people's helplessness amidst the cruelties of daily life, as families covertly medicate loved ones, as heartbreaks, crop failures and exam failures push farmers and young people to suicidal leaps, youth are murdered to defend family 'honour' … tales of never-ending loops of injustice, which only connect with one another in seamless continuity, offering no respite, no exit and no deliverance.

Is 'mad' only a word, not experience?

We all know the word 'mad' as an inherited construction from earlier generations and with it a way to look at people. It is not like the word 'cloud', or 'rainbow', or 'flower'. There is a disturbance inherent in it. Is it anger, or deep suffering? It seems to reveal an attitude of incomprehension and impatience, rather than an attempt at understanding someone. It is certainly not a noun, only an adjective; an emotion, not a state of being. Someone may have a mad moment, or a mad phase– they don't *become* mad. They do not change permanently into a phase. They remain who they are at a fundamental level. I seek that core in everyone and rejecting the word

DOI: 10.4324/9780429465444-39

'mad' in all its variants comes to me from that heartfelt location. Naturally now, it seems a great dilemma to encounter 'Mad' politics, or to embrace it.

Ever since I entered the domain of Mad Studies, trying to understand the field and its players due to doctoral research, I am troubled and puzzled by the long history it comes with. Had I not had this opportunity, would I ever have known about the resistance against psychiatry, which is hardly present in the world I come from? Two decades of patient-hood never made me question psychiatry, for I believed it would bring me to a clearing. Even when I 'recovered', among the first acts I performed was to write about myself, in the belief that possibly I was one of those rare exceptions who could. So it became a little bit of an identity assertion – and carving a new identity, instead of a patient's identity. The next thing was to look for others who trod the same path. That proved a little humbling, for it brought me down a notch or two to know that I was not so unique after all. It also pointed at a fork in the road – from a personal to a social project. This makes me think at times that if I took such a long path to unravel the colonial nature of a medical specialty, how many others will have to labour alone, and for how long, before they come to similar clarity? How can people look beyond a hegemonic discourse? Who will understand that the discourse is what dominates and not a solution to their suffering? Rather than being embraced as an equal, asserting one's identity as 'Mad' in such a scenario can only lead to further isolation, or further domination from above.

Searching a name to call myself

I never look upon myself as a psychiatric survivor, because in 'survivor-hood' I hear a victim's voice. I see myself as someone who, by dint of labour expended over decades, emancipated herself. There were passing friends but not a single peer. Later when peers appeared, I could not comprehend their ideas, for mine seemed such a personal journey to overcome suffering and rehabilitate. It was a much longer journey of inquiry whose path appeared through the labyrinth of research that introduced the radical perspectives going around the globe, research I have done alone at home, for decades. I write this to highlight the relative lack of a social movement questioning psychiatry, which can reach most psychiatric patients. And considering the size of India, the geographical separation between people and the social differences due to education, worsened by local factors like caste, religion, language, gender, and other identity-based conflicts, keep people away from one another more so, while radical ideas remain confined to a minuscule few.

As I write this, I think of scores of people, and wonder who among them would like to echo the word 'Mad' back to me. The only images that come to mind are the well-heeled, sophisticated, globally mobile, urban Indians; the tiniest minority among them. When I remember the crestfallen faces of people standing in long queues in government hospitals at the crack of dawn, of parents fervently struggling to get medicines in the hope of a relief for their children, of young people craving to be heard, of fathers/husbands who are fearful of their child's/wife's 'psychotic' fury, I know what the word 'mad' means to them. I doubt any one of them would want to claim it for themselves or their loved ones. Everyone wants to distance themselves from the experiences, or from even a hint of any experiences that could associate them with a stigmatizing identity.

Few have the courage or wind in their sails to first identify, then fight oppression at a personal level, and thereafter social. The struggles of being alive in a decent manner in the third world[1] are so big, that to think of dealing with any systemic violence is not only beyond our comprehension, but also beyond the scope of our resources. As a society in which a majority struggle for the essentials of food, shelter, safety, livelihoods, clean water, air, housing and so much more, day-to-day living produces enormous challenges. If anyone perchance overcomes a diagnostic oppression while being aware of it, in all likelihood whatever it will take us to rebuild our life from that shattering is by itself such a daunting climb, that we would be vary of doing anything with mental health ever again.

All that I am saying is that 'Mad' as an idea or as a response to an oppression has only a symbolic presence in our society, and then not in a truly radical, emancipatory or visionary manner; it is an identity category that a few uphold. And sadly enough when we choose 'Mad' as an identity or self-representation in a society where the business of living produces an absurd/mad behaviour at every juncture, it does not evoke camaraderie, respect or solidarity, but rather a fear and a distance from those who truly need the emancipatory vision of 'Mad' politics.

There are two issues that I set out to distinguish here: the issue of 'Mad' as an identity category and the politics of Mad Studies. Whereas I reject and steer clear of the former, I resonate with the latter, without feeling a need to position myself as a 'Mad' person. Neither do I accept 'Mad/mad' as a description for others nor myself. I believe, in the context where I am situated, and possibly other locations, the 'mad' word evokes what Fricker (2007:4) calls an 'identity prejudice': a label for prejudices against people of a certain social type. 'Mad' clearly produces a certain 'othering'; based on cultural stereotypes and the majority of people distance themselves from anyone labelled 'mad'. Where they don't adopt a social distance, a benevolent paternalism often enters into in their descriptions of 'such' people – 'poor … unfortunate him/her/them'. I prefer to use the word 'mad' within inverted commas, along with other words that label a person in different categories of 'madness'. I believe 'mad' is someone's view of another, not an objective truth about anyone – nor is it permanent or unchangeable. There are many complexities in the day-to-day lives of people who negotiate the micropolitics of mental health, often struggling to be heard. Having personally experienced these individual and group struggles makes me desist from using 'Mad' as an identity label, or even a tool of resistance anywhere.

Experience teaches me that in India the community of mental health activists who oppose psychiatry in India, is somewhat fractured, and frequently people do not support, embrace or even recognize one another unequivocally. This makes a number of us seem like lone wolves or solitary warriors, speaking a language with limited social recognition or connect. For example, in response to one of my published pieces of writing one person wrote in a social media message – '*Excellent … It is up to each of us to change perceptions and change the world*'! The attitude that words like these reveals is what I have called the 'lone wolf syndrome' above. It lacks a realization that organizing together is the most important resistance we need to focus on. If we really believe that singlehandedly we can change perceptions or change the world, this only indicates our deeply entrenched neoliberal individualism and self-aggrandisement. This does not augur well for collective action, and betrays our collective capability for organized struggle.

It is from this personal self-reflection that I derive the sensibility of resisting the 'Mad' label in India. I also wish to urge caution about our organised resistance. We could respond to every idea as an act of concern, caution, foresight and cultural meaningfulness, lest we end up choosing precisely that which distinguishes us as the very category we fight against.

Micropolitics of mental health

'*My wife Kirti is bipolar Madam,*[2] *and I think you may be able to help us*'- Sameer,[3] 41.

'*Madam, I do not have anything, but my husband doesn't understand*' Kirti, 37.

'*I feel lighter after talking to you, …(for)nobody asked me in all these years why I jumped into the lake. It seems as though nobody wants to know*'. Yash, 25

'I never wanted to specialize in pediatrics, but my father wanted me to. In me he sees the fulfillment of his dream of becoming what he could not. So he started sabotaging every decision I wanted to make for myself, including taking an exam to enter into a specialization of my own choice. When I took up an internship in a hospital he informed my seniors that I was on drugs for schizophrenia. One senior resident asked me quietly whether I was on medication. When I asked him why, he said, "your father called and told us about it." He made it impossible for me to work there'. Ajit, 26

As a peer therapist[4] I am not listening for any hints of 'illness', but looking for the roots of suffering. Everyone who watches a loved one suffer, suffers thus and wonders what they can do. A majority take the familiar road of 'treatment', and when in years it does not produce the outcomes hoped for, another search for alternatives begins. This is how some knock at my door. In the beginning it is difficult for anyone to understand why I say they are not 'mad '– for them their actions and behaviours, or those of their loved ones certainly seem to fit the description.

By the yardstick of where I am, neither the idea of 'recovery' nor the term 'peers' mean much. Few believe that people can 'recover', or that it is feasible or within everyone's reach. The landscape resounds with simplistic, biomedical representations of mental 'illness', or at most, a rights driven perspective to delivering mental health services,[5] another guise for pushing the Global Mental Health agenda. The vast majority of stakeholders within mental health, which includes psy-professionals led by psychiatrists, and other groups such as patients, caregivers, non-governmental organizations (NGOs), bureaucrats, legal experts, etc. demand more psychiatric knowledge, information, access to treatment, and enhanced infrastructure. People unquestioningly believe the organized rhetoric of the 'treatment gap' which ominously points towards a rising incidence of mental illness or panic mongering that we are socially under-equipped to deal with the vast numbers who are going to be afflicted. In 2017, our Mental Healthcare Act was passed in the Parliament, a seemingly democratic legislation, which few understand, has only given more power to the psychiatric profession. The word 'recovery' does not appear in the Act at all. The social clock ticks audibly and everyone from politicians, the media, the youngsters and kin of those labelled are scouring the internet – self-diagnosing, or looking at others through diagnostic lenses. The anxiety to be diagnosed, medicated and educated is all pervasive.

What are they all looking for? For confirmation or for signs of an 'illness'? The influx of the internet in a society with limited education and a nominal ability to question authority has made the task of global psychiatry rather congenial. Any mental health issue is just a google search away, and there is an avalanche of patient groups on the internet and social media, parroting psychiatric propaganda and knowledge with zest, confidence and belief. Moreover, the internet is full of self-administered tests so that '[w]ith self-help quizzes and professional diagnostics mirroring each other, we may be "quizzing ourselves sick"' (Reynolds, 2018:9). Many of the young people I interact with have first been 'diagnosed' by their families, or themselves, via these 'helpful' internet quizzes and have later consulted psychiatrists, seeking confirmation of their beliefs.

Challenges of traditional societies

Traditional societies often have a set of problems stemming from tradition, which is of the essence here. To question tradition is to threaten social order. India has traditionally been an agrarian society in which village communities formed the social ecosystem and everyone who was part of that network was taken care of. Villages often had common resources, a village doctor or '*vaidya*' among them. They would take care of all health needs of the people and make appropriate recommendations to deal with illness or other health conditions. A doctor's occupation was accorded an honourable status due to this ability to relieve suffering and bring healing. Doctors and teachers have been venerated in our society, and both have been very closely integrated within the communities they lived in. Somewhere at the back of the collective unconscious of Indians we still believe in these values. With biomedicalization further accelerated by the neoliberal agendas that recently independent countries have eagerly embraced, most patients and families still look up to doctors as saviours, healers and ultimate arbitrators of their wellbeing (see Nagarajan 2018). One cannot argue with another that their doctor is wrong, misleading, or does not know how to deal with their problem; it is quite unthinkable.

> Me: '*You never questioned whether the medicine is working for you or not?*'
> Megha: '*Oh no not at all definitely, not at all I haven't questioned the medicine … but … what is happening, what is happening?*'
> Me: '*I mean but listen … you have been on medicine for long time, right? It's almost 25 years … do you see that it has worked for you in any meaningful way or do you…*'
> Megha: '*Yeah, yeah I trust my doctors and I think this has worked for me.*'

Psychiatrists in India have few critics. Violations and inhuman stories about their treatments are audible if not rampant, yet the scale of numbers is such that their numerical insufficiency becomes a bigger issue than the day-to-day violence their methods inflict (see Davar 2012, 2015). This is the micropolitics I refer to, which individual patients/families have to negotiate, surrounded by a macro environment that offers next to no alternatives for them, other than what they are already oppressed by. This is the backdrop to our cogitations about 'Mad' politics.

Carving a 'mad' identity

'Mad' activism, scholarship and views occupy a tenuous position in society. Whereas in the Global North (North), where 'Mad' struggles have incubated and germinated, they appear to have gained a modicum of respectability, presence, recognition, following and possibly bargaining power,[6] this is not the case for rest of the world. It is beyond the scope of this writing to analyse the cultural differences that lead to such disparities between the North and the South, but it may be remembered that societies of the South are highly unequal societies, unlike the North where centuries of industrialization and planned development have facilitated access to a relatively decent, dignified life for a majority of people. In the midst of such diversities, any representation of 'Madness' in one part of the globe cannot simply mirror the social complexities of another part of the globe.

In India there is a relative absence of social critique of psychiatry, and this cannot be stressed enough. In fact, psychiatry commands pride of place in the public mind, and appears quite unassailable. But our society being as unequal as it is, brings in many interlinked issues in aspects of social representation, in particular class privilege. In a fragmented, iniquitous and class-conscious society when someone dares to adopt a label that is otherwise a social taboo, they do not usually belong to a socially oppressed or marginalized segment of society. Their ability to defy social mores is usually an outcome of class privilege, which goes unrecognized. If a humble, small town or economically necessitous person thinks of calling herself 'Mad' publicly, she would in all likelihood end-up being lampooned and ostracized further. But if the same thing is done by a person who is in a more powerful position, due to education, financial resources, family connections and/or global mobility, people would just shrug and think, '*well this is what she wants to do*'. While there is no doubt that the identity model contains some useful insights, it can also end up reifying group identities and obscuring the fact that we need distributive justice in society.

Fraser (2000:109) reminds that identity is constructed dialogically, through a process of mutual recognition. Recognition from others is essential to the development of a sense of self. To be denied recognition – or to be 'misrecognised' – is to suffer both a distortion of one's relation to one's self and an injury to one's identity. There is no doubt that in the initial decades when 'identity' became a tool of resistance, it empowered millions of people worldwide on grounds of race, colour, ethnicity, gender and much else. But that phase seems over. We are at a juncture where the politics of identity has reached a phase of maturation; voices once at the margins are increasingly being heard. In mental health, this moment has still to come in all parts of the world. But when we look at this issue within the large umbrella of identity politics, it must be borne in mind that there are no level playing fields. There are major differences between and within the North and the South; differences due to other interlocking variables such as class privileges, as I noted earlier. People within the North or South are not equally marginalized, neither can any group in any location represent all.

Identity politics inadvertently undermines group cohesion among marginalized populations and entrenches social class, confusing vast numbers of people about its message. A lack of consensus about one's social location and identity mostly ends up further consolidating psychiatry's powerful position in society. Fraser fortifies this argument saying that

> the identity model serves as a vehicle for misrecognition: in reifying group identity, it ends by obscuring the politics of cultural identification, the struggles *within*[7] the group for the authority – and the power – to represent it. By shielding such struggles from view, this approach masks the power of dominant factions and reinforces intragroup domination. The identity model thus lends itself all too easily to repressive forms of communitarianism, promoting conformism, intolerance and patriarchalism.
>
> *(Fraser, 2000:112)*

As a researcher explicit about her ex-patient status, I am either met with caution, confusion or curiosity. To some I seem suspect and possibly in remission. If not, then it is attributed to other things such as my classical music training that I have recovered. If in such a milieu I were to further suggest I am 'Mad' I doubt anyone would see me as anything but 'mad'. Is it even remotely feasible for me to operate here as a researcher or peer-'therapist' and call myself a 'Mad' person? I have noted elsewhere (Sharma, 2019) the prejudice associated with 'mental illness' is not confined to current patients; ex-patients are well within its ambit. If an ex-patient additionally goes around calling herself 'Mad' – would anyone understand what it implies in a milieu where psychiatry's wisdom and leadership is unquestioned, hegemonic and a beacon of hope for the vast majority? On the other hand, if I were to position myself as 'Mad', who would understand the subversion and not think *here is another 'mad' person*. Since I offer support and services to peers the least I can do is to reveal my calm and healed side to the world, not necessarily the anti-oppressive radical I may be, who brings that approach to understanding their oppressions and not to identity politics.

How 'mad' are you – 'mad' or 'Mad'?

'Mad' as represented by those who oppose psychiatric hegemony, is a subversion of the labelling or condemning as 'mad' and an invitation for scholarship, activism and an alternative representation. Le Francois et al. (2013:10) affirm that 'madness talk and text invert the language of oppression, reclaiming disparaging identities and restoring dignity and pride to difference'. It is symbolic of collective anger against a dominant, socially embedded worldview. It makes sense at a philosophical level, and I feel a resonance in spirit. But coming from a part of the world where the word 'mad' has many synonyms in any number of languages,[8] it is not possible to distinguish between 'mad' and 'Mad' in my plural linguistic landscape. Here the label 'mad' may be seen to be the same as the angry, reclaiming, collective, challenging 'Mad'. Being in India or possibly anywhere where English is not the only language spoken, one may have to think again before claiming publicly that we are 'Mad' scholars, activists, researchers or that one can take pride in a 'Mad' label. We don't raise our voices here by changing the case alone; we need to build a syntax of resistance. But before that we first need to establish the contours of a framework within the scope of which all resistance is carried out and within which we can locate our positions.

People who can look beyond psychiatric rhetoric are a minority anywhere. Barring pockets of visible resistance in industrialized countries, those opposing psychiatry, far from locations of such organized opposition, either remain silent, withdrawn or outnumbered to such an extent that their resistance becomes invisible. The larger community of mental health ex/'patients', caregivers and/or stakeholders may not understand what they are talking about or why. To confound the picture further, since they also want acknowledgement, inclusion, recognition and support of the same people as the more dominant and well-resourced psychiatric community, they find themselves on the same fora as the dominant groups. Unfortunately, in this dissonance their voices compete with many others 'representing' mental health issues. Few are able to discern or even engage with ideas that reject 'madness' as a category, or the challenge such voices offer to psychiatry as a whole. One can imagine this marginalization of radical views to be widely present in the South, especially now that global psychiatry, under the wingspan of the Global Mental Health Movement is projecting a benign, humanistic, human rights oriented perspective – claiming that in treating people 'respectfully' it is restoring their dignity, which was taken away by previously inhuman and 'unscientific' ways of treating the 'mentally ill'.

There could be two levels of resistance, even within a 'Mad' framework. The first, as I note above, is a collective challenge to psychiatry – an opposition established in the Global North for at least a few decades. The second from my perspective is a need for caution among those who resist psychiatry in the South. I propose that as former colonial subjects, we may also have to be wary of the 'Mad' perspectives of our peers from the North – a naïve mirroring of their language, tools, methods and ways is not likely to cut much ice here, if to include our local peers is one of our goals. Here people balk at the mention of the 'mad' word, for it evokes a deep cultural stigma. Moreover there is, as yet, no opposition to psychiatry here – to build that opposition, by spreading awareness is perhaps the first act of resistance we need to consider, towards an emancipatory goal of restoring epistemic justice to ourselves and our peers.

And how could such a resistance come about? For a people colonised by biomedical psychiatry, we live a reality where identification with the coloniser is axiomatic. A question of resistance can arise only with an awareness of colonization. This knowledge about colonization, or the ability to recognise one's ongoing oppression, is a goal whose pursuit is the need of the hour. Unless the subjects of a particular worldview understand their oppression, unravel how they are not safe in their relationship with the coloniser, they can never understand why they continue to suffer whilst the coloniser prospers. Instead, they continue their self-acceptance of subject-hood and submit, in effect, to a perpetuity of psychiatric practices. Finally, it comes down to the idea of education, or as the social reformer and framer of India's constitution, Dr.B.R.Ambedkar[9] said, 'educate, agitate, organize'.

De Lissovoy (2010:203) warns of the problem one has to tackle in an inhuman world, to raise 'a voice against the truth of power, the dead and finished truth of what is decided, the truth of the inert and incontrovertible'. And though everyone who shares an emancipatory agenda understands power, more significantly he adds that,

> [t]he problem of education is the problem of unwinding the human body and soul from this intricate clockwork of not merely the correct and commendable but also the apparently self-evident and inevitable. It is the problem of rescuing *being* from *what is*, a *what is* that has conquered every other possibility to give itself the status of fact and truth. This *what is* not just an apparatus of painful training; it is a machine of assimilation and destruction.
>
> *(De Lissovoy, 2010: 203)*

For those of us who offer a resistance to psychiatry, this 'being' translates as *being* subjects of psychiatry. Accepting it as a truth people accept *what is* and that which requires 'treatment'. The acceptance of mental illness is what needs to be questioned foremost. In what manner can we rally others around this by calling ourselves 'mad', 'Mad' or 'Mad proud' is something I am concerned about, for I know its polarizing potential in my location.

Holding the hands of peers

A personal passage is a point of entry into emancipatory resistance; but it need not be the only one. Personally speaking, this spectrum has *being* a patient at one end, to becoming a healing-oriented collaborator at the other. It passes through stages of becoming an ex-patient, progresses as one slowly starts questioning *what is*, and learning to distance oneself from the reductionism of mental illness. I wonder whether the differences people have in their self/representations come from the position/s we occupy on this spectrum of psychiatric persecution. There are some who have met the benign arm of psychiatry who completely believed it would bring deliverance someday. There are others who have been violated and coerced into psychiatric subjugation, never believing their labels, yet outnumbered to fight back alone. Perhaps a majority of our peers in the North belong to the latter and a majority of us in the South to the former groups? No two peoples have identical situations, yet we can all find something in common, without privileging anyone and remaining cognisant of our social differences. Perhaps we could make that a starting point for a common struggle?

Being a peer-therapist has been a complex experience and has entailed coming to terms with new realities, for there are social differences even here that I am beginning to understand. One of my findings is that the road to supporting one person make the crossover, from a refugee of psychiatry to questioning psychiatric finality takes time, patience, support and careful mediation of crises. Time and again I have understood how the struggle of a person spills over into their family.[10] In India, you don't usually work with solitary individuals, but with families closely enmeshed with all aspects of a person's life. To support one, you interact with all, and help everyone see the situation differently.

Just like a boatman (also called '*majhi*' in India) helps people cross a river on his boat, a peer who works in supporting others does likewise, by helping those passing through stormy passages of their lives. The boatman in India is also presented as a guide who leads you to the other side of the river, giving you a new direction in life.[11] Just like a boatman we hold one person, one family at a time and help them tide over their turbulence, trying to keep ourselves calm through it, for we have waded through the waters many times ourselves.

Embracing politics, leaving the label

At least we can learn about the power of a label from our experiences of psychiatry, and how that label can rob us of our selfhood. Would I take another label, also framed in psychiatric language, to resist? Do I even want to counter psychiatry? If one believed that psychiatry is only a consensus among certain people whose interests are served by viewing human suffering through a diagnostic lens, can we create another consensus as a viable alternative? Certainly there is no harm trying, but do we want to expend effort in fighting it? What sort of resources would such an enterprise require? Will we ever be able to come close to the kind of resources psychiatry has at its disposal, and the institutional mechanisms to enable them? Would we rather not create an alternative which does not pathologise distress and call it names? This is the invitation from 'Mad' politics I have taken up.

To embrace politics means to recognise the polarity of power, and on what axis it rests. If it is oppression, does it merely emanate autonomously from a so-called medical specialty, standing alone by itself? Or does it arise and get bolstered by the global flow of capital? To weave all these disparate ideas together we need an overarching frame, towards which 'Mad' Studies appears to nudge us.

The personal as political?

Without political consciousness and an emancipatory vision, the personal does not become political. In the initial feminist rallying cry this phrase was used as a consciousness-raising activity, 'a form of political action to elicit discussion' (Napikoski, 2019). Until people are philosophically convinced that something is the matter with their treatment regimens, nobody will raise a voice against wrongdoing, for they wouldn't understand it as wrong. No political consciousness that is unaware of its economic base can have a clear or radical vision, because its goal is not universal but person–centric.

If social emancipation be our goal, then personal empowerment is only the inauguration of a longer struggle. To continue that journey by embracing others, for the personal to become political, we need to challenge the individualism inherent in it. Otherwise narcissism may not permit us to go beyond identity politics. By collaborating with each other will we be ready to build a global axis of resistance. But until we work in that direction with a plan and a path, we underestimate those who we resist. The forces we oppose continue to organise more and more, with a capital base we can never fathom. To oppose them what else do we have? It has to be more than an assemblage of ideas and words from the labels they imposed on us.

We create an alternative to this scale of power by arriving at another social construction, and work out pathways to disseminate it. The new lexicon could respond to the material differences between the North and the South, which are not financial resources alone. These include knowledge, and access-related issues, inherent social inequalities, multiple axes of social injustice in the South, (possibly in also the North in a different manner). Assuming a lexicon is underway, we would be wise to be cautioned by Morrison (2008:xi) who notes that, '"[m]ental patients" who resist treatment and insist on speaking for themselves against mental health practices are particularly feared and misunderstood'. We need not imperil ourselves further by being feared by both our peers and oppressors. Instead the task ahead, as I see it, is to build solidarities against all forms of oppression – whatever is possible wherever, and struggle for a universal emancipation. Nandy (1983:xiii) reminds that, 'the meek inherit the earth not by meekness alone. They have to have categories, concepts, and, even, defences of mind … within the traditional world views still outside the span of modern ideas of universalism'. Our task appears clear; for among us lie the seeds of the future.

Notes

1 I prefer this to the more sophisticated 'Global South' which is spoken of to represent the 'developing' countries.
2 It is customary in India to address a woman in a formal role as 'Madam' or 'Ma'm/Ma'am' instead of using first names. Ordinarily first names are used only within families and friends.
3 Names and other identifying information have been changed
4 Even though I use this phrase, it is to indicate a professional position, which foregrounds my experiential knowledge. Neither am I a peer nor my work has a clinical connotation or therapeutic claims of psy-professionals. I work with an emancipatory sensibility towards 'recovery', while ensuring that people do not linger on as 'patients'/clients with me for too long.
5 The only services available are pharmacological treatments.
6 Though by all standards from all that I have read, studied and understood this is not the case even in the North.
7 The italics are original.
8 India has 22 official languages, in addition to English, from http://mhrd.gov.in/sites/upload_files/mhrd/files/upload_document/languagebr.pdf.
9 Taken from https://en.wikipedia.org/wiki/B._R._Ambedkar, on 26 January 2019.
10 My personal experiences see the engagement of family as the predominant social network of a person in a vast majority of cases. The role of friends, or any other networks does not appear so significant. I say this with observing both my social, research and counselling experiences. In all cases I have interacted with families.
11 Taken from Archives and Research Center for Ethnomusicology, via vmis.in/ArceCategories/music_in_context_innercat/97. Accessed on 7 October 2018.

References

Davar B V (2012). Legal frameworks for and against people with psychosocial disabilities. *Economic and Political Weekly, Vol* XLVII, *No 52*, 123–131.

Davar, B V (2015). Narratives of Coercion: Law as a social determinant of clinical interactions in mental hospitals. *CUSP – The Journal, Vol.1, No.1.* http://www.cuspthejournal.com/47.html. Accessed: 24 June 2019.

De Lissovoy N (2010). Rethinking education and emancipation: Being, teaching and power. *Harvard Educational Review*, 80 (2), 203–220.

Fraser N (2000). Rethinking recognition. *New Left Review*. https://newleftreview.org/issues/II3/articles/nancy-fraser-rethinking-recognition. Accessed: 16 March 2019.

Fricker M (2007). *Epistemic Injustice: Power and the Ethics of Knowing*. New York: Oxford University Press.

LeFrançois, B A, Menzies, R and Reaume, G. (2013) Introducing Mad Studies. In B A LeFrançois, R Menzies and G Reaume (eds.) *Mad Matters: A Critical Reader in Canadian Mad Studies*. Toronto: Canadian Scholars Press, 7–22.

Morrison L J (2008). *Talking Back to Psychiatry: The Psychiatric Consumer/Survivor/Ex-patient Movement*. New York and London: Routledge.

Nagarajan R (2018). Healthcare corruption – A consumer's view. In S Nundy, K Desiraju, S Nagral (Eds.). *Healers or Predators? – Healthcare corruption in India*. New Delhi: Oxford University Press, 293–310.

Nandy A (1983). *The Intimate Enemy – Loss and Recovery of Self Under Colonialism*. Delhi: Oxford University Press.

Napikoski L (2019). The personal is political. https://www.thoughtco.com/the-personal-is-political-slogan-origin-3528952. Accessed 17 March 2019.

Reynolds J F (2018). A short history of mental health rhetoric research (MHRR). *Rhetoric of Health and Medicine*, 1(1–2), 1–18.

Sharma P (2019). Shades of silence – Doing mental health research as an 'insider'. *Journal of Ethics in Mental Health*, Open Vol.10, 1–12.

34

'MADNESS' AS A TERM OF DIVISION, OR REJECTION

Colin King

Introduction

This chapter examines the political and theoretical role of 'Mad studies' and its possible contribution in supporting the liberation of black mental health survivors, including survivor researchers. Such liberation needs to extend to exposing the racialised processes in the biomedical quantitative Euro-centric diagnosis of schizophrenia, which has led to the over-representation of black men in the mental health system (Mental health Foundation, 2015; Government UK, 2018). In line with principles of 'Mad Studies', this chapter explores how to make possible a transformational position for an authentic black survivor; the research method, models and theories that can offer such a critical strategic position. This needs to be a position that enables the first person 'black experience' to challenge how it is objectified through the third person 'white' researcher, offering a radical critique of the political and economic forms of exclusion legitimated through unchallenged traditions of white dominance in co-production in mental health work. The chapter examines the ethics of joint collaboration across the colour line, and the potential for a truly inclusive anti-racist 'Mad Studies', Beresford (2015), Ingram (2008) and Russo and Sweeney (2016) as an important analytical position in relation to race and mental health. The chapter is thus concerned with the changes needed to recentralise the experiential knowledge, from a position of rejection to acceptance of the life experiences of black men currently in the mental health system (Chase, 2014; Cummins, 2015; Gajwani et al., 2016). I consider how helpful 'Mad Studies' can be in ensuring European values work more effectively alongside Afro-centric values to remove the classification, 'schizophrenia'. I want to see if there can be a form of 'Mad Studies' that breaks the hierarchy of race, from its eugenic position, to one that has a central transcultural role in dismantling and reforming biomedical scientific processes that have long perpetuated rejection and divisions in relation to the role of the black survivor researcher.

Mad studies, the unlived and unrecognised black survivor researcher

It's important to ensure that 'mad studies' is not about division and rejection. This is to break its perceived association with a privilege given to white, middle-class survivors who have become academics, a privilege defined by (Eddo-loge, 2017) as 'white privilege is an absence of the

DOI: 10.4324/9780429465444-40

negative consequences of racism ... it is an absence of funny looks directed at you because you're believed to be in the wrong place...' (Eddo-Lodge, 2017:119). Mad studies makes a moral commitment to incorporate the black voice. Its reference to the importance of a connection to social movements and activism, inclusivity and anti-oppressive practice, with a commitment to shared lack of resources and survivor ownership and the role of the allies, is crucial. I share this vision, of a dynamic change in mental health work, through the radical potential of 'mad studies' and survivor research as a critique of psychiatry, which I see as extending to a critique of 'white European psychiatry'. These are the challenges that 'Mad studies' must embrace to analyse mental health and race, particularly the role of its own whiteness. This is an important ethos, to foster strong relationship towards a counter-discourse to biomedical 'white' psychiatry as referenced by Beresford and Wallcraft 'The psychiatric system is unpromising ground for reform, but many survivors are held within it. It cannot be ignored' (1997:79).

Mad studies in moving towards acceptance and collaboration, as opposed to rejection and division, faces including the 'first person experience' of the black mental health survivor as institutionally significant through all its work. A practice of understanding and interpreting these experiences, as social injustice and a form of political control (Drapetomaina) that has become economic capital for current research, (NSUN, Reignite the space, Advancing race equality in Mental health work, Mind) is likely to improve the experiences of black men in the mental health system. It is a position that recognises the 'first person black experience' through the Afro-centric approaches of (Fanon, 1967) and (Du Bois, 1903), in terms of the use of the 'white mask' and 'veil'. These are theoretical and methodological approaches that translate the black mental health survivor research position in relation to the biomedical philosophical and psychiatric approaches to mental health work. Despite recent publications in relation to race and mental health, (Fernando, 2017) and (Kalathil, 2008) the concept 'madness' has to be considered more seriously as a method of reform in the area of racism in mental health. It needs to be reconceived to open up the possibility of a radical examination of the racialisation of the label 'schizophrenia' as a form of madness in current methodological and theoretical studies. In this way it may distinguish between studies that now examine forms of madness in their investigation into racism in mental health work, rather than colluding with the term madness that has been negatively associated with black men (Ritchie, 1994).

Consequently, it's important that 'mad studies' is conceived in a way so it's not associated with the historical link between race and madness (Cartwright, 1851; Jung, 1930; Freud, 1949), framing black men as primitive, noble savage (James and Harris, 1993). It is thus crucial to adopt integrated methodological and theoretical tools across the colour line that changes the systems, as opposed to changing how black men's experience is understood in a racist biomedical system. This is an approach to 'mad studies' that moves from the *service use* co-production model (Needham and Carr, 2009) as discussed by (Gillard et al., 2010), to a position suggested by mad studies, in advancing ethics and knowledge *through a civil rights* approach to co-production (Khan, 1967 cited in Needham and Carr, 2009). This would be co-production built on black survivors researchers having ownership and true intellectual capital, as discussed and promoted by Russo (2016) and Sweeney (2010), in relation to participation, ownership, values and methods that challenge dominant ideas about mental health and race.

I believe, not the title, but the concept of 'mad studies' is a radical critical approach to biomedical symptom's approach that has the collective potential to change how historical European theories contributed to the madness experienced by black men such as me. This is an approach to 'mad studies' that moves to a political positioning of empowering and ensuring whiteness is examined as part of a culture (Said, 1994) from both a methodological (Ladman, 1972) and social activist positioning. It is also an important challenge for white survivors within 'mad studies' to reflect on the way their whiteness influences their own position when truly working with black survivor researchers, that is not about moral obligations, patronage, or cosmetic representation.

Consequently, 'mad studies' has an analytical responsibility to explore the role of whiteness amongst its white academics in relation to race and misdiagnosis. This promotes the concept 'mad studies' as one that is reflective and has empathy with the lived experience of the black mental health survivor in their reaction to white psychiatry. This has been a form of white psychiatry that produces studies of madness in which black men (Littlewood and Lipsedge, 1981; Bromberg and Simon, 1968; Metzl, 2009) are constructed. In this chapter I see 'mad studies' as new ways of collectively making sense of the biomedical diagnosis of schizophrenia associated with Euro-centric models of race; a shared, collective and political methodological approach to race in mental health work as being linked. Linked and associated with external structures; the family, school, mental health systems and research. For 'mad studies' to be credible for black mental health survivor research, it must represent the interpretations of the experiences of African man over-represented in the mental health system as an important priority. This is a priority that connects to the principle of 'centralizing experiential knowledge', that ensures that African men and their historical past are given recognition as integral to the politicisation of both the method and methodological approach to race and mental health (Keating and Robertson, 2004; Kalathil, 2008).

I believe that 'mad studies' should have an important shared, strategic approach to social justice and race equality in exposing both the biomedical approach and the role of White European psychiatry. The challenge for 'mad studies' for developing a purposeful inclusive and anti-racist practice is situated in the following statement, 'critiquing our lived experiences of the manifestation of 'goodness and whiteness' (LeFrancois et al., 2013). This is a critique that should aim to reshape how whiteness in psychiatry understands the experience of black men like me diagnosed with schizophrenia. The possibility then is that 'mad studies' can contribute to the decolonalisation (Mbembe, 2015) of the hegemonic power of whiteness to re-establish 'the first person experiences of African men as normal inside the English psychiatric system'. This would be a form of 'mad studies' that repositions a radicalisation of whiteness in shaping how academics, researchers and practitioners can support the emancipation of black men from the biomedical approach to mental health. This chapter thus aims to examine the principles of 'mad studies' that enhances how we analyse madness within the historical theories of race and racism in mental health diagnosis that black men endure.

Mad studies and the European theorists: Epistemic justice

The literature on race, mental health and the diagnosis of African men appears to attend to institutional poor practice without any reference to the importance of epistemic justice, one of the central principles of 'Mad studies'. From Cartwright's (1851) diagnosis of African slaves running away from their slave masters, i.e. 'Drapetomania', to (Bromberg and Simon 1968; Metzl, 2009) the study of schizophrenia as a 'protest psychosis', in relation to black men during the civil rights movement. Both fail to recognise the oppression within their studies; a simplistic reductionist position in relation to understanding the complexities of and inequalities in the relationship between the white practitioner and the black patient. They formulate a conspiracy of race in mental health as an attack on European biomedical science (Metzl, 2009; Fernando, 2017) without any analytical examination of what is happening between the actors: the practitioners and patients involved in the drama of the misdiagnosis of black men.

As mentioned earlier, it's important not to be tempted to associate the narrative, 'mad studies' with the negative connotation of madness, a term associated with insanity, mental illness and the dangerousness of black men (Ritchie, 1994). These negative terms are often made in reference to the experiences of black men assessed within the conventional mental health framework and create divisions with white professionals (Littlewood and Lipsedge, 1981). The notion of 'cultural schizophrenia' (Littlewood and Lipsedge, 1981:17), that is the social distance between white psychiatrist and black patient, restricts the potential to work within a collaborative approach to 'mad studies in a new conceptualised approach to race. This is the central inclusive anti-racist principles of 'mad studies' the possibility of working across the colour-line and professional lines towards a shared understanding of how racism operates in the diagnosis of African men born in British society.

The philosophical position of 'mad studies', is to liberate and empower in resistance to the biomedical framework, through the political role of black men's interaction with a mental health service (Chase, 2014). It offers the opportunity of a politicised methodological approach to the experiences of black men inside the mental health system rather than just their stories of their experiences of the services. 'Mad studies', can equip black mental health survivor researchers to act on the assertions made by Aggarwal (2012) 'that white psychiatry is an inherently racist culture as regards the clinical assessment of black men'. Such assertions are further reinforced by researchers such as (Fernando, 2017) with his inquiry into schizophrenia. Both keeps alive the view that black survivor research can only be reliable, valid and creditable if it is done by black academics. White academics have tended to depoliticise the authentic black experience in mental health care.

Mad studies' can prevent divisions and rejections of the black survivor research movement, if it challenges the way European philosophers have created eugenic theories of race. The theories of race by Hobbes (1661) and Kant (1788) reduced the African to a non-human status. The challenge here is to expose the discrimination in the process of assuming African people are mad, primitive, and dangerous. The challenge is to politicise race within 'mad studies' to change the ideas made about African people through traditional research methodology and process and acknowledge the primary importance of first person Black experiential knowledge. To develop a more structural and ethnical analysis to schizophrenia in relation to African men, 'Mad studies' as a radical critique of the biomedical approach must critique alongside black-survivor researchers how white European models have produced perceptions of race and madness. 'Mad studies', must stand outside of a tradition of white academics and stand up for changes in European philosophy, to work in collaboration with the Afro-centric approaches of Fanon (1967), Asante (1985) and Wilson (1993). This is the conceptual collaboration to disempower the way Euro-centric models as values emerge inside the diagnosis of schizophrenia and African men. This is an approach to 'mad studies' based on a commitment to change historical white models as European perceptions of African men when diagnosed with schizophrenia. It lies at the heart of Mad Studies, which rejects the medical model that gives rise to the diagnostic category of schizophrenia.

Mad studies, developing a radical critique of white European diagnosis

I suggest that the tradition of 'mad studies', built on diverse and marginalised groups being heard, adopting the explicit approach of survivor research, can move towards equality and inclusion as opposed to being tied to rejection and division. It must raise political and methodological curiosity to understand the deficiency of the definition of schizophrenia that black men like me have fallen victim to. 'Mad studies' as a project of enquiry enables an examination of how diagnostic frameworks, such as ICD and DSM, as being biomedical reveal features of cultural madness. Adopting 'mad studies' is also to critique white psychiatry, and the impact on my experiences as an African mental health survivor. 'Mad studies' in alliance with black survivor research needs can go beyond the biomedical approach and also challenge how European philosophers need to review the global impact of European models. This must lead to understanding the changes in the practices of whiteness necessary to radically dismantle the diagnosis of schizophrenia in relation to black men like me.

If 'mad studies' are to achieve parity with traditional positivism and quantitative 'science' in the areas of schizophrenia and racism then they have to normalise black survivor research as transcending the colour line. It has to integrate black mental health survivor research as lacking access to the privileges it takes for granted as handed down to white survivor academics. This makes possible co-production of political and methodological equality that enables me as a Black survivor researcher to examine why the diagnosis of schizophrenia is so polarised between the African and European experience. 'Mad studies' suggest the importance of co-produced research (Gillard et al., 2012). To do this it must challenge 'whiteness' both in its approach and its focus.

This requires a 'mad studies' that begins to conceptualise how race from the fifteenth century to the eighteenth century constructed black men as mad (Foucault, 1967). For 'mad studies' to develop a co-production of equality with black mental health survivor research it needs to develop a new conceptual approach to race that looks at the range of factors in relation to African men who have died in the psychiatric system. Such co-production and conceptual collaboration is essential to refute the idea (LeFrancois et al., 2013:13) that 'mad studies' is similar to race studies as a shared response to the dominant biomedical model. The absence of understanding of whiteness as a feature within the biomedical models is then reduced to what (Diangelo, 2018) describes as 'white fragility'. This thus contributes towards an emotional fear and silence that reinforces what (Diangelo, 2018) describes as ('racial equilibrium') (Diangelo, 2018:57). 'Mad studies' has the conceptual potential as a tool to move beyond this fear or emotional silence.

The first stage of moving beyond emotional silence is seeing black mental health survivor researcher as more than one dimensional. This is to engage in a co-production where white academic survivor researchers must focus on changes in patterns of behaviour that stems from a fear of examining whiteness. As part of this, 'Mad studies' must start with an investigation into the experiences of their first person accounts. This calls for a form of enquiry (LeFrancois et al., 2013) that leads to understanding whiteness as experience, and developing a range of theories to produce a new way of looking at how whiteness is formed in relation to understanding how African men are excluded. Consequently, it is important that 'mad studies' addresses how the experiences of African men born in England can re-educate assumptions of whiteness.

Consequently, for 'mad studies' to avoid perpetuating existing divisions between black men and white psychiatry, it must give serious consideration to a framework that enables it to conceptualise the African experience through a new radical, methodological approach. This is to enable whiteness to see its purposive contribution to race and mental health (Beresford, 2005, 2015). The challenge for 'mad studies' is to develop an understanding of whiteness that is not simply related as an invisible normative standard, but one that makes whiteness visible and accountable. This is the introspective approach to whiteness as an experience that should re-define its dominant professional norm to work in a more equitable way. 'Mad studies' must make transparent the potential of whiteness beyond Said's (1994) reference to it as a 'secret cultural weapon'. This enables an approach to challenging whiteness to manage new inclusive political organisational cultures within current research; a reflective culture of change in the structures of whiteness from the school to the wards in relation to the experiences of African men.

Challenging pre-production biomedical white psychiatry through 'mad studies'

For black survivor researchers to seek true authentic equality through the principles of 'mad studies', there has to be an agreement to the critique of the biomedical approach within white psychiatry and the historical practices of racism that impact on African men. These practices can only be changed if the eugenic theories of whiteness are dismantled. This means the dismantling of theorists such as Freud (1949), drawing on eugenic values that reduce African men to having no emotional qualities to experience 'mental health'. 'Mad studies' is the radical responsibility to expose the most intrusive features of the biomedical approach; to expose how founding theories of eugenics shape how white psychiatry assesses madness in African men. Thus to avoid rejection and division with black survivor research, 'Mad studies' must engage with the importance of the pre-production stage – the stage in which white European models implicitly and unconsciously had been used as a form of scientific racism. This is to engage with a political position that is reconciled with the importance of alterative cultural heritages, best represented in the Afro-centric approaches of Fanon (1967), (Tchandela, 2008; 2011) and (Wilson, 1993). These are approaches that must be central to 'Mad studies' going forward to disempower Euro-centric models from the pre-production periods (Cartwright, 1851). These were key models and theories that emerged as historical European perceptions of African men through which they have become disempowered and demoralised.

'Mad studies' through its principle of a 'radical potential for survivor research', and the principle of developing a 'counter-discourse' to biomedical psychiatry has a responsibility to show how the pre-production stage has institutionalised a definition of schizophrenia that black men like me have fallen victim to within white psychiatry. This commitment then enables a form of 'mad studies' that is inclusive and sensitive to alternative voices and experiences within the mental health survivor movement. It allows us to understand how unconscious values from the historical pre-production stage contributes towards a white psychiatry.

This would mean exploring how the pre-production stage in which white psychiatry emerged and revealed its power created methodological divisions between black and white survivor research. It entails examining how the period of slavery and post-colonialism have contributed to theories that reject the first-person account of African men as discussed in the work of Garvey (1925). Garvey and other African philosophies offer a form of liberation, an alternative radical position that offers equality to African voices. This is the voice of the Afro-centric (Welsing, 1991), that examines the impact of the pre-production stage. Addressing this enables 'Mad studies' to move to a collaborative form of whiteness in working and empowering black men in relation to changing the biomedical approach to mental health.

'Mad studies' has a critical role in exposing a biomedical white psychiatry that has legitimised both the overt medication and sectioning of black men, and the legal powers given to white professionals to classify the black male experience as a mental disorder. 'Mad studies' in an alliance with a new critical race theorising must then position the period of slavery as an important ideological contribution to the patterns of behaviour within current psychiatric practices in the restraint and killing of black men. 'Mad studies' thus has an ethical position to re-evaluate – white psychiatry and the theories of mental illness used to translate the African experience as victims of white injustice. Thus the potential of a civil rights model of co-production with radical black survivor researchers producing a range of theories and new ways of looking at changing how African men have been constructed through the pathways of white philosophy.

If 'Mad studies' is to continue in its vision of offering a radical critical position to biomedical psychiatry then it will need to show how white philosophy and white psychiatry have served as a form of racialised injustice. It means for 'Mad studies' to move from an 'ivory tower' third-person structural analysis of race in mental health to a personal and individualised reflective consideration of whiteness. Practitioners within 'mad studies' will have to examine their power and privilege, their behaviours and values of whiteness and the roles and structures they will need to create to address the serious disempowerment of a black survivor research position.

For 'mad studies' to be effectively accountable to real inclusive anti-racist practice is to truly challenge the whiteness that emerges as a consciousness (Frankenberg, 1993), a cognizance, a powerful influence in 'mapping cultural' changes for white academic survivor researchers to advocate for a 'mad studies' to challenge inequality in mental health and race. Consequently, 'Mad studies', to avoid being a term of division and rejection, must make its own whiteness explicit in the co-production process in order to produce new collaborative perspectives with black survivor researchers. 'Mad studies' then has an important civil rights position a co-production model where whiteness gives up the power it was afforded in pre-production stages. This can lead to important changes in a new perspective that leads to challenging changes in psychiatry and the mental health treatment of black men in the British care system.

'Mad studies' has to begin to develop new theories of race equality for a new type of co-production in the British health care system that affects the relationship between the clinical professional and the black patient. Consequently, black survivor researchers make a plea for a 'mad studies' that engages with the challenges for a co-production process that does not restrict black men to a statutory identity, and that only white academics or black academics with no lived experience can research this. It is a demand for an approach that can conceptualise my departure from Maudsley Hospital by exposing the back-stage cultures of whiteness (Goffman, 1961). This is the backstage in which whiteness in psychiatry develops its power and its identity through a range of white philosophers with the privilege to define me through its discharge and care planning. 'Mad studies' has to make visible the privilege of white biomedical psychiatry to diagnose schizophrenia in relation to me. In this context, 'mad studies' is the method of making visible the importance of the pre-production period, in which Goffman (1959) assumes the ward setting gives African men like me access to white people they would not have encountered in the outside world.

'Mad studies' has the potential for a co-production for black survivor researchers to access a political alliance towards equal access to change the present power imbalance. The power imbalance taken for granted as forms of privilege from the pre-production stage that has stripped African men of their identity and exposed them to therapies, medications, and procedures that are built on the pre-production values of white biomedical psychiatry.

'Mad studies' in alliance with the lived experience of black survivor research can change the ability of whiteness to empathise with the cultural other, that is, African men. It can pressure white psychiatry not to collude with the pre-production past in which black men have simply been seen as suffering from a form of madness brought about by a failure to integrate into the cultural demands of white British culture (Littlewood and Lipsedge, 1981). 'Mad studies' in deconstructing a diagnosis that reflects Western psychiatry privilege, is in a position to empathise with the outcomes for black men currently inside the mental health system, who are seventeen times more likely than their white counterparts to be diagnosed as schizophrenic, (Mental Health Foundation, 2015).

'Mad studies' has a responsibility to halt the transition from the pre-production to co-production stage in the ways in which the power of Black men within white psychiatry is denied. It has an analytical role to recognise how these powers have contributed to what Littlewood and Lipsedge (1981) refer to as 'cultural schizophrenia'. Such a cultural schizophrenia makes visible how the pre-production period has created a social and political distance between white psychiatry and black men based on a form of irrationality rarely studied. The success of 'mad studies' is then to look at strategies to address the cultural distance between the white psychiatrist and black men; between white survivor and black survivor researchers and activists. It offers the possibility of a joint strategy that challenges psychiatric, medical and social work professionals to locate whiteness as a practice rooted in a period in which black men were denied basic civil rights.

For co-production to be successful, it needs to engage with the principle of inclusivity in relation to race equality, and whiteness must take full account of its privileges, economically, politically and culturally. The challenge for 'mad studies' in a collaboration with black survivor research is to ensure that whiteness is not accepted as the 'professionalised norm'. It needs to address and change the norms of whiteness that have played a pivotal role in relation to the psychiatric profession in terms of how white professionals act. It is the cultural values within white psychiatry – and their complex forms of whiteness (Basso, 1979) – that are portraits, coded and performed in different ways to construct schizophrenia in African men. This has huge and complicated complex implications if 'mad studies' is to relocate the power between black men and white psychiatry by exposing these codes, behaviours and portraits.

Mad studies, a joint political venture with black survivor research to dismantle the injustice of biomedical white psychiatry

The major political and theoretical challenge for 'mad studies' is the complete dismantling of the privileges ceded to white psychiatry in the assessment of schizophrenia in relation to black men during the last 60 years. This is a challenge that requires a radical reform of co-production that empowers white survivor researchers to address how the heritage of European philosophy connects to its lived experiences within race and mental health. This is a 'mad studies' that challenges European white psychiatry and the power of European philosophy to reinterpret the human experiences of racism in relation to black men. It is getting 'mad studies' and white psychiatry to change its cultural lenses in order to review how African men have been constructed by systems that were formed through racialised practices of rejection and division.

These practices of rejection and division can be addressed by a 'mad studies' that includes the perspectives of black men within a new narrative of race that redresses the power of white psychiatry. A new type of co-production based on an equitable collaboration, that facilitates and promotes greater equality in working across race. It would be based on a new racial contract (Mills, 1997) in which the voices of black men are recognised as contributing towards legitimate theories and models inside the practices of mental health care in modern Britain. Consequently, I am advocating for a type of 'mad studies' that recognises the experiences of black men as representing the foundations of a new approach to race in mental health beyond that of being a patient/survivor.

I suggest 'mad studies', in line with its principles of co-produced research, particularly in the area of race and racism in mental health work, has to examine the power given to it (Freud, 1949) to define 'Schizophrenia' and the lack of power given to the black experience to define this diagnosis. It needs to be co-produced research that examines the historical biomedical origins of the term schizophrenia without any compromising of the 'first person accounts' of black men. This will help to expose the value judgements made about black men which fail to question why the African contribution to the reality of schizophrenia has never been properly acknowledged and why it has been excluded from consideration in the construction of 'schizophrenia'. For 'Mad studies' to embrace its radical critique of biomedical psychiatry it must promote a collaboration in terms of how the African reality is rejected as an experience.

Consequently, to be effective, collaboration between white and black survivor research within the principles of 'Mad studies' needs to work to redress the historical power imbalance, first between black patient and white psychiatry, and second, in relation to black and white survivor research. It will need to adopt the 'white masks' (Fanon, 1967:4) to illuminate the racialised lenses that can be used; methodologically investigate the social injustice and the civil right of communities of an African heritage. 'Mad studies' thus must remove the expert knowledge attributed to white clinical models that has colluded with studies that create perceptions of madness within the black patient. This can challenge the impact of biomedical European Psychiatry by questioning how symptoms are constructed and connected to racialised values of 'mental disorder'. White academics have rarely disclosed or analysed the impact this has on the black community in the modern age of western psychiatry. The challenge of a joint venture between white and black survivor research is to analyse the ways in white psychiatry has listed psychotic symptoms without any reference to an Afro-centric approach, or the Afro-centric reality to what is considered 'mental health'. Consequently, 'mad studies' needs to examine how the legacy of past classification systems (DSM, ICD) has constrained African men within a system that has denied their own lived experiences. The crucial question for 'mad studies' is giving communities of an African heritage the opportunity to respond to a classification system that is outside of its cultural heritage. This is the commitment to engage an African classification system which both white survivor research, and black academic institutional researchers need to embrace (Ladman, 1972).

Consequently, there is a need for 'mad studies' to adopt the principles of Mills (1997), to examine, develop and enforce a racial contract that redefines the position of white psychiatry and white survivor researcher. One that is able to work in cooperation with other cultural worlds. This is the cooperation that reflects a new pattern where white men's relationship to African men is based on a new equitable 'Race Construct' 'that challenges the assumption of the European world'

> an agreement, originally among European men in the beginning of the modern period, to identify themselves as "white" and therefore fully human, and to identify all others, in particular the natives with whom they were beginning to meet, as "other" non-white and therefore not fully human.
>
> *(Mills, 1997:27)*

Therefore, 'Mad studies' occupies a significant position to ensure a new approach to whiteness within European psychiatry, collaborating within a changed racial contract. This is a contract that reflects and accepts equality with African men, in terms of practice, assessment and the African contribution towards a new diagnostic framework. This equality must consider the central significance of race and power; the power given to African men that can influence white psychiatry in understanding how mental disorder is experienced in British health care. I am an advocate for a transcultural approach to a 'race contract' that elevates the African experience so that it has real meaning within a cultural co-production approach to mental health from research to practice.

Conclusion

In concluding this chapter, let me say that I have an affinity to the purpose of 'mad studies' as a radical critique of the biomedical approach and the principles of empowering survivor research in the specific area of race justice in mental health. I have argued here that it must force race, racism and whiteness to address its impact and the legacy of its classification system in relation to the African experience. It must try and develop a reflective approach to whiteness that considers how features of race emerge in relation to the diagnosis of schizophrenia during the last sixty years, similar to the protest psychosis developed in the work of Bromberg and Simon (1968) and Metzl (2009). Because of this, there is a need to dismantle current International Classification of Diseases and the Diagnostic Statistical Manual that has contributed to the over-representation of black men as prisoners to a 'protest psychosis' and to institutionalised racism in the wider structures of British society. 'Mad studies' must then develop an approach that incorporates the perspectives of black mental health survivors across both the colour and gender lines. 'Mad studies' must have as one of its central principles, developing a critical methodology for reading the perceptions of whiteness that exists within current research and mental health practices. This mission should be to change the road map of mental health research that places Black survivors' research at the bottom, (subjects) as opposed to the centre of research (the facilitator), as crucial to a new form of co-production. Co-production can only be effective if the reality of the African experience is translated through the subjectivity of whiteness. This is the ideological challenge of making transparent the subjective nature of whiteness in the research into classification systems and the impact this has on people of African descent.

To conclude here, Husserl's (1973) phenomenological approach has the potential to evaluate the impact of how whiteness operates within a co-production relationship within 'mad studies'. What is needed is a 'mad studies' that can operate to change its negotiations with black men within the co-production process of a new empowerment framework. Husserl (1973) suggests that intuition, description, the process of articulating one's symptoms, can all reshape how our experiences can be reconfigured to a new approach. This should inspire a new model of co-production, one that recognises black men's subjective experiences as being important in the dialogue round diagnosis within and through white psychiatry. We must move away from a form of 'cultural silence' that appears to operate inside white research in both philosophy and survivor research, to consider a new radical inclusive approach within a partnership of understanding based on trust that is formed through a new definition of 'mad studies'.

In the development of the 'Whiteness and Race Equality Network Conference' St George's University, 2019, a collaboration of representatives from Professional Kendall, national lead for Mental Health, Peter Beresford, Mad Studies, Akiko Hart, National Survivor User Network, Lancet Psychiatry, Professional Fulford, Oxford University, Lorraine Marke, carer, Michael Bennett, PFA, and Steve Gillard, St George's University, this process of cultural silence was broken in relation to the following:

1. To expose whiteness as a critical approach to research into race and racism in mental health work.
2. To embrace working across lines of colour and historical tribal differences to achieve real negotiated race equality in mental health work.
3. To extend the concept, 'lived experience by expertise' to all individuals and groups working in the area of race equality and mental health work.
4. To ensure black survivor research is central and institutional to research, practice and models of change.

5. That we work towards dismantling areas of rejection and division from the pre-production stage of race and eugenics in white psychiatry.

6. To develop integrated methodologies and methods of investigation that recognise and incorporate Afro-centric theories, methods and classification systems.

7. To recognise the imprisonment, restraint and murder of black men in the mental health system is civil and human rights concern.

8. To dismantle as opposed to attempt to improve a system that has not improved the lives of black men and other marginalised groups.

9. To recognise change is economic, political and cultural in destroying the social injustice of modern slavery in the mental health system.

10. That we can work together towards change.

It can be done. The enduring mission of 'Mad Studies' is to work to make it happen.

References

Aggarwal, N K (2012) Adapting the Cultural Formulation for Clinical Assessments in Forensic Psychiatry. *J Am Acad Psychiatry Law* 40(1), 113–118.

Asante M K (1985). Afrocentricity and Culture. In M K Asante and K W Asante (eds). *African Cultures: The Rhythms of Unity*. Greenwood Press, Westport CT, ix–a.

Basso K H (1979). *Portraits of the Whiteman: Linguistic Play and Cultural Symbols among the Western Apache*. Cambridge University Press, Cambridge.

Beresford P (2005). Social work and social model of madness and distress. Developing a viable role the future. *Social work& Social Sciences Review*, 12 (2), 59–73.

Beresford P (2015). Speaking as a survivor researcher. *MadInAmerica.com* https://www.madinamerica. com/2015/03/speaking-survivor-researcher/. Accessed: 16 July 2020.

Beresford P and Wallcraft J (1997). Psychiatric System Survivors and Emancipatory Research: Issues, Overlaps and Differences. In C Barnes and G Mercer (Eds.). *Doing Disability Research*. Leeds, UK: Disability Press, 66–87.

Bromberg M D and Simon F (1968). The "Protest" Psychosis. A Special Type of Reactive Psychosis, *Arch Gen Psychiatry*, 19 (2), 155–160.

Cartwright S (1851). Report on the Diseases and Peculiarities of the Negro Race. *DeBow's Review* XI.

Chase L (2014). Ethnic Inequalities in Mental Health: Promoting Lasting Positive Change. *A Consultation with Black and Minority Mental Health Service Users*. Lankelly Chase Foundation, London.

Cummins I (2015). Discussing Race, Racism and Mental Health: Two Mental Health Inquiries Reconsidered. *International Journal of Human Rights in Healthcare*, 8(3), 160–172.

Diangelo R (2018). *White Fragility. Why It's so Hard for White People to Talk about Racism*. London: Penguin Random House UK.

Du Bois W D (1903). *Souls of a Black Folk*. Dover Publications, New York.

Eddo-Lodge R (2017). *Why I'm No Longer Talking to White People About Race*. London, Bloomsbury.

Fanon F (1967). *Black Skin, White Mask*. Penguin, London.

Fernando S (2017). *Institutional Racism in Psychology and Clinical Psychology. Race Matters in Mental Health*. Palgrave Macmillan, London.

Foucault M (1967). *Madness and Civilisation*. Routledge, London and New York.

Frankenberg R (1993). *White Women, Race Matters. The Social Construction of Whiteness*. Routledge, New York and London.

Freud, S (1949). *An outline of psychoanalysis*. Norton. New York.

Gajwani R, Parsons H, Birchwood M and Swanran P S (2016). Ethnicity and Detention: Are Black and Minority Ethnic (BME) Groups Disproportionately Detained Under the Mental Health Act 2007? *Soc Psychiatry Psychiatry Epidemiology*, 51, 703–711.

Garvey M (1925). *Philosophy and Opinions of Marcus Garvey*. Edition 1977 Atheneum, New York.

Gillard S, Borschmann R, Turner K, Goodrich-Purnell N, Lovell K and Chambers M (2010). "What Difference Does it Make?" Finding Evidence of the Impact of Mental Health Service User Researchers on Research into the Experiences of Detained Psychiatric Patients. *Health Expectations*, 13(2), 185–194.

Gillard S, Simons L, Turner K, Luckock M. and Edwards C (2012). Patient and Public Involvement in the Coproduction of Knowledge: Analysis of Qualitative Data in a Mental Health Study. *Qualitative Health Research*, 22, 1126–1137.

Goffman E (1959). *The Presentation of Self in Every day Life*. Pelican Books, England.

Goffman E (1961). *Asylums. Essays on the Social Situations of Mental Patients and Other Inmates*. Pelican Books, England.

Government UK (2018) The Independent Review of the Mental Health Act. https://assets.publishing.service.gov.uk/government/uploads/system/uploads/attachment_data/file/703919/The_independent_Mental_Health_Act_review__interim_report_01_05_2018.pdf Accessed: 16 September 2020).

Hobbes T (1661). *Leviathan*. In C B Macpherson (ed.) (1985). Penguin Books, London.

Husserl E (1973). *Zur Phänomenologie der Intersubjektivität: Texte aus dem Nachlass. Erster Teil. 1905-1920*. Springer, Netherlands.

Ingram R (2008). *Mapping "Mad Studies": The Birth of an in/Discipline*. Disability Studies Conference. San Jose, CA.

James, W and Harris, C (1993). *Inside Babylon. The Caribbean Diaspora in Britain*. Verso: London and New York.

Jung C G (1930). Your Negriod and Indian Behaviour. *Forum*, 83(4), 193–199.

Kant I (1788). *Critique of Practical Reason (Kritik der praktischen Vernunft)*.

Kalathil J (2008). Dancing to Our Own Tunes Reassessing Black and Minority Ethnic Mental Health Service User Involvement; Network for Mental Health. *National Survivor User Network*.

Keating F and Robertson D (2004). Fear, Black People and Mental Illness: A Vicious Circle. *Health and Social Care in the Community*, 12 (5), 439–447.

Ladman J (1972). *The Death of White Sociology*. Routledge, London.

LeFrançois B A, Menzies R and Reaume G (Eds.) (2013). *Mad matters: A critical reader in Canadian Mad Studies*. Canadian Scholars' Press, Toronto ON.

Littlewood R and Lipsedge M (1981). *Aliens and Alienists: Ethnic Minorities and Psychiatry*. Routledge: London.

Mbembe A (2015) Decolonizing Knowledge and the Question of the Archive. https://wiser.wits.ac.za/system/files/Achille%20Mbembe%20-%20Decolonizing%20Knowledge%20and%20the%20Question%20of%20the%20Archive.pdf. Accessed: 16 July 2020.

Mental Health Foundation (2015) Fundamental Facts about Mental Health. https://www.mentalhealth.org.uk/sites/default/files/fundamental-facts-15.pdf Accessed 16 September 2020).

Metzl J M (2009) *The Protest Psychosis. How Schizophrenia Became a Black Disease*. Beacon Press, Massachusetts.

Mills C (1997). *The Racial Contract*. Cornell University Press, Ithaca, NY.

Needham C and Carr S (2009). SCIE Research Briefing 31: Co-production: An emerging evidence base for adult social care transformation, Social Care Institute for Excellence, London.

Ritchie J H (1994). *The Report of the Inquiry into the Care and Treatment of Christopher Clunis*. Stationery Office Books, London.

Russo J (2016) Towards our own framework or reclaiming madness, part two. In Russo, J and Sweeney, A (eds.) *Searching for a Rose Garden. Challenging Psychiatry, Fostering Mad Studies*. Monmouth: PCCS Books, 59–68.

Russo J and Sweeney A (2016) (eds.) *Searching for a Rose Garden. Challenging Psychiatry, Fostering Mad Studies*. Monmouth: PCCS Books.

Said W (1994). *Culture and Imperialism*. Vintage Books, New York.

Sweeney A (2010). *Exploring Mental Health Service Users' Perspectives on and Experiences of Continuity of Care* (Doctoral dissertation). King's College London, UK.

Tchandela (2008) *Jah Rastafari Visions of Faith*. Jahlove Publishing, Brighton.

Tchandela (2011) *Jah Rastafari. Volume 2 The Babylon System*. Jahlove Publishing, Brighton.

Welsing F C (1991). *The Isis Papers. The Key to the Colors*. Third Generation Press, Chicago.

Wilson A (1993). *The Falsification of Afrikan Consciousness: Eurocentric History, Psychiatry and the Politics of White Supremacy*. African Research Publications, USA.

AFTERWORD
The ethics of making knowledge together

Jasna Russo

At the end of a long process to put together and edit this book, the fact that it will now be out there does not feel like an accomplishment in itself. It seems much more to me that the work behind this book is just about to begin and that the most important task is still ahead of us: that is, to bring the many ideas of this collection forward rather than let them stay within the confines of a publication that will not be affordable to many. Or in the words of Audre Lord:

> [W]e do not learn from what goes on in the book. We learn from that interaction that takes place in the spaces between what is in the book and ourselves.
>
> *(Kraft, 2018:81)*

It is our hope that both authors and readers will carry on sharing, deepening and extending the body of knowledge that this handbook seeks to reveal. That 'revelation' can only ever be partial, but we do hope that the chapters provide a glimpse into the kind of scholarship that Mad Studies makes possible. If I were to choose one single key characteristic of that scholarship, I would quote from the brief guidance we sent to the contributors. One of our requests was:

> [P]lease don't be afraid to open up complexities – we don't expect answers and solutions, but seek to advance our thinking and offer agendas for action on many different levels.

This having-no-fear-of-complexities is something that connects all contributions, including challenging the concept of Mad Studies itself. There would probably be no particular need to even mention this if many of us were not familiar with having to strategize and compromise in our scholarly work and experiencing firm limits to the amount of complexity that our respective disciplines can bear. Mad Studies will hopefully keep proving it is capable of demanding and fostering daring in our thinking, and in our practice.

Summarizing the learnings from single contributions or prioritizing their core messages could never do justice to their rich and multi-layered content. The authors and the readers can now speak directly to each other, our main job as editors is to bring them together. It has been a

DOI: 10.4324/9780429465444-41

pleasure and a privilege to witness and gently accompany the birth of the authors' manuscripts, as well as to experience how they gradually and together brought this handbook into its current shape. At the proposal stage, we did have a list of topics that we aimed to include but that plan started to change as soon as we started receiving the first contributions: many times, authors made us think of an issue that we initially did not consider and then sought to include. That was the exciting part of the editing adventure but also part of the reason why the making of this collection took so long and could certainly take even longer. The learnings and the dynamics of the editing process are a topic in itself, that might be worth documenting and reflecting upon one day. Nevertheless, I am writing this afterword with hardly any distance from everything that has happened (and hasn't happened) along the way. First, I will take another look at the collection as a whole and the ways in which its main sections relate to each other and to Mad Studies. I will then move on to my thoughts and feelings from the side of the reader and focus on just two major questions that struck me through this work. The first one is about how we approach differences and move forward; the second is about the room for Mad Studies in this world and where to seek that room.

Note on 'we'

To me, Mad Studies is a collective effort. When I use 'we' I mean anybody who is interested in joining and advancing Mad Studies.

Reversing the microscope

Lucy Costa's text "What is Mad Studies – What is it and why you should care" (2014) is one of the first writings that describes some core characteristics of Mad Studies in an accessible and inviting manner. She uses an effective metaphor of flipping the microscope that is traditionally directed to people deemed mad and turning it instead towards the so-called normal world that surrounds us and people embodying 'normality'. In this sense, Mad Studies is much more about thinking and theorizing from the designated social place of the 'Other' (in this case, the place for those considered 'mad') than it is about explaining any specific kind of 'otherness' that is currently largely being framed in the language of 'mental health'. But as we know, 'madness' is not exhorted into a single social place. Its social (dis)location is always an intersection of several other social positionings. The authors in this collection are not only writing from different parts of the world; they also write from particular interfaces of their lives. Given the multi-issued nature of their contributions – ordering the chapters in book sections was not an easy task. However, the flow of the sections follows in a way that gradually reverses the microscope that is at the heart of Mad Studies.

In Part 1, activists from Canada, Great Britain, India, Japan, New Zealand, Peru, Uganda, USA and former Yugoslavia reflect on knowledge accumulated in our respective movements and the (potential) use of that knowledge. In this section we aim the microscope at our own political organizing, our collective self-definitions, various scope of our joint actions, past achievements and failures as well as future prospects. This section ends with Wilda White's clear call to "expand our gaze beyond psychiatry and the mental health system" that is largely shared throughout the book.

Part 2 begins with an account of the circumstances in which the term Mad Studies was coined and the authors subsequently turn the microscope towards the work of those who have similar goals to ours in order to explore commonalities and differences as well as situate Mad Studies scholarship in relation to its neighboring fields (anti-psychiatry, critical psychiatry and disability studies). This section ends with making a case for the chronically missing piece and the need to "weaponize absent knowledges" (Beaupert and Brosnan, Chapter 14).

In Part 3, the "absent knowers" rise to speak and address the topics that are traditionally governed by psychiatry and mental health as well as characterized by white supremacy. The contributions not only challenge and question but also re-define and re-arrange hegemonic approaches. Knowledge-making is put on an equal footing and the authors chart counter epistemologies to the dominant ones: they take racialized subjects out of oblivion and erasure and move on to de-psychiatrize the prevailing approaches to experiential knowledge, co-production, motherhood, professional work and stigma.

In Part 4 that we entitled "Doing Mad Studies" the microscope moves further away from psychiatric and mental health discourse. Beginning with the call to de-medicalize our lives the authors in this section depart from discourse and disciplines that specifically govern "mad" people's lives and explore a spectrum of topics ranging from violence, war, colonial technologies, incarceration, architecture, "planetary well-being" and spirituality to communities' potential to deal with human crises and find collective responses to suicidality.

In the last section, the microscope makes a full circle, turning back to us and our own doings – this time the focus is on the project of Mad Studies itself and the ways in which it has been taking shape so far. The authors discuss how we conceptualize Mad Studies, how we seek to establish it in the academic world, including the notion of 'teaching'. Furthermore, the very concept of Mad Studies is being challenged and critical questions arise about how adequate this concept proves when attempting to travel across geographical and other borders. The authors make clear demands to decolonize activism, expose Whiteness in our work, disrupt the tradition of Euro-centrism, foster full equality and work across North/South borders and most importantly across the color line of 'race'. Colin King's concluding statement that this can be done and that "[t]he enduring mission of 'Mad Studies' is to work to make it happen" carries optimism but also responsibility and is kind of the essence of this whole collection. This last section is where the book actually starts again, handing the microscope over to the reader and inviting us to keep reversing it and digging deeper under the surface of what we see.

I will now use the opportunity to briefly engage with the main issues that have resurfaced for me. As said earlier, those are the questions of *how* and *where* we shall work together to "try to give a sense of what is possible within Mad Studies that is not possible elsewhere" (Lauren Tenney, Chapter 29).

Welcoming difference, finding sameness

The question of how to turn the story of falling apart into the story of coming together (Garza, 2020) is not a new question. It is there on every corner of what we do together or attempt to do together and is always about – who is 'we', who is in and who is out, where is the border and most importantly, where is that place where our experiences edge so close to each other that the division lines dissolve and we step into a whole new territory. And even though these questions remain pretty much the same, we do move on. Perhaps carrying them with us at all times and always searching for what connects us is the only way to avoid remaining stuck in the divisive legacies that we were born into.

Compared with the colonial and racist heritage, the othering based on the line of sanity/ madness seems easier to confront and resolve. This is perhaps because the institutions to introduce this kind of separation and the whole industry employed to maintain it – historically arose later. However strong the so called psy-complex has grown and wherever it seeks to expand, it seems that we are starting to challenge and erase the identities that it produces, rather than reclaim them. Even though this is not a consensus in Mad Studies as this issue was never put up to any kind of 'vote', it is a standpoint convincingly presented in several contributions in this collection and something to thoroughly consider. There are different ways however to work against the deepening of this particular demarcation line that inevitably accompanies liberation projects that reclaim and celebrate single, socially ostracized identities. On one hand, there is the rights-based approach as described by Tina Minkowitz (2020):

> Nobody – certainly not I – chooses to occupy space as a mad person, as the mythologized stigmatized other created by societies and augmented by psychiatry. I put myself forward to represent this collective as an affirmation that nobody deserves to be placed in that role – to erase the identity by claiming our rights in the context of the CRPD. It deserves to be a disappearing identity, is not one that I have any desire to hold onto or make meaningful. I suppose I differ in that regard from those who claim 'mad' as a positive identity meaning something like, resisting society's normality. […] My work on CRPD is a bearing witness, an act of reparation and transformative justice, that calls for the opening out of those labelled as mad, into simple humanity, really a spectrum of intense and often painful experiences that are unintelligible until the way is found to articulate them.

On the other hand, challenging the "universality that is embedded in the CRPD" and the shortcomings of its applicability to non-Western contexts, Femi Eromosele (Chapter 32) argues for a broader, *Ubuntu* approach that preserves human dignity as "simultaneously political, ethical, and spiritual". By providing these two approaches side by side, I do not intend to bring them into conflict but instead highlight the magnitude of knowledge that is out there, when not lessened according to the ruling, Western parameters of what constitutes knowledge. Understanding and dismantling the established hierarchies of knowledge is one of the major tasks for Mad Studies as clearly expressed by several authors. This task is greater than the task of visibilizing and legitim-izing knowledge of people deemed mad. As soon as we dig deeper into the issues of absences and dominances in official knowledge-making processes, the initial scope of Mad Studies becomes outpaced. This is, in my view, one of the many arrival points that this handbook brings us to: the necessity to illuminate and work against the divisive forces that precede the sanity/madness line and are ingrained deeper in our ways of being and knowing. Since many emancipatory projects create their own comfort zones and collapse precisely at this juncture, the question is whether Mad Studies is up to also confronting the colonial and racial division lines, and in particular their effect on 'social science' and the ways we conceptualize 'knowledge'? And even when willing to take up the challenge, how are we going to actually do this and work *together* on something as big as pain and injustice that are not a thing of the past but are being constantly refreshed and nurtured by current regimes of our unequal lives? How are we to recognize and dismantle those division lines each time they appear and bring us all together on one side? Proving that madness doesn't exist seems like a piece of cake compared to this kind of an undertaking.

In the absence of viable answers, I always come back to the saying that some paths can only be made by walking. And some questions are better answered through the actual joint work than in theory. Or in the words of the editors of the first collection to introduce Mad Studies, "the full story of Mad Studies has yet to be acted out, much less written down" (LeFrançois et al., 2013:11) But before handing over the responsibility to the reader, I will share some rare, wise advice that I found on how "the creative use of difference will help us really move toward change, toward that future we can share" (Audre Lorde in interview with Marion Kraft, 2018:83).

In their excellent article "The Contours of Anti-Black Racism: Engaging Anti-Oppression from Embodied Spaces" that is based on their own working experiences, four authors (Kumsa et al., 2014) ask themselves "[h]ow do we foster collaboration among oppressed groups and creatively engage the reality of competition that they are set up for?" (p.31), and "[w]ithout homogenizing our experiences, though, how do we sit down and work together?" (p.33). One of their answers is:

> We need anti-oppressive practices that honour all experiences without homogenizing them, honour differences without isolating them into separate cocoons, and reclaim that 'we' of our multiplicity without collapsing it into 'I' of our individuality or vice versa (Ahmed, 2000; 2009).
>
> *(Kumsa et al., 2014:31)*

This interplay of *I* and *we* that is able to enlarge both, rather than curl them up so that they can apparently fit each other better, seems to be at the heart of progressing towards those new territories, unlike the places of impossibilities we've already been to many times. Achieving such 'we' in the world that keeps positioning us on the opposite of each other, including long before we are born is an ongoing, never-ending process. To me it means always finding a common ground on which to stand and work from, it means taking off the baggage that we carry alone and understanding that it is *our* baggage that we are to carry together. It means committing to share the burden of oppression that unequally lands on each of us and approaching it as the burden of us all that we can get rid of together. Most of all, this means learning to be and work with differences, as beautifully explicated by Audre Lorde (1982):

> You do not have to be me in order for us to fight alongside each other. I do not have to be you to recognize that our wars are the same. What we must do is commit ourselves to some future that can include each other and to work toward that future with the particular strengths of our individual identities. And in order to do this, we must allow each other our differences at the same time as we recognize our sameness.

Reflections from the doorstep of the Master's house

Thinking in terms of room for marginalized epistemologies within socially recognized, institutionalized sites of knowledge production inevitably opens up the question of whether these distinct knowledge-making traditions are at all compatible with each other. Entering the academic realm is not only dependent on a good command of its ruling conventions but also requires willingness and capability to apply them in our own work. Those conventions are not just about the notions of 'objectivity' and positivist approaches to social science that are slowly but firmly beginning to ease off. The academic standards range from the compulsory anonymization of participants' contributions as a guiding ethical principle, to competitiveness and battling one another over the number and impact of scientific publications. The established rules also include profiting from (or suffering under) unfair division of labor and credentials made possible by institutional, gender and cultural hierarchies, including in what is known as survivor-led projects. Adhering to these conventions can certainly help establish flagship carriers of individuals that have made it *despite* their 'outsider' status and by virtue of "using experience and identity as a commodity to gain entry into systems of power" (Voronka, 2016:199). However, re-defining and re-arranging the academic structures so that they can open up to everybody *because of* and not despite of their diverse ways of knowing is a whole different matter. As Jijian Voronka observes:

> Yet once in, being and staying in cannot be the end goal; inclusion into systems of power is never enough.
>
> *(2016:199)*

Applied to Mad Studies this means that we don't need to wait for the future in order to understand that seeking scientific recognition from disciplines that are based on our epistemic exclusion will not stop the wheel of exclusion. If we aspire to more than launching academic niches to secure a greater number of places inside the 'master's house' (Lorde, 1984), then we need other strategies and other tools. In one interview Audre Lorde explains how she understands these other tools in academic contexts:

> It means different tools in language, different tools in the exchange of information, it means different tools in learning. It means that we use the tools of rationality, but we do not elevate it to the point that it is no longer connected to our lives. It means that we do not require from each other the kinds of narrow and restricted interpretations of learning and the exchange of knowledge that we suffered in the universities or that we suffered in the narrow academic structures. It means that we recognise that, while we are functioning in the old power, because we must know those tools, we cannot be ignorant of them. We are also in the process of redefining a new power, which is the power of the future.
>
> *(Kraft, 2018:81)*

Unfortunately, not everybody chooses that kind of process. The 'master's house' has its seductive power and many of those who move into it have no difficulties to start using its tools as soon as they have them at their disposal. Attaining positions of power is certainly a matter of urgency for all oppressed and marginalized groups but solely occupying those positions will not open up and democratize the existing structures.

Reflecting on her position as an 'outsider within', as an "African American woman from a working-class background, and an academic, who has experienced considerable upward social mobility", Patricia Hill Collins writes:

> Challenging power structures from the inside, and working cracks in the system, requires learning to speak multiple languages of power convincingly.
>
> *(2013:38)*

Not everybody is up to this task. More often we are inclined to celebrate individual (academic) achievements rather than (publicly) consider their price or reflect on the associated losses. It is certainly up to each individual to find their own ways, but it cannot be expected that everybody will commit to working cracks in the system. Despite all the laments about its precarious neoliberal situation (that are most eloquent in the richest parts of the world), the Master's House is still a cozy place to be. Could it be the time to take an honest look at our own definitions of achievement? At the time when Mad Studies is largely standing at the doorstep to universities, it might be the right moment to ask whether its success can be measured by the number of courses that will take off at different places and the number of academic positions and degrees that those courses will produce? Thinking about the future life of this handbook, I wonder whether the number of university libraries that will have it on their shelves will truly be an indication of how far we got? It is not my intention to belittle any achievement, but every achievement also sets new standards and brings about new responsibilities.

Finally, I want to believe that Mad Studies can importantly contribute to 'epistemologies of the South' (Santos, 2014, 2018). This concept divorces Eurocentric critical tradition that "excels in knowing about, explaining and guiding, rather than *knowing with*, understanding, facilitating and walking alongside" (Santos, 2014:ix, emphasis added). In the introduction to his book "The end of the cognitive empire" Santos explains:

> The epistemologies of the South concern the production and validation of knowledges anchored in the experiences of resistance of all those social groups that have systematically suffered injustice, oppression, and destruction caused by capitalism, colonialism, and patriarchy. The vast and vastly diversified field of such experiences I designate as the anti-imperial South. It is an epistemological, nongeographical South, composed of many epistemological souths [...].
>
> *(2018:1)*

This author believes that epistemologies of the South will transform the conventional university and envisions *pluriversity* and *subversity* as new institutional forms (2018: 269–291). My hope is that room for Mad Studies can and will be found at many different places, in and outside of official 'educational' sites. I hope that this collection will serve as a helpful source to move this way and that its content will break free from the confines of this particular publication and disperse in many different directions.

References

Collins, P H (2013) Truth-Telling and Intellectual Activism. *Contexts*, 12:36–41.

Costa, L (2014) Mad Studies – What it is and why you should care. https://madstudies2014.wordpress.com/2014/10/15/mad-studies-what-it-is-and-why-you-should-care-2/ Accessed: 24 February 2021.

Garza, A (2020) *The Purpose of Power. How to Build Movements for the 21st Century*. London: Penguin Random House UK.

Kraft, M (2018) *Empowering Encounters with Audre Lorde*. Münster: UNRAST Verlag.

Kumsa, M K, Mfoafo-M'Carthy, M, Oba, F and Gaasim, S (2014) The Contours of Anti-Black Racism: Engaging Anti-Oppression from Embodied Spaces. *The Journal of Critical Anti-Oppressive Social Inquiry* 1:21–38.

LeFrançois, B A, Menzies, R and Reaume, G. (2013) Introducing Mad Studies. In LeFrançois, B A, Menzies, R and Reaume, G. (eds.) *Mad Matters: A critical reader in Canadian mad studies*. Toronto: Canadian Scholars Press. 7–22.

Lorde, A (1982) "Learning from the 60s" a speech delivered at the celebration of the Malcolm X weekend at Harvard University. https://www.blackpast.org/african-american-history/1982-audre-lorde-learning-60s/ Accessed: 24 February 2021.

Minkowitz, T (2020) Identities and who gets to have them https://tastethespring.wordpress.com/2020/12/17/identities-and-who-gets-to-have-them/?fbclid=IwAR0GvqlMZbqzcqjJfmzG7RmNSJT4DQT_jWANGc79n3rrNONBsDJC_8YZifw Accessed: 24 February 2021.

Santos, B (2014) *Epistemologies of the South. Justice against Epistemicide*. Boulder/London: Paradigm Publishers.

Santos B (2018) *The End of the Cognitive Empire: The Coming of Age of Epistemologies of the South*. Durham: Duke University Press.

Voronka, J (2016) The Politics of 'People with Lived Experience'. Experiential Authority and the Risks of Strategic Essentialism. *Philosophy, Psychiatry, & Psychology,* 23 (3/4): 189–201.

POSTSCRIPT
Mad Studies in a maddening world

Peter Beresford

As we have come to the end of this project and assembling this book, it has been difficult not to be struck by the powerful insights contributors have offered. As Jasna made clear in her last chapter, the struggles of survivors, their intellectual and emotional journeys and discoveries, have highlighted complexity, pluralism and diversity. They do not offer one simplistic or straightforward theory or understanding. That is except insofar as the insights they offer come from their diverse experiences of madness and of both the systems that humans have set up in response to it or what can befall you in such circumstances. Jasna raised two big questions in that chapter. The first one is about how we approach differences and move forward; the second is about the room for Mad Studies in this world and where to seek that room. Building on that, in this chapter I particularly want to focus on actual and potential relationships between madness, Mad Studies and the politics and ideology that we are subject to and which are the context of our lives.

The social relations of madness

The book highlights both the social relations of madness and the inventiveness of those experiencing it in confronting and trying to make sense of it. What survivors strongly contest are longstanding interpretations and prevailing notions of madness as a condition restricted to particular 'special' or 'damaged' individuals or groups, which is unconnected to the wider world we live in. They have also challenged whether madness is always essentially negative, reiterated its creative as well as destructive potential and have sometimes seen it as an expression of diversity and responses to it, rather than problem or defect. Instead they make the social relations of Madness much more clear. A pioneer in doing this was the survivor thinker and activist Peter Sedgwick (Beresford, 2016a) We can see both madness and conventional responses to it as ideological and political as well as personal issues. Some things may drive any of us mad; for example, bereavement and loss, personal conflict, war, family breakdown, disempowerment, impoverishment, abuse, neglect, physical loss or change and other forms of trauma that relate primarily to us and our relationships.

We cannot assume there will ever be a perfect world where people are saved from such precipitating misery and hardship. But also, as we have seen, there are societal and political pressures that can both be maddening in their impact and also be different in degree both in

DOI: 10.4324/9780429465444-42

different societies, at different times and in relation to different groups. In feudal times, human beings did not have the ability to control their environments. In times of dearth, famine and other natural disasters lords and rulers could suffer just as serfs and slaves went hungry. The modern world and modern industrialised societies however, do have that ability, but we have seen their continuing unwillingness to ensure that all people and all parts of the world benefit from it.

Madness's political relations

The two political ideologies that came to dominate the first half of the twentieth century bear early and sharp witness to this: Soviet Communism and German Nazism. The Nazis murdered many disabled people and mental health service users in its Aktion T4 programme 'as lives unworthy of life' and Soviet dissidents from 1960–1986 were detained as patients in its psychiatric system (Beresford, 2021).

Madness then clearly has ideological and social relations connected with how we are treated and how we behave to each other in society. Thus the discrimination and abuse experienced by people who face structured and institutionalised oppression – whether as poor, women, Black and minoritized ethnic groups, disabled, older, etc. etc., by virtue of living in low-income countries or because of a combination of the two. Madness is not only to be understood as an internal act, but a much more situated one, as contributors to the book begin specifically to articulate in Part 4.

The twentieth century was a time when social, political and economic forces exerted an unprecedented influence on the individual. For the first time, much broader forces could have a far greater and more extensive reach, with mass media, mass production and consumption, mass conscription, mass bombing, mass produced drugs. But it was also the century of the rise of psych sciences, their rolling out of individualising explanations for people's troubles and difficulties, despite the visibly structural issues generating them.

Thus, for example, the French sociologist Durkheim's study Suicide (1951), highlighted the social nature of suicide. He suggested that there were different kinds of suicide and evidenced the way that suicide rates for different groups, in different societies at different times varied. Suicide is not a random individual act. In 1947 the French actor and writer Antonin Artaud, himself a psychiatric system survivor, who like Van Gogh was ultimately to end his own life and who also experienced electroconvulsive therapy (ECT) among other 'treatments', argued that Van Gogh's work so disturbed society that it shunned his art and led to his despair and suicide (Artaud, 1947). He concluded that Van Gogh was a man *'suicided by society'*. Artaud dismissed crude psychiatric assessments of Van Gogh that even now continue to obscure his life and work. Instead what he offered was a pre-figurative 'social model of madness and distress'.

Maddening consequences

The world in the early twenty-first century continues to be a heavily conflicted and threatening place. It is characterised by international unrest, local and proxy wars, conflicts between faiths and ethnic groups, economic and forced migration, rising 'natural disasters' including flooding and famine associated with climate change and human interventions and pandemics originating with the mistreatment of animals. All these have consequences for our lives and wellbeing, including our emotional and mental wellbeing and these consequences affect groups differently, as contributors to the book highlight, according to the status and treatment afforded them under different political ideologies and systems.

As we have seen with Covid-19 globally human beings apart from a few politicians and other Covid deniers do not seem to find it hard to understand the social relations of pandemics and understand the need therefore for public health measures as opposed to narrowly individualised approaches. Yet in the context of madness and distress, despite the constant assertions that they are best understood in bio-medical and illness terms, the same barely seems to apply. There is little formal recognition of the way different social and political structures impact on such 'mental health', very few community or public health measures in western societies address that impact beyond the individual currently being encouraged 'to tell their story' when in terms of accessing employment or where applicable access to welfare benefits, it may not be a good idea. There is minimal provision for social responses or understandings. The only significant exception is the development of the psychiatric diagnostic category Post Traumatic Stress Disorder (PTSD) as though such a response is pathological rather than a predictable and entirely rational one to the appalling horrors of war, conflict, bombing, combat and violence.

Making connections

The broader connections between 'mental health problems' and political systems have now been well rehearsed by social epidemiologists. The dominant global politics in the twenty-first century has been neoliberal; that is to say based on globalized free market-driven economics with reduced expenditure on supportive welfare services (Beresford, 2016b). High profile concerns have been expressed about this ideological approach and its consequences. This has been evidenced most notably in the work of Wilkinson and Pickett. They argue that inequality in societies, which is particularly associated with free market ideology and politics, is damaging for health, including mental health. They argue that it is bad for all, rich and poor and ultimately damaging to societies suggesting that more equal societies are more successful (Wilkinson and Pickett, 2009; Pickett and Wilkinson, 2018). As they conclude:

> Societies with more equal distribution of incomes have better health, fewer social problems such as violence, drug abuse, teenage births, mental illness and obesity, and are more cohesive than ones in which the gap between the rich and poor is greater.
>
> *(University of York, 2011)*

Thus political and social systems may have the potential to drive us mad by imposing pressures that are maddening and/or to force us into categories that are conceived of in terms of madness.

Leaders and madness

However, societies which create and perpetuate the conditions for madness and distress through their harshness, inequality and divisiveness may also be led by people who seem to fit the same description as those they oppress. As we have seen, for example the leaders of both the Soviet Union and Nazi Germany have been subjected repeatedly to long-distance diagnoses and both have been identified as 'mentally disordered' (Langer, 1972 [1943]; Snow, 1967). More recently enormous international attention has been paid to the mental state of Donald Trump as US president, with major texts, articles and video calling it into question. One book compiling the views of psych professionals described what it called the 'clear and present danger' his 'mental health' posed to the 'nation and individual wellbeing' (Lee, 2017).

It is not being suggested here that maddening politics result from mad politicians, but rather that harsh and conventional politics and policy, including responses to madness, may tell us less about the people oppressed by them than about the nature, aims, assumptions and attitudes of the regimes and individuals who impose and perpetuate them. Given that the term mad is so often used to describe what is seen as appallingly bad, it is perhaps not surprising if sometimes the vicious and cruel acts associated with powerful leaders are not redefined in crude psychiatric terms, just as the disempowerment and distress of those they may oppress is. Perhaps more interesting and using their own terms, are the questions raised about the 'mental health' of those individuals and structures which support such leaders to come to and stay in power?

Prevailing neoliberal politics seems to have developed a powerful informal alliance with the psychiatric system with both placing an emphasis on individualized explanation, which increasingly frames social problems in terms of individual pathology and deficiency, creating more and more psychiatric diagnostic categories in the process and extending the authority and reach of psychiatry. Marginal medicalized services and enforced employment are offered as the primary response in the global north and self-help and the legacy of colonialist institutionalization in the global south.

As links between ideology, politics and madness begin to emerge it may be helpful to remind ourselves about how madness tends to be defined. Of course definitions vary over time, place and culture. The medicalization of madness and distress has also created complexities and greatly added to the range of phenomena, experience and perception included in the category. There have also been and continue to be faith-based and spiritual conceptions of madness. Having said that, madness tends to be associated with a range of phenomena and behaviours, including loss of reason, unpredictability, threat, violence possession, irrationality, failure to anticipate consequences, confusion, fearfulness and dangerousness.

The madness of politics

At this point it is interesting to note the massive gap there seems to be between the world we prepare our children for and the one they can expect to inhabit. At school, children acquire social and technical skills. They learn to get on with each other, and respect the needs and rights of others. They are taught one or other moral code, perhaps secular or faith based, which outlaw killing and stealing and instead are likely to encourage kindness and generosity, giving to charity and those less well off than yourself, while seeking to contribute to society through your abilities and skills. Children are encouraged to treat animals with love and kindness or at least to keep their distance from them, the environment with care and concern, to be aware of the potentially damaging effects humans have on the ecology, the climate, rainforest, animals and their habitats

At home, as parents and guardians, we are encouraged to reinforce what our children learn at school to help them in turn become good citizens and parents. This includes treating others with equality, valuing our brothers and sisters and our elders, to learn and abide by a moral code, be polite and have good manners; to play our part in running the home, taking turns cleaning and washing up, going shopping, looking after pets, understanding and accepting responsibility, respecting the rights of others, telling the truth, taking on increasing responsibilities.

However the world we can expect to take our place in after childhood (if it allows us a childhood) is a very different one – as the Black Lives Matter and #MeToo, environmental and peace movements currently highlight. In the US it is one where Black people run a disproportionate risk of being killed by the police who are meant to be there to protect them. Internationally it is a world where women routinely run a disproportionate risk of sexual and physical attack, rape and murder. Ours is a world:

- Of endless destructive war, fighting and killing, where people are expected to kill others by all means possible, sometimes including children, sometimes as children;
- Of massive damaging pollution and inadequate action against it putting the future of the planet and more and more species and fauna at risk. Some of the biggest and most powerful nations have the worst records in relation to the environment;
- Where people are increasingly required to be in damaging alienating employment while the constant aim is to cut jobs to reduce costs;
- Where an 'underclass' of impoverished people has long been highlighted and vilified as deviant and destructive but where in reality there is a small over-powerful 'overclass' beyond the constraints of conventional law, moral, ethical and behavioural codes;
- Where large numbers and increasing proportions of traumatized and oppressed people are maintained by a massive pharmaceutical industry, which is related to the destructive arms and agribusiness industries, or turn to a massive exploitative, destructive and criminal illicit international drugs industry to sustain themselves;
- Where far more is spent on armed forces and the arms industry than support to look after each other;
- Where millions die from diseases that can be controlled, hunger and poverty that is created rather than alleviated and from 'natural' disasters that are originated and perpetuated by human hands, rather than averted by them.

Maddening the world

Perhaps this lack of fit between the expectations placed on us and on the ideologies our lives are subject to is just a means to ensure our conformity and to maintain our obedience to our governments and rulers. Perhaps it just tells us something about the shortcomings of human beings in organizing and governing themselves, with the logic of political processes an amoral and Machiavellian one. While it is important to avoid simplistic assumptions and oversimplifying rhetoric, it is, however, difficult to see how the resulting world makes any rational sense or relates helpfully to the principles we are widely brought up to value and respect. Free rein has been allowed to a global neoliberal system that puts profit and production before saving the planet and all dwelling on it. It is more a world of Dr. Strangelove complete with 'mutually assured destruction' (MAD) than one based on any notion of human progress, sustainability and cooperation. This would be described as madness if it were associated with any individual rather than with states and statesmen, ideology and global politics. Put simply, in ordinary understanding, it also looks like both a mad and maddening world.

My hope is that this book may help us think beyond this. Contributors have helped make so many connections; between abuse, trauma and disempowerment and discrimination, between the personal and the political, the psychological and the social. But perhaps most important are the disjunctions and inequalities they highlight between us and our struggles and the importance of challenging them. And what I have learned is that Mad Studies may be a particularly helpful and necessary lens to do this, however helpful others may also be.

The future for Mad Studies

I have also learned from the global south, in being involved in this book, the importance of Mad Studies refusing to stay within boundaries imposed by psychiatry and the medicalizing of madness in the Global North. Mad Studies can be invaluable as a critique and rejection of this, but it also needs to be and extend much further. The true focus of Mad Studies should be one beyond the psych system and psychiatrization of everything. It will also benefit by learning from the linking of material struggles in the global south to challenge the maddening nature of our world and our often irrational political and economic structures and assumptions more generally. We have already had wise warnings in this book about pitfalls Mad Studies should avoid; becoming narrowly associated with the academy, perpetuating the inequalities and oppressions of white privilege and failing to renew itself through a determinedly inclusive and reaching out approach to its task.

But there are also the positives which cumulatively this book's contributors highlight for us as critically important. We are still at an early stage in the history of Mad Studies so we need to work hard on developing it, building on resources like this book to do so. This will include:

- Coming to see Mad Studies as a perspective on the world not just on 'madness';
- Conceiving of Mad Studies not as one badged view from mad people but as the wide range of emancipatory insights that they/we and our allies may bring to bear;
- Collectively developing our own ideologies and conceptual frameworks in participatory ways rather than accepting ruling ideologies, and the exclusionary ideas and explanations imposed upon us;
- Exploring politics, organizational structures and forms of collectivity that build on the humanistic, accessible qualities, aspirations and nature of the disabled people's, survivors and other service users' and new social movements;
- Exploring and developing personal and other relationships based on equality;
- Exploring key current issues like climate change denial, artificial intelligence, sustainable economics, care and support from a Mad Studies perspective;
- Developing inclusive participatory approaches to making change based on working in equal coproductive ways;
- Developing our own ideas, schemes and funding for survivor-led holistic approaches to preventing and supporting madness and distress;
- Treating experiential, minoritized and indigenous knowledges with at least equal value and respect as professional, experimental and so-called 'expert knowledge';
- Connecting and building alliances with other emancipatory, rights-based new social movements, which will almost certainly have positive links with our own, to share insights and extend our strength and power.

We hope this book helps refine and take forward these and other tasks prioritized by our movement, offering encouragement, practical guidance and theoretical support and evidence.

References

Artaud, A. (1947), *Van Gogh: The Man Suicided by Society*, Paris, publisher not known.
Beresford, P. (2016a), From Psycho-Politics To Mad Studies: Learning the legacy of Peter Sedgwick, *Critical And Radical Social Work*, Volume 4, Number 3, November 2016, pp. 343–355(13).
Beresford, P. (2016b), *All Our Welfare: Towards Participatory Social Policy*, Bristol, Policy Press.
Beresford, P. (2021), *Participatory Ideology: From Exclusion to Involvement*, Bristol, Policy Press.
Durkheim, E. (1951), *Suicide: A Study in Sociology*, New York, The Free Press.
Langer, W. C. (1972 [1943]), *The Mind of Adolf Hitler: The Secret Wartime Report*, New York, Basic Books.
Lee, B.X. (2017), *The Dangerous Case Of Donald Trump: 27 Psychiatrists and Mental Health Experts Assess a President*, New York City, Macmillan.
Pickett, K. and Wilkinson, R.G. (2018), *The Inner Level: How More Equal Societies Reduce Stress, Restore Sanity and Improve Everyone's Well-being*, London, Penguin.

Snow, C.P. (1967), On Stalin's Triumph, On Stalin's Madness, *Esquire,* 1 May, https://classic.esquire.com/article/1967/5/1/on-stalins-triumph-on-stalins-madness accessed 30 March 2021.

University of York (2011) Influential Book by York Academics Wins Top Award, 30 November, https://www.york.ac.uk/news-and-events/news/2011/quality/spirit-level-award/ accessed 29 March 2021.

Wilkinson, R.G. and Pickett, K. (2009), *The Spirit Level: Why Equality is Better for Everyone*, London, Allen Lane.

INDEX

Note: Page numbers with italic *f* indicate Figures; those with italic *t* indicate the Table.

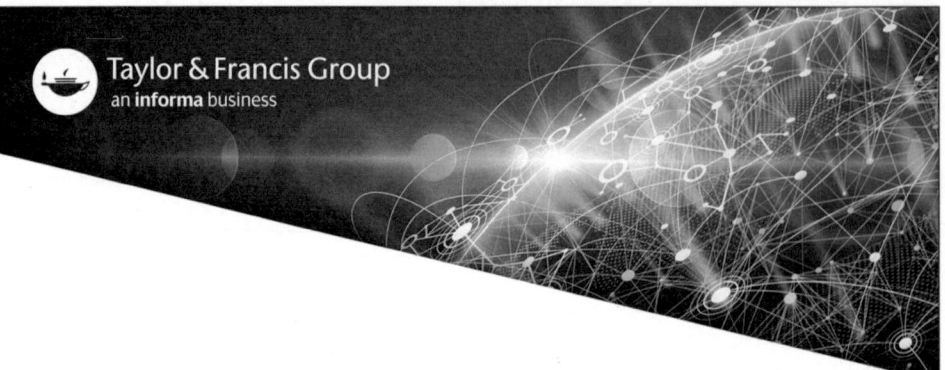
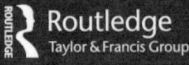
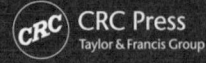